The Practical Management
of
Low-Grade Primary Brain Tumors

The Practical Management
of
Low-Grade Primary Brain Tumors

Editors

Jack P. Rock, M.D.
Department of Neurosurgery
Henry Ford Hospital
Detroit, Michigan

Mark L. Rosenblum, M.D.
Department of Neurosurgery
Henry Ford Hospital
Detroit, Michigan

Edward G. Shaw, M.D.
Department of Radiation Oncology
Wake Forest University School of Medicine
Winston-Salem, North Carolina

J. Gregory Cairncross, M.D.
Department of Clinical Neurological Sciences and Oncology
University of Western Ontario and London Regional Cancer Centre
London, Ontario, Canada

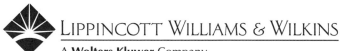

LIPPINCOTT WILLIAMS & WILKINS
A **Wolters Kluwer** Company
Philadelphia · Baltimore · New York · London
Buenos Aires · Hong Kong · Sydney · Tokyo

Acquisitions Editor: Elizabeth Greenspan
Manufacturing Manager: Kevin Watt
Production Manager: Robert Pancotti
Production Editor: Emily Harkavy
Cover Designer: Sandy Mohandru
Indexer: Linda Fetters
Compositor: Lippincott Williams & Wilkins Desktop Division
Printer: Maple Press

Printed in the United States of America

9 8 7 6 5 4 3 2 1

Library of Congress Cataloging-in-Publication Data
 The practical management of low-grade primary brain tumors / editors,
   Jack P. Rock ... [et al.].
      p.   cm.
   Includes bibliographical references and index.
   ISBN 0-7817-1101-0 (alk. paper)
   1. Brain—Tumors.   I. Rock, Jack P.
   [DNLM: 1. Brain Neoplasms—therapy.   2. Glioma—therapy.   3. Brain
 Neoplasms—diagnosis.   4. Glioma—diagnosis.   WL 358 P895 1999]
 RC280.B7P72 1999
 616.99′481—dc21
 DNLM/DLC
 for Library of Congress   98-44542
                                                                                   CIP

Care has been taken to confirm the accuracy of the information presented and to describe generally accepted practices. However, the authors, editors, and publisher are not responsible for errors or omissions or for any consequences from application of the information in this book and make no warranty, expressed or implied, with respect to the contents of the publication.

The authors, editors, and publisher have exerted every effort to ensure that drug selection and dosage set forth in this text are in accordance with current recommendations and practice at the time of publication. However, in view of ongoing research, changes in government regulations, and the constant flow of information relating to drug therapy and drug reactions, the reader is urged to check the package insert for each drug for any change in indications and dosage and for added warnings and precautions. This is particularly important when the recommended agent is a new or infrequently employed drug.

Some drugs and medical devices presented in this publication have Food and Drug Administration (FDA) clearance for limited use in restricted research settings. It is the responsibility of the health care provider to ascertain the FDA status of each drug or device planned for use in their clinical practice.

To our patients

Contents

Contributing Authors   ix
Acknowledgments   xi

Section I: General Overview

1. General Perspectives   3
   Jack P. Rock

2. Imaging of Low-Grade Primary Brain Tumors   5
   William P. Sanders and Gregory A. Christoforidis

3. Classification and Pathobiology of Low-Grade Glial
   and Glioneuronal Neoplasms   33
   Jorge A. Gutierrez

Section II: Management Alternatives

4. Surgery for Adult Low-Grade Primary Brain Tumors   71
   Jack P. Rock, Marianne E. Naftzger, and Mark L. Rosenblum

5. Role of Radiation Therapy in the Management of Low-Grade
   Glioma in Adults   81
   Edward G. Shaw

6. Chemotherapy and Alternatives for Adult Low-Grade Glial Tumors   99
   Tom Mikkelsen

7. Management of Cerebellar Astrocytomas in Children   103
   Paul M. Kanev

8. Uncommon Low-Grade Primary Brain Tumors   111
   S. Ather Enam and Jack P. Rock

Section III: Common Management Issues for the Practitioner

9. Adult Low-Grade Gliomas: Natural History, Prognostic Factors,
   and Timing of Treatment   135
   *Joseph O. Bampoe, Glenn Bauman, J. Gregory Cairncross,
   and Mark Bernstein*

10. Epilepsy and Low-Grade Gliomas   149
    Kost Elisevich

11. Genetics and Genetic Counseling   171
    Paula M. Czarnecki and Daniel L. Van Dyke

12. Practical Case Scenarios 181
Tom Mikkelsen, Edward G. Shaw, Mark Bernstein, J. Gregory Cairncross,
Jae Ho Kim, Mark L. Rosenblum, and Jack P. Rock

Section IV: Research and Future Directions

13. Development, Molecular Genetics, and Gene Therapy of
Glial Tumors 193
Steven P. Dudas and Sandra A. Rempel

14. Low-Grade Glioma: Guidelines and Outcomes Analysis 231
Jack P. Rock, Beverly C. Walters, and Edward G. Shaw

Subject Index 235

Contributing Authors

Joseph O. Bampoe, M.B., Ch.B, F.R.C.S.(I), *Staff Scientist, Division of Neurosurgery, The Toronto Hospital, Western Division, University of Toronto, Suite 2-405, McLaughlin Pavilion, 399 Bathurst Street, Toronto, Ontario M5T 2S8 Canada*

Glenn Bauman, M.D., *Department of Clinical Neurological Sciences and Oncology, University of Western Ontario and London Regional Cancer Centre, 790 Commissioners Road East, London, Ontario N6A 4L6 Canada*

Mark Bernstein, B.Sc., M.D., F.R.C.S.C., *Professor, Division of Neurosurgery, The Toronto Hospital, Western Division, University of Toronto, Suite 2-405, McLaughlin Pavilion, 399 Bathurst Street, Toronto, Ontario M5T 2S8 Canada*

J. Gregory Cairncross, M.D., *Professor, Department of Clinical Neurological Sciences and Oncology, University of Western Ontario and London Regional Cancer Centre, 790 Commissioners Road East, London, Ontario N6A 4L6 Canada*

Gregory A. Christoforidis, M.D., *Department of Diagnostic Radiology, Henry Ford Hospital, 2799 West Grand Boulevard, Detroit, Michigan 48202*

Paula M. Czarnecki, M.S., *Certified Genetic Counselor, Department of Medical Genetics, Henry Ford Hospital, 2799 West Grand Boulevard, Detroit, Michigan 48202*

Steven P. Dudas, Ph.D., *Post-Doctoral Research Fellow, Department of Neurosurgery, Henry Ford Hospital, 2799 West Grand Boulevard, Detroit, Michigan 48202*

Kost Elisevich, M.D., Ph.D., *Associate Professor of Neurosurgery, Case Western Reserve University; Department of Neurosurgery, Henry Ford Hospital, 2799 West Grand Boulevard, Detroit, Michigan 48202*

S. Ather Enam, M.D., Ph.D., *Consultant Neurosurgeon, Department of Neurosurgery, Henry Ford Hospital, 2799 West Grand Boulevard, Detroit, Michigan 48202*

Jorge A. Gutierrez, M.D., *Department of Pathology (Neuropathology), Henry Ford Hospital, 2799 West Grand Boulevard, Detroit, Michigan 48202*

Paul M. Kanev, M.D., *Associate Professor of Surgery and Pediatrics, Division of Neurosurgery, Penn State University College of Medicine; Department of Neurosurgery, Hershey Medical Center H110, P.O. Box 850, Hershey, Pennsylvania 17033*

Jae Ho Kim, M.D., Ph.D., *Chair, Department of Radiation Oncology, Henry Ford Hospital, 2799 West Grand Boulevard, Detroit, Michigan 48202*

Tom Mikkelsen, M.D., *Departments of Neurology and Neurosurgery, Henry Ford Hospital, 2799 West Grand Boulevard, Detroit, Michigan 48202*

Marianne E. Naftzger, PA-C, *Neurosurgical Physician Assistant, Department of Neurosurgery, Henry Ford Hospital, 2799 West Grand Boulevard, Detroit, Michigan 48202*

Sandra A. Rempel, Ph.D., *Director of Molecular Neuro-oncology Research, Department of Neurosurgery, Henry Ford Hospital, 2799 West Grand Boulevard, Detroit, Michigan 48202*

Jack P. Rock, M.D., *Codirector of Surgical Neuro-oncology, Department of Neurosurgery, Henry Ford Hospital, 2799 West Grand Boulevard, Detroit, Michigan 48202*

Mark L. Rosenblum, M.D., *Chairman, Department of Neurosurgery, Henry Ford Hospital, 2799 West Grand Boulevard, Detroit, Michigan 48202*

William P. Sanders, M.D., *Senior Staff Neuroradiologist, Department of Diagnostic Radiology, Henry Ford Hospital, 2799 West Grand Boulevard, Detroit, Michigan 48202*

Edward G. Shaw, M.D., *Professor and Chairman, Department of Radiation Oncology, Wake Forest University School of Medicine, Medical Center Boulevard, Winston-Salem, North Carolina 27157*

Daniel L. Van Dyke, Ph.D., *Professor of Medical Genetics, Case Western Reserve University; Department of Medical Genetics, Henry Ford Hospital, 2799 West Grand Boulevard, Detroit, Michigan 48202*

Beverly C. Walters, M.D., *Department of Clinical Neurosciences, Brown University School of Medicine, Providence, Rhode Island 02912*

Acknowledgments

*The Editors gratefully acknowledge
the editorial support of Sarah Whitehouse, M.A.W.*

SECTION I

General Overview

The Practical Management of Low-Grade Primary Brain Tumors, edited by Jack P. Rock, Mark L. Rosenblum, Edward G. Shaw, and J. Gregory Cairncross. Lippincott Williams & Wilkins, Philadelphia, © 1999

1

General Perspectives

Jack P. Rock

Department of Neurosurgery, Henry Ford Hospital, Detroit, Michigan 48202

Primary brain tumors are tumors that histologically arise from cells comprising the parenchyma of the central nervous system (i.e., neurons and their supporting cells). The term low-grade has been used to describe these tumors because of their relatively slow growth rate as compared with their malignant counterparts. Unfortunately, low-grade brain tumors have been referred to in the past as benign brain tumors, based on this slow growth and in an effort to emphasize this indolent course. Although slow growth may characterize the biologic behavior of these lesions as a group, individually they still retain the potential for malignant conversion. Therefore the term *benign* is incorrect and should no longer be used. The median 5- and 10-year survival rates of many of these patients after treatment vary from 32% to 68% and from 19% to 39%, respectively.

Incidence rates measure the occurrence of newly diagnosed cases of disease and are expressed in a standard unit of person-years (usually 100,000 person-years, with each person-year reflecting one individual over 1 year). The generally accepted annual incidence rate of adult and pediatric low-grade gliomas in North America is thought to be approximately 12% to 15% (1,500 cases) of all diagnosed primary brain tumors. The histologic subtypes occurring most frequently are astrocytoma, oligodendroglioma, and mixed oligoastrocytoma. The cumulative incidence of the other, less common low-grade tumor types adds another 5%. Thus, the tumor types

discussed in this book account for approximately one-fifth of all primary brain tumors. Because of the low incidence of these lesions, definitive studies of natural history and management outcomes have not been effectively undertaken. Therefore, clinicians have had to rely on the numerous uncontrolled, retrospective reviews of patient series in the medical literature. These reports present varying options for management, frequently with conclusions not fully supported by the data. The treating physician must therefore choose from several strategies determined not from evidence-based information but from pure consensus and remain uncertain about the ultimate best plan for the management of each patient. This necessarily leads to controversy about many of our everyday treatment recommendations. What we have attempted to do in this book is to bring together the information that is known in the literature and balance it with what is unknown in this same literature. Accordingly, we hope to present an amalgamated view of patient management that, although perhaps leaving the reader in a persistent quandary, will at least create a greater awareness of the limitations of our current knowledge and the critical need for further study.

Section I serves as a foundation and includes detailed reviews of radiologic and pathologic features of low-grade brain tumors. In Chapter 3, Dr. Gutierrez has added many insightful ideas to the fundamental pathologic issues.

Section II presents the various aspects required for management of patients with low-grade brain tumors, including observation without intervention, surgery, radiation therapy, and chemotherapy. Issues regarding pediatric brain tumors and the uncommon primary brain tumors are presented. In addition to emphasizing what is generally known or at least accepted in the literature, the authors have attempted to clarify what is not known regarding critical matters of diagnosis and treatment so that the reader can understand why there are several strategies for management in many of these lesions.

Section III includes discussions on epilepsy and genetics, two commonly expressed concerns of patients with low-grade brain tumors. The practical case scenarios present expert opinion about the management of several cases. It will be apparent from these discussions that not all experts agree and that opinions vary in patient management.

Section IV presents a comprehensive review of the molecular biology of brain tumors and is followed by a discussion of outcomes and guideline issues. This final chapter presents the results of an evidence-based effort to develop a set of management guidelines involving certain patients with low-grade brain tumors. As opposed to the traditional consensus-based (i.e., generated by acknowledged experts in the field) guidelines we currently rely on, efforts of this kind utilize a careful assessment of the literature in an attempt to determine a more scientifically relevant guideline. The effort is well intentioned, but as many practitioners will note, the literature does not contain enough well-designed and implemented studies to form a basis for definitive conclusions. We must still rely on expert opinion until future studies lead to improved information, and this is not as easy as one might think. The low incidence of low-grade brain tumors makes it absolutely imperative that multi-institutional studies be carried out. Even if this can be done, it may prove daunting to overcome the individual physician and patient biases with which we all contend.

In this book we have tried to incorporate the available information into a form that will aid the practitioner in the management of patients with low-grade brain tumors. The literature is unclear on important questions. Should patients be treated immediately after diagnosis, or can treatment be deferred? Is biopsy worth the risk? Does radical surgery improve outcome? What is the place of radiation therapy in the management of patients with low-grade brain tumors? Does chemotherapy play a role? What is the natural history of untreated patients? Many of these questions remain unresolved. It is the task of physicians and patients interested in improving our understanding of these tumors to find the answers.

The Practical Management of Low-Grade Primary Brain Tumors, edited by Jack P. Rock, Mark L. Rosenblum, Edward G. Shaw, and J. Gregory Cairncross. Lippincott Williams & Wilkins, Philadelphia, © 1999

2

Imaging of Low-Grade Primary Brain Tumors

William P. Sanders and Gregory A. Christoforidis

W. P. Sanders and G. A. Christoforidis: Department of Diagnostic Radiology, Henry Ford Hospital, Detroit, Michigan 48202

Imaging of neoplasms of the brain has progressed in recent years similarly to imaging of all lesions of the brain. Computed tomography (CT), first developed in the 1970s, has continued to progress and in many cases has been replaced by the more sensitive images obtained by magnetic resonance imaging (MRI). Although the sensitivity of MRI has been shown to be greater than that of CT (13), the overall specificity for distinguishing low-grade from high-grade primary brain neoplasms has not reached initial expectations (4,6,38,40,61,64,73,74,91,153,158). Measurement of T1 and T2 values and enhancement patterns of high-grade and low-grade tumors overlap considerably, although general trends are seen in most cases; these are discussed later in this chapter. Research interest currently is in the realm of functional MRI, in which the metabolic activity of tumors as portrayed on perfusion and diffusion imaging, as well as the chemical composition as seen with MR spectroscopy, shows promise for greater specificity in the diagnosis of various types of tumors. However, there will likely always be considerable overlap in the imaging and biochemical signatures of these tumors, because the imaging reflects the physiologic and chemical makeup of these tumors. It is well known that within a single tumor there may be areas of high-grade tumor alongside areas of low-grade neoplasm. There may also be more than one histologic tumor type within a single mass. Thus the imaging and metabolic appearance of these tumors will reflect the variegated composition of these lesions, making an absolutely definitive diagnosis by imaging alone unlikely.

LOW-GRADE ASTROCYTOMA

The most commonly used pathologic description of primary brain tumors is based on the World Health Organization (WHO) classification, which consists of low-grade astrocytoma, low-grade astrocytoma with anaplasia, and glioblastoma multiforme (163). A common method used previously was the Kernohan classification in which astrocytomas were divided into four grades (grades I–IV) followed by glioblastoma multiforme (68). Although these differences in classification have relevance to clinical prognosis, treatment, and histologic diagnosis, the change in classification has little bearing on the imaging characteristics. Since it has always been difficult to separate grade I from grade II of the Kernohan classification on imaging studies alone, the WHO classification fits better with CT and MRI appearances.

Low-grade astrocytomas are often divided into two general categories on imaging appearances. One type is a well-defined focal lesion that is typically low density on CT examination with little or, more often, no contrast enhancement (17,65) (Fig. 1). On MRI examination the lesions remain well-defined and are low signal intensity on T1-weighted

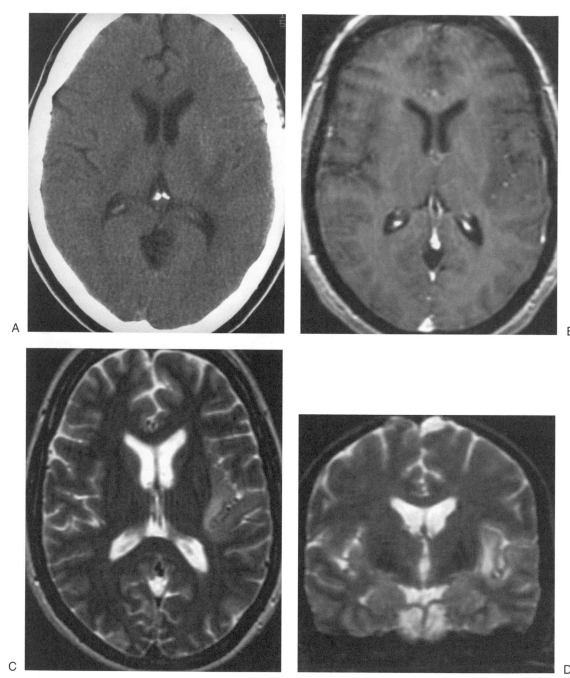

FIG. 1. Low-grade astrocytoma. **A:** Nonenhanced CT shows subtle low density in the left subinsular white matter. **B:** Axial gadolinium-enhanced T1 MR image shows nonenhanced low signal in left subinsular region. Axial (**C**) and coronal (**D**) T2 MR images reveal typical subinsular high signal with minimal mass effect.

images and high signal on T2-weighted images. Similar to CT, on MRI the lesions typically show no or only minimal contrast enhancement (4,6,38,40,61,64,73,74,91,153, 158). These lesions may exhibit mild local mass effect, which usually is minor.

The second type of low-grade glioma is a more diffuse infiltrating type of lesion. These lesions are notoriously difficult to identify on CT examination and may present with slight density difference and typically with no contrast enhancement (4,6,38,40,61, 64,73,74,91,153,158). Similarly, the MR characteristics are slightly low signal on T1 and high signal on T2. Both on CT and MRI examination, these lesions show nearly zero mass effect on any sequence because of their infiltrative rather than expansile nature. Again, as with CT, these lesions show little or no contrast enhancement on MRI. Both the discrete and the infiltrative lesions are typically seen in the white matter of the supratentorial compartment. However, the abnormal tissue may extend into deep gray matter structures or into the cortex, with the signal abnormalities spreading from the white matter to the gray matter. This pattern is best appreciated on MRI because of the superior tissue contrast properties inherent to the modality (Fig. 2).

These descriptions account for most low-grade astrocytomas, especially those in the supratentorial compartment. However, atypical findings are seen with low-grade gliomas. Significant contrast enhancement has been uncommonly reported (Fig. 3) (6,74,158). Cystic changes within the supratentorial astrocytomas are also uncommon (Fig. 4). When cystic change is seen, it is usually in the pilocytic form of low-grade astrocytomas (131). Significant mass effect is uncommon but has been reported.

A specific type of low-grade astrocytoma occurs in the cerebellum, typically in children. Histologically, this is a pilocytic astrocytoma and presents as a midline cystic cerebellar mass, with an enhancing mural nodule (Figs. 5 and 6). These lesions are biologically benign, and resection of the nodule usually results in cure. For unknown reasons these cystic pilocytic astrocytomas are uncommon in the supratentorial compartment (138).

Although low-grade astrocytomas have typical imaging appearances, there is signifi-

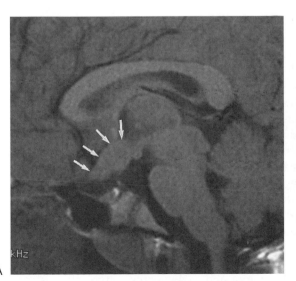
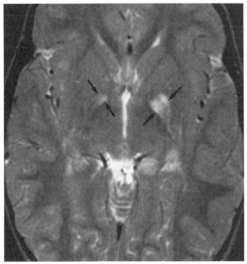

A
B

FIG. 2. Optic glioma. **A:** Sagittal T1 MR image shows the enlarged optic chiasm, nerves, and proximal tracts (*arrows*). **B:** Axial T2 cephalad to the tumor demonstrates hyperintense signal due to infiltration into the optic tracts (*arrows*).

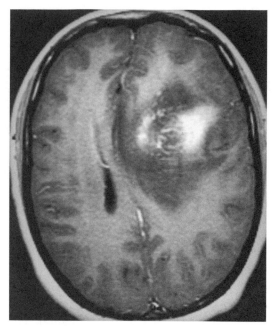

FIG. 3. Left frontal astrocytoma showing central enhancement on this axial gadolinium-enhanced T1 image.

cant overlap with the more aggressive primary and metastatic neoplasms. There are more than a few reports of high-grade astrocytomas and even glioblastoma multiforme neoplasms that presented with low density seen on CT, no enhancement, and little to no mass effect, and T1 and T2 changes similar to low-grade tumors (20). Therefore, based on these findings, a truly accurate histologic diagnosis cannot be obtained with imaging alone, and thus adequate biopsy samples must be obtained to arrive at a correct diagnosis. However, a single biopsy specimen may also be inadequate because of the often variable histology within a given lesion. MRI and CT appearances are helpful in directing the surgeon to areas of the tumor that will give a higher yield for accurate diagnosis (10, 38,40,64). CT and/or MR images obtained with a stereotactic biopsy frame in place or fiducial markers for nonstereotactic three-dimensional localization are often the preferred methods for localizing the best areas for biopsy.

Although standard imaging technology remains unable to differentiate in all cases between high- and low-grade neoplasms, research continues into newer ways to understand both the biology of neoplasms and their histologic identity. So-called functional MRI (*f*MRI) assesses to a greater degree the metabolic activity of all types of brain abnormalities (5,10,97,118). With regard to brain neoplasms, studies have shown greater metabolic activity in high-grade versus low-grade primary brain tumors (5). This activity is most commonly seen with imaging dependent on blood oxygenation level. Although imperfect, this type of sequence does add specificity toward a histologic diagnosis. Probably of more clinical significance, perfusion and diffusion imaging techniques utilize the unique abilities of MR to study blood flow and spontaneous fluid transfer, respectively, within a given brain lesion (5,118,159). However, although these sequences do have application in separating high- and low-grade neoplasms, they are more useful clinically in the differentiation of recurrent neoplasm versus radiation-induced necrosis (5,118,159). In general, the areas of radiation necrosis show a lower metabolic activity than the abnormally high metabolic activity in recurrent tumor, similar to positron emission tomography (PET).

Radionuclide imaging of the brain has been performed for many years. However, with the advent of new agents there has been a resurgence in activity and usefulness of this procedure. The largest number of reports on radionuclide imaging for brain neoplasms stem from PET imaging in which radiolabeled brain metabolites are used to evaluate areas of high or low metabolic activity. The most commonly used agent is fluorodeoxyglucose (FDG), which measures glucose uptake in the evaluated area. In general, low-grade brain neoplasms show an area of hypometabolism compared with normal brain parenchyma, and high-grade neoplasms tend to be hypermetabolic on FDG studies (26,32,48,62,119). Radiation-induced necrosis typically is hypometabolic, compared with normal brain (15,33).

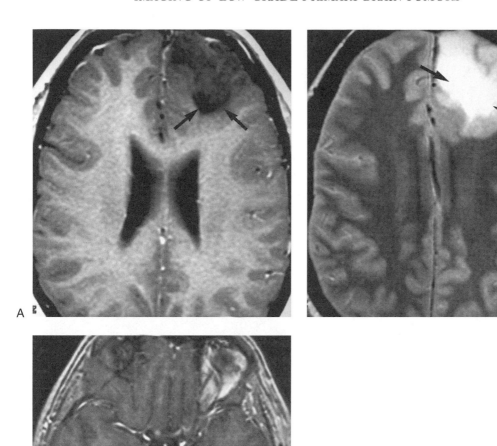

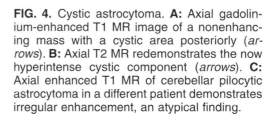

FIG. 4. Cystic astrocytoma. **A:** Axial gadolinium-enhanced T1 MR image of a nonenhancing mass with a cystic area posteriorly (*arrows*). **B:** Axial T2 MR redemonstrates the now hyperintense cystic component (*arrows*). **C:** Axial enhanced T1 MR of cerebellar pilocytic astrocytoma in a different patient demonstrates irregular enhancement, an atypical finding.

Another frequently used agent is ^{11}C-L-methylmethionine, a radiotracer that measures amino acid uptake in actively metabolic cells (31,119). Interestingly, with low-grade astrocytomas, methylmethionine uptake is either lower than or equal to that of normal brain and rarely mildly greater than normal brain parenchyma (31,119). However, oligodendrogliomas, another type of low-grade glioma, show significantly increased levels of methylmethionine uptake (31).

Another amino acid analog, ^{18}F-fluoro-2-deoxyuridine ([18]FudR), has been studied in high- and low-grade gliomas. High-grade lesions showed high activity with [18]FudR, compared with no abnormal uptake in low-grade gliomas (62). A third radionuclide agent, thallium-201, has been used to evaluate primary brain tumors as well as to differentiate recurrent tumor from radionecrosis (110,139). One study showed that thallium-201 single-photon-emission computed tomography (SPECT)

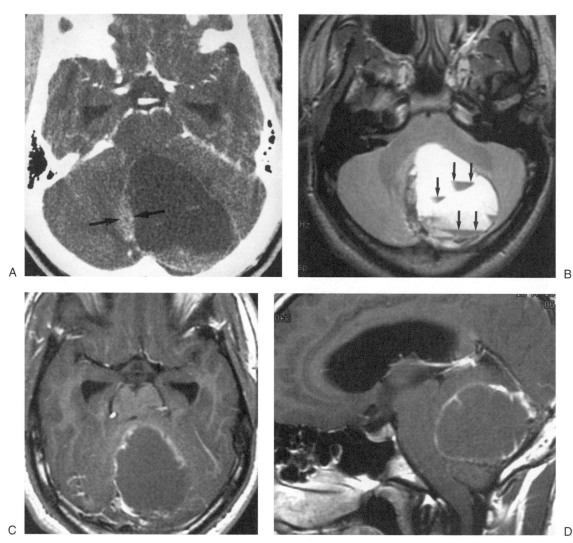

FIG. 5. Pilocytic cerebellar astrocytoma. **A:** Contrast-enhanced CT shows a large cystic mass with nodular enhancement medially (*arrows*). **B:** Axial T2 MRI reveals fluid-fluid levels (*arrows*) due to layering of various protein elements within the cyst fluid. Axial (**C**) and sagittal (**D**) T1-enhanced MR images confirm the nonenhancing cavity with their peripheral enhancement, more prominent medially.

is more sensitive and more specific than CT examination in separating recurrent neoplasm from radiation changes (15). The ratio of thallium-201 uptake in neoplasm to that of the contralateral normal brain (the thallium index) has been useful in predicting tumor biology and thereby separating high-grade versus low-grade neoplasms (110). Other agents are currently being investigated, most of which are analogs of amino acids that are incorpo-

rated during various cell division stages. These agents include ^{11}C-pet, [111]indium-DTPA-octreotide SPECT (92), and [18]FudR PET (62). Although all these modalities show promise in statistically differentiating high-grade from low-grade neoplasms, each reported series does show some degree of overlap between the two tumor grades, which reinforces that the imaging characteristics cannot entirely predict tumor biology but can

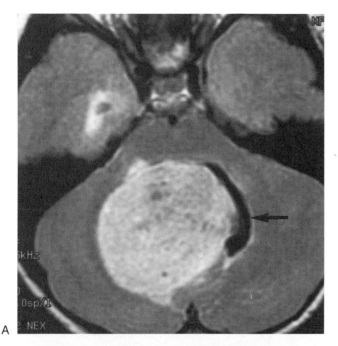

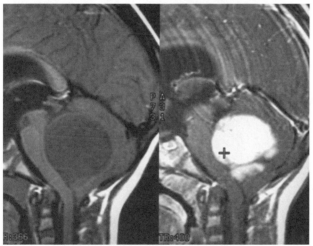

FIG. 6. Pilocytic cerebellar astrocytoma, unusual case with large area of solid tumor and a small cystic component. **A:** Axial T1-enhanced MR image demonstrates a large enhancing mass (nodule) with a small cystic component on the left (*arrow*). **B:** Sagittal T1 without (left) and with (right) contrast demonstrate that the bulk of the abnormality is solid enhancing tissue.

only reflect the variable tumor histology within any single lesion.

Before the advent of clinical MRI, MR was used as a tool for analysis of biochemical substrates in *in vitro* samples. *In vivo* spectroscopy has been used extensively for investigations into a variety of central nervous system (CNS) lesions, including neoplasia. Although investigational units are used to measure phosphorus (for stroke research, for

example), spectroscopy for neoplasia is geared to the resonance frequency of hydrogen (Fig. 7). Various signals are measured, including *n*-acetylaspartate (NAA) as a neuronal marker; choline, which is a cell membrane component, presumably increases in proliferating tumor tissue; lactate, a marker for glycolysis, which is sparse in normal brain but is increased in tumors; and creatine/phosphocreatine, which are markers for energy

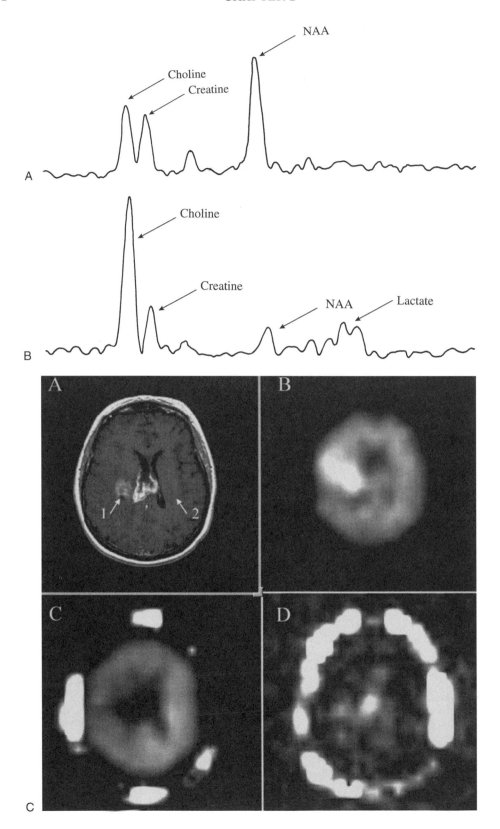

metabolism (52). Briefly, the NAA concentration in tumors is decreased compared with that of normal brain, whereas lactate is increased in high-grade but not in low-grade tumors (46,50,52,113,120,125). Choline tends to be increased in both high- and low-grade tumors but localized in the periphery of the more aggressive lesions (52). Spectroscopic imaging is a new way to look at these spectra. Many points of interest throughout the area being studied (e.g., a single axial slice of a brain MR with some tumor tissue and some normal tissue) have spectrographic data acquired, and a gray scale is assigned to the calculated areas under the peaks of the various elements being studied (e.g., NAA, choline, etc.). The images are maps of the relative concentrations of these various chemicals. Also, an image can be generated showing various ratios calculated, such as NAA/choline (see Fig. 7). Grading of neoplasms using spectroscopy is promising, but, like PET and other imaging studies, there is considerable overlap between the low-grade and high-grade lesions, as well as differences in the spectral analysis within regions of a single tumor (50,113). The most useful parameters appear to be the ratios of choline to creatine and NAA to creatine (50). Response to therapy, with definite prognostic implications, can be measured with MR spectroscopy, as high-grade lesions responding to treatment tend to assume spectra similar to normal brain or low-grade tumors (52). Elevated choline values with MR spectroscopy correlate with [18f]FDG uptake seen with PET scanning

(46). This suggests that the hypermetabolic rate of tumors (elevated [18f]FDG uptake) corresponds to increased cell turnover, as evidenced by the choline elevation on MR. Although no single study can accurately predict a tumor's biologic behavior, the combination of MR imaging, MR spectroscopy, PET, and *f*MRI may be able to discriminate between tumor types. Such correlation studies are ongoing, and their results may be exciting.

PLEOMORPHIC XANTHOASTROCYTOMA

Pleomorphic xanthoastrocytoma (PXA) is a rare glial neoplasm, characterized histologically by cells with varying appearances, often in a fascicular pattern, with globular lipid-containing cells predominating (49,67). These tumors occur typically in children or young adults with a long history of seizures, with a mean age of 14 years (49,67,115). These tumors are peripherally located in the supratentorial compartment, with approximately half involving the temporal lobe (115,160). They usually involve the leptomeninges but uncommonly involve the outer dura (49,67,115).

The typical imaging features of a PXA are that of a peripheral tumor, associated with a prominent cyst (in 89%), uncommonly demonstrating significant edema (Fig. 8) (49, 67,87,115,160). Calcifications are rare. Significant contrast enhancement is seen on both CT and MRI (87,115,160). T1 and T2 images are nonspecific, with T1 values similar to the surrounding brain and T2 hyperintense to

---

FIG. 7. Right hemisphere oligodendroglioma. **A:** Normal proton spectra (*arrow 2* in gadolinium enhanced T1-weighted image in image A of **C**). Note the high NAA peak and similar heights of the choline and creatine peaks. **B:** Proton spectra of enhancing tumor (*arrow 1* in image A of **C**). Note the height of the choline peak compared with creatine, strongly suggestive of neoplasm, along with the minimal NAA peak reflecting the lack of neurons. Note the prominent lactate couplet, possibly due to anaerobic metabolism. **C:** Four images at same level throughout tumor. A = gadolinium-enhanced T1-weighted MRI of an enhancing right-sided oligodendroglioma with callosal involvement. B = spectroscopic imaging (SSI) map representing high choline levels as the bright area on the right side. C = SSI map of NAA, showing low signal on the right due to the lack of NAA present in the tumor. Note that the low signal area is larger than the abnormal enhancement seen in A. D = Lactate SSI map showing relatively high lactate levels, likely due to anaerobic metabolism within the tumor or possibly in an area of necrosis.

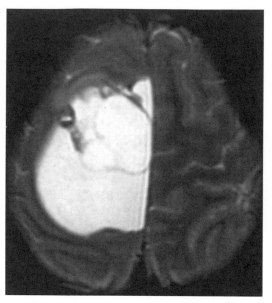
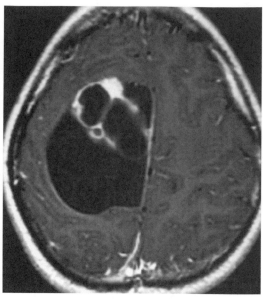

A   B

FIG. 8. Pleomorphic xanthoastrocytoma. **A:** Axial T2 MR image shows a large, septated cystic mass abutting the falx, with no significant surrounding edema. **B:** Axial enhanced T1 MR reveals the enhancement of the septations and a small nodule anteriorly.

brain (87,115,160). Despite the intracellular lipid material, no cases of high-signal PXAs on the T1-weighted MR images have been reported. Although these lesions are generally relatively benign and slow growing, aggressive growth and recurrence have been seen (151). The presence of necrosis is a strong predictor of aggressive behavior (115), and careful evaluation of the solid component of the tumor for necrotic areas is warranted.

The differential diagnosis for a peripherally located intra-axial mass includes a ganglioglioma and meningioma. Meningiomas are characterized by their extra-axial location and possible adjacent osseous hyperostosis. A ganglioglioma is difficult to differentiate from PXA, and these lesions have been found to coexist (44,81,117,165).

OLIGODENDROGLIOMA AND MIXED OLIGOASTROCYTOMAS

Oligodendrogliomas are glial neoplasms arising from oligodendrocytes; however, an astrocytic component is commonly present within these tumors (8,133,167). The distinction between oligodendroglioma and mixed oligoastrocytoma is made based on the relative percentage of neoplastic astrocytic cells within the tumor (133,167). These tumors are almost always supratentorial and distributed equally in all lobes on the basis of the size of the lobe. They have also been found in the posterior fossa and within the ventricular system (8,34,114). Oligodendrogliomas tend to involve both the gray and white matter (8,14, 16,133,140,167). Subarachnoid spread and multifocality have been described (112,140). These tumors are found in children and adults (from 3 to 80 years of age) with a mild peak in the fourth and fifth decades and a slight male predilection (8,167).

CT typically demonstrates a peripherally located tumor that is hypodense in 57% to 70% of cases (83,149). However, intraventricular oligodendrogliomas have a tendency toward hyperdensity (34). Calcifications are common, seen in 40% to 90% of cases (Fig. 9) on CT (34,83,149,156). Although calcifications tend to be coarse, more punctate or

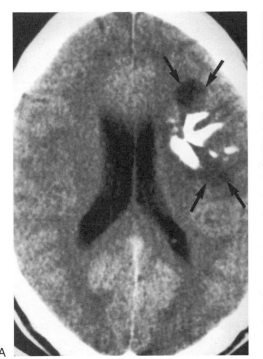
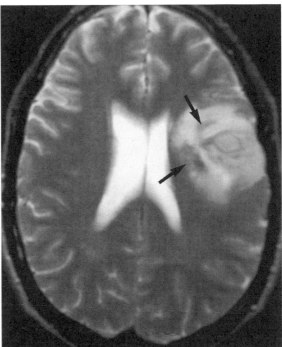

A   B

FIG. 9. Oligodendroglioma. **A:** Enhanced CT reveals the typical hypodense tumor (*arrows*) with obvious dense calcifications. **B:** Axial T2 shows the hyperintense mass with ill-defined hypointensities due to the calcifications (*arrows*).

linear calcification may also be present. Although calcifications have been correlated with a better prognosis in small radiologic series (103,156), this finding has been disputed in larger pathologic series (16,104). Cysts have been identified in 20% of oligodendrogliomas on CT (83) and in 32% in pathologic series (104). Oligodendrogliomas are well circumscribed in 49% to 57% of CT examinations, and enhance in 24% to 66% of cases (83,149). Calvarial erosion, indicative of long-standing tumor, has been identified in 17% of CT examinations (83).

On MRI the tumor is usually hypointense on T1 (Fig. 10) and hyperintense and heterogeneous on proton density and T2-weighted images (Fig. 11). The tumor is usually found to be well circumscribed (83) and foci of enhancement are readily visible. Marked enhancement tends to be associated with anaplastic grades, whereas mild or nodular enhancement does not appear to have a predilection for any grade (24). Calcifications are not as readily visible on MRI (see Fig. 9B) as with CT but may be more conspicuous on gradient-echo acquisitions (7,55). In our experience of 28 patients, we found cystic components following cerebrospinal fluid (CSF) on all pulse sequences associated with an oligodendroglioma in 21% of cases (24). Histologically proven microcysts, which have been correlated with a better prognosis on pathologic series (103,104,137), give a high signal intensity on proton density, T2- and T1-weighted imaging. Oligodendrogliomas tend to spread along white matter tracts and occasionally into and through the corpus callosum, but this does not correlate with tumor grade (24). Although hemorrhage has been noted to occur within these tumors, it is not common in the literature or in our personal experience (83,133,149,156,167). Recurrence is not unusual, and especially in lower-grade tumors nonenhancing recurrence may be dif-

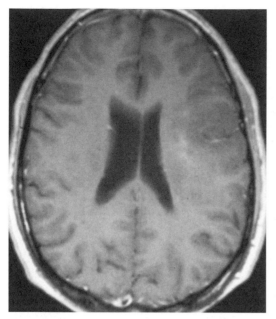

FIG. 10. Oligodendroglioma (same patient as in Fig. 9). T1-enhanced MR shows hypointense nonenhancing mass in left frontal lobe.

ficult to distinguish from postoperative or postradiation changes on CT or MRI. Rarely, distant metastases have been reported (93).

The differential considerations of low-grade oligodendrogliomas and low-grade mixed oligoastrocytomas on imaging include anaplastic astrocytoma, ganglioglioma, gangliocytoma, and dysembryoplastic neuroepithelial tumor. Distinguishing features of oligodendrogliomas include a combination of gray and white matter involvement, the presence of calcifications, and signal heterogeneity on MRI.

SUBEPENDYMOMA

Subependymomas are biologically benign, slow-growing peri- and intraventricular tumors with a male predilection that occur in adult patients with a mean age of 48 years. These tumors rarely produce symptoms and are commonly identified incidentally in autopsy series. Based on critical location and

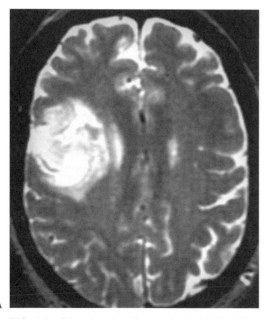
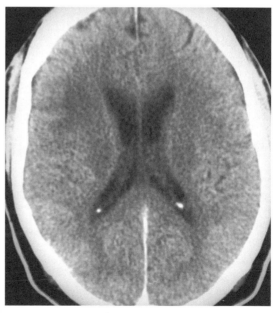

A   B

FIG. 11. Oligodendroglioma. **A:** Axial T2 MR demonstrates the typical heterogeneous hyperintensity. **B:** CT of same patient (3 years prior to the MR in **A**) reveals subtle hypodensity without mass effect.

size, hydrocephalus is the most common presentation (8,22). Subependymomas are most commonly found in the fourth ventricle and lateral ventricle (8,22), although they have also been identified in the third ventricle and even in the spinal cord (54).

The imaging appearance of subependymomas varies according to location (22). CT of fourth ventricular subependymomas demonstrates variable density compared with gray matter with calcifications in 50% to 100% of cases (Fig. 12) and enhancement in 62% to 92% (22,60,80,89). Conversely, lateral ventricular subependymomas vary in density but are more often hypodense, usually do not enhance, and show calcifications in less than 10% (22,80). Unlike subependymomas, other lateral ventricle tumors such as ependymoma, choroid plexus papilloma, and central neurocytoma are more likely to demonstrate calcification and contrast enhancement.

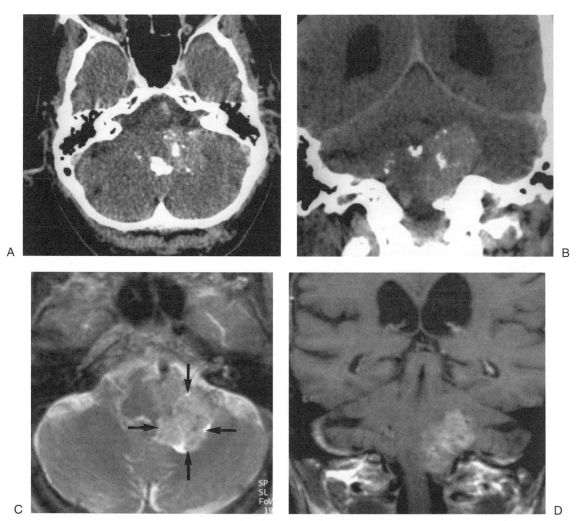

FIG. 12. Subependymoma. Axial (**A**) and coronal (**B**) enhanced CT shows a mildly enhancing posterior fossa mass with scattered calcifications. **C:** Axial T2 MR demonstrates a minimally hyperintense mass (*arrows*) with no significant surrounding edema. **D:** Coronal enhanced T1 MR image reveals the enhancing mass and resultant hydrocephalus.

MRI of fourth ventricular subependymomas demonstrates the origin to be from the floor of the fourth ventricle with frequent extension through the foramina of Lushka or Magendie. They are either hypointense or isointense to gray matter on T1, and isointense or hyperintense to gray matter on T2. Fourth ventricular subependymomas almost always demonstrate heterogeneous enhancement on MRI. Therefore, it is difficult to distinguish subependymomas from more aggressive tumors of the fourth ventricle based on imaging alone unless the tumor is demonstrated to invade the adjacent brain parenchyma, which is distinctly unusual for subependymoma (43). Fourth ventricular subependymomas have a close relationship to the brain stem and nearby cranial nerves and thus should be carefully scrutinized prior to surgery because, even with incomplete excision, recurrence or CSF dissemination is unusual (22,43). Although MRI may demonstrate encasement or displacement of adjacent blood vessels, these tumors can usually be dissected away from blood vessels at surgery (54). Lateral ventricular subependymomas are typically hypointense to gray matter on T1 and hyperintense on T2. As with CT, they seldom demonstrate enhancement and are thus readily distinguished from other lateral ventricular tumors that typically do enhance (22,54,70).

SUBEPENDYMAL GIANT CELL ASTROCYTOMA

Subependymal giant cell astrocytomas occur almost exclusively in 10- to 20-year-old patients with tuberous sclerosis. The intracranial manifestations of tuberous sclerosis are imaged by both CT and MRI, although MRI is more sensitive for detecting many of the lesions (3,45,56). The subependymal giant cell astrocytoma is a neoplasm that arises from subependymal tubers found along the sulcus terminalis and bulge into the lateral ventricles (12,41). These tubers are composed of fibrillated gemistocytic astrocytes that are thought to dedifferentiate into a true glial neoplasm

and occur in approximately 10% of patients with tuberous sclerosis (12,41). Because they arise from the subependymal tubers, these giant cell astrocytomas are predominantly intraventricular and classically located near the interventricular foramen of Monro, causing outlet obstruction of one or both lateral ventricles. Treatment is usually restricted to surgery, with good long-term survival rates (99).

CT of subependymal giant cell astrocytomas usually shows a nonspecific intraventricular mass that is often calcified, with moderate contrast enhancement, and that may have areas of nonenhancing necrosis (3,45,56,99,102). MRI reveals a nearly isointense mass on T1-weighted images, with heterogeneous high signal intensity on T2-weighted sequences (3,56). As with CT, these lesions enhance to a moderate degree but may show areas of nonenhancement resulting from calcification or necrosis. The identification of an enhancing intraventricular mass in a patient with known tuberous sclerosis makes the diagnosis relatively simple. The presence of nonenhancing cortical and subependymal tubers confirms the diagnosis of tuberous sclerosis.

CHOROID PLEXUS PAPILLOMAS

Approximately 10% of all CNS neoplasms involve the ventricular system (150). Many of these are glial neoplasms or parenchymal metastases that invade the ventricular walls. However, truly intraventricular neoplasms do occur. Meningiomas and choroid plexus papillomas comprise most of these tumors, with neurocytomas also included but less abundant.

Choroid plexus papillomas are usually seen in children under 10 years old and are slightly more common in males (66,98,133,150). In children, the atrium of the lateral ventricle is the most likely site of occurrence, whereas in adults, the fourth ventricle is the more common site of origin (66,133).

Imaging of choroid plexus papillomas usually reveals hydrocephalus resulting from overproduction of CSF, causing nonobstructive ventricular enlargement. CT of these lesions usually reveals a well-marginated intraventricular mass that is iso- to slightly hyperdense compared with brain (25,58,106, 133) (Fig. 13). Calcification is unusual in the pediatric tumors but occurs in up to 25% of adults with these tumors (66). Contrast enhancement is typically dense and homogeneous. However, the malignant choroid plexus carcinomas often show a heterogeneous enhancement pattern (25,58,106,133), with edema often seen in the adjacent brain parenchyma.

MR of choroid plexus papillomas is variable, with T1 signals typically isointense to brain and T2 showing variably bright signal intensity, depending on tumor vascularity, calcification, cyst, or hemorrhage. Typically, there is intense enhancement with gadolinium, similar to the CT findings. MR is extremely sensitive for identifying peritumoral edema and seeding of tumor in the ventricular system, which may happen with both benign and malignant tumors (25,98,133).

Angiography demonstrates an intensely enhancing tumor, fed by enlarged tortuous vessels (66). The pattern and degree of tumoral enhancement distinguish these lesions from the typical moderate diffuse enhancement seen with meningiomas. Choroid plexus carcinomas similarly are densely enhancing, although the feeder arteries may not be as large and tortuous, as these malignant lesions are faster growing, with less time available for vessel enlargement.

DYSEMBRYOPLASTIC NEUROEPITHELIAL TUMOR

Dysembryoplastic neuroepithelial tumor (DNT) is a recently described cortically based tumor defined by a multinodular architecture that may include specific glioneuronal elements, a nodular component of glial cells, and cortical dysplasia (28). Approximately 7.5% to 14% of intractable epilepsy cases have been attributed to DNT (28,126). Patients typically present in childhood, although DNT has been found in patients up to age 61, and there

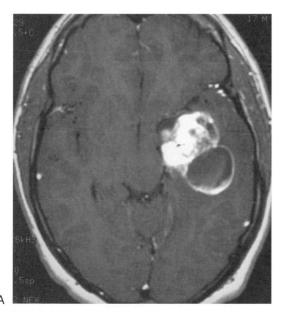
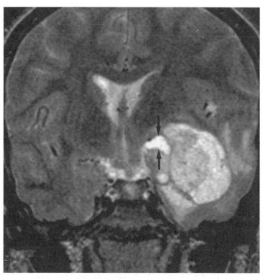

A B

FIG. 13. Ganglioglioma. **A:** Axial enhanced T1 MR image demonstrates the enhancing temporal lobe mass with a large cyst posteriorly. **B:** Coronal T2 MR shows the high signal mass with a small medial cyst (*arrows*).

is a slight male predominance (127). In their original description of DNT in 39 epilepsy patients, Daumas-Dupont et al. (28) found the tumor in the temporal lobe in 62%, the frontal lobe in 31%, and the parieto-occipital lobe in 9%. Subsequent series (72,78,84,126) have found an incidence of 40% to 91% in the temporal lobe with a predominance in the mesial temporal lobe (79% in one series) (126), and 6% to 40% in the frontal lobe. Cerebellar involvement (127) and multifocal involvement of thalami, pons, basal ganglia, and third ventricle have also been described (85).

CT typically demonstrates a well-circumscribed hypodense lesion with a pseudocyst appearance (26,84,126), although CT has been found to be normal in approximately 10% of cases (28,72,126). Occasionally, these tumors are isodense to gray matter, or even mixed density (1,28,79). True cysts have been noted in 28% of cases (146), and calcific hyperdensities occur in 20% to 36% (72,78,126), although calcospherites are seen on histopathologic examination in 81% of cases (126). Focal contrast enhancement on CT was noted in only 18% of patients (126). Calvarial scalloping or temporal fossa erosion, which are signs of chronicity, is reported with peripheral tumors in 9% to 60% of cases (28,78).

MRI usually demonstrates a well-circumscribed, cortically based tumor with gyral or nodular configuration, which is hypointense on T1 and hyperintense on T2 relative to gray matter (1,28,72,78,79,84,126,127) and homogeneous in 57% of cases (126). Signal on proton density is increased in 66% and decreased in 33% relative to gray matter (126). MRI identifies cystic components in 31% of cases (126), and focal and punctate enhancement in 16% to 66% of cases (72,78,126,127), although diffuse enhancement has been reported in 33% of lesions in one series (126). The cause of the punctate contrast enhancement is unknown; however, vascular arcades are seen on microscopic examination (78). White matter extension is noted in 43% of cases, and blurring of the gray/white interface has been attributed to edema, invasion, cortical dysgenesis, and dysmyelination noted on

pathologic examination (8,126). The nodularity of the tumor has been speculated to be related to the histopathologic architecture of the tumor, with nodular foci of cortical dysplasia and hypercellularity (126, 127). Microcystic change accounts for at least some of the focal hyperintensities (78). Angiography has typically been unremarkable, with no neovascularity, although occasionally avascular mass effect can be demonstrated (28). Radionuclide SPECT imaging has demonstrated marked hypoperfusion and no thallium uptake, unlike with other low-grade gliomas that demonstrate moderate hypoperfusion and low thallium uptake.

Differential considerations on MRI include low-grade gliomas such as astrocytoma, oligodendroglioma, ganglioglioma, and pleomorphic xanthoastrocytoma. Distinguishing features of DNT, compared with these other tumors, include a thick nodular or gyral configuration with little or no white matter extension, rarely seen in other glial tumors (1,78, 79). Well-demarcated lobulated tumor margins without mass effect are seen in 80% of these tumors (78). The surgeon should submit the entire specimen to the pathologist because the pathologic diagnosis depends in part on the multiple nodular components of this tumor (28), as cortical dysplasia, a congenital nonneoplastic entity, must be distinguished from DNT. On MRI, cortical dysplasia follows the signal intensity of gray matter on all pulse sequences (8,78,126). Thin-section volume acquisition with multiplanar reformatting in patients with intractable epilepsy may help identify the tumor's relationship to the mesial temporal structures. This technique may also demonstrate small DNT in areas difficult to discern on routine MRI examination such as the upper convexities. Furthermore, this approach may help identify foci of cortical dysgenesis, areas of cystic degeneration, and calcifications (126).

GANGLION CELL TUMORS

Tumors containing neoplastic ganglion cells are termed *ganglion cell tumors* and include gangliogliomas, ganglioneuromas, and the more malignant ganglioneuroblastoma (133,167).

Gangliogliomas are formed by an admixture of neoplastic ganglion cells along with glial cells. Unlike DNTs, in these tumors the primary component is predominantly astrocytic and involves both gray and white matter (141). Patients affected range in age from 3 months to 80 years (59,82), with a median age at diagnosis reported among different series to be 14–25 years, with a slight male predilection (18,30,35,53,82,145,166). Gangliogliomas are the most frequent tumor to produce chronic intractable seizures, although cranial nerve deficits and headache are not uncommon presenting symptoms (23,53,82,105). These tumors represent from 0.3% to 0.6% of all brain tumors and 1.2% to 7.8% of pediatric brain tumors (30,133,167). A recent retrospective review of pediatric spinal tumors and adult cerebral gliomas using immunohistochemical neuronal markers revealed that the tumor may be more common than previously thought in the spinal cord and brain stem (101). These two locations have an increased risk for recurrence (53,82). Intracranially, the most common location is the temporal lobe, variously reported to occur in 30% to 84% of cases. Other frequently reported sites include the floor of the third ventricle, cerebellum, and brain stem, although any part of the brain, including the optic nerves, may be affected (18,23,35,53,88,90,133,141,166).

CT of gangliogliomas exhibits a hypodense tumor relative to gray matter in 50% to 75% of cases (18,35,166), with 38% to 47% of the gangliogliomas appearing cystic (18,35,145, 166). This cystlike component has often been found to be solid intraoperatively (30,59). A mildly hyperdense tumor is identified in up to 23% of cases (18,35,145). Calcifications are identified in 31% to 41% of cases examined with CT (18,35,141,166). Contrast-enhanced CT exams demonstrate enhancement in 18% to 70% of cases (18,35,145,166). CT was negative in 0 to 33% of cases (18,141,145,166).

MRI is superior to CT in demonstrating the full extent of the tumor, its location, and the presence of cysts; however, calcification is much better demonstrated on CT. At least two reported cases of patients who had normal MRI exams underwent temporal lobectomy for partial complex seizures (145). MRI of these tumors typically exhibits a well-defined cystic component and a less well-defined solid component (18) (see Fig. 13). Lesions that are primarily cystic occurred in 31% to 57% of large series, whereas completely solid lesions occurred approximately half of the time (18,145,166). Cystic components are hypointense on T1- and hyperintense on T2-weighted images; however, the proton density signal may be variable (18,166). The solid components of these tumors typically are low or intermediate signal on T1, high signal or intermediate signal on T2, and proton density (18,166). Homogeneous gadolinium enhancement has been variously reported in up to 44% of cases (166). Diffuse leptomeningeal spread of ganglioglioma on gadolinium-enhanced MRI is rare (157). Gangliogliomas are typically avascular on angiography, although a case of a highly vascular ganglioglioma has been reported (11).

Differential considerations for gangliogliomas include dysembryoplastic neuroepithelial tumor, pleomorphic xanthoastrocytoma, low-grade astrocytoma, oligodendroglioma, and gangliocytoma. Suggestive imaging features for ganglioglioma include temporal lobe or posterior fossa location, involvement of both gray and white matter, combination of well-defined cystic and ill-defined solid components, calcifications, and an enhancing nodule.

Gangliocytomas are extremely rare, purely neuronal tumors that can occur anywhere in the CNS. Intracranially, those typically occurring in the cerebral hemispheres and brain stem are distinctive from intrasellar gangliocytomas and dysplastic gangliocytomas of the cerebellum (Lhermitte-Duclos disease) described later. The age range is 5–52 years, with an average age of 11 years at presentation and a slight male preponderance (167).

Only limited imaging analysis has been reported for cerebral gangliocytomas. They tend to be slightly hyperdense on CT with little or no contrast enhancement, and no mass effect. These tumors usually are difficult to identify on T1-weighted MRI, although if detected they are of mixed signal intensity. Signal intensity is intermediate to high on proton density MRI and intermediate to low on T2-weighted MRI (2,42). Because of these signal characteristics, the lesions can thus be confused with hemorrhagic lesions. The intermediate and low T2 signal has been speculated as being related to dense congregations of large nuclei with prominent nucleoli with long-chain fatty acids, causing an increase in the T2 relaxation rate (2,111,134). The hyperdense appearance on CT and the hypointense T2 signal of gangliocytomas may serve to differentiate them from most other CNS neoplasms, which tend to be hyperintense on T2 and hypodense or isodense on CT. Cortical heterotopia can be distinguished based on its tendency to follow gray matter signals on all MR pulse sequences (8). Gangliocytomas have also been observed to possess cystic components and enhancing nodules that may appear similar to gangliogliomas, PXA, or low-grade astrocytomas (57,63).

When they occur in the sellar region, gangliocytomas should be distinguished from hypothalamic hamartomas, which are congenital. Gangliocytomas, unlike hamartomas, demonstrate neoplastic cells and growth and are associated with pituitary adenomas in 65% of cases. Acromegaly is the most common presenting symptom in these patients. Sellar gangliocytomas cannot be distinguished from pituitary adenomas with imaging alone. They are hyperdense on CT in 90% of cases, enhance with contrast, and demonstrate calcifications in 8% of cases. On MRI they are round, typically intrasellar masses, although they may involve the hypothalamus (77,100).

Dysplastic cerebellar gangliocytoma (DCG, Lhermitte-Duclos disease, purkingioma) is a mass characterized by thickened cerebellar folia due to hypertrophy of granular cell neurons, hypermyelination in the molecular layer, and Purkinje cell loss with white

matter atrophy (77,167). It is considered by some to represent a hamartomatous, not a neoplastic, lesion (27,100). Conditions coexisting with DCG include holoprosencephaly, neurofibromatosis, Cowden's disease, and multiple hamartoma syndrome (86,128,129, 142,148). Patients typically present with headache and hydrocephalus and range in age from newborn to 74 years, with an average age of 34 (77).

No large series of this entity is available in the imaging literature. CT usually demonstrates a hypodense cerebellar lesion (Fig. 14A) (77,100), with alternating layers of isodensity and hypodensity relative to gray matter involving the cerebellar cortex (77,100). Calcifications are rarely present, and there is usually no enhancement (77,100,142). MRI demonstrates the lesion to better advantage, especially since beam-hardening artifact can hinder posterior fossa imaging on CT. The lack of clearly distinctive color, consistency, and structure relative to normal cerebellum makes it difficult to identify the lesion's margins intraoperatively. MRI can thus help define the resection margins (142). MRI demonstrates a laminated lesion of T2 hyperintensity and T1 hypointensity with mass effect involving the cerebellar hemisphere, often with involvement of the vermis (Fig. 14B,C). Hydrocephalus is a frequent finding in these patients, but chiari I and syrinx have also been observed with this lesion (77,95,100). The striated appearance represents an isointense molecular layer, with sulcal effacement observed along the cerebellar folia with signal abnormality (increased on T2, and decreased on T1) in the granular layer, deep molecular layer, and underlying white matter (77,100). Vascular proliferation is thought to represent the source of calcification and enhancement occasionally observed in these patients (9,27,77,100). Recurrence after resection has been observed up to 12 years after initial resection; thus long-term follow-up is suggested (51,77,94, 100,124,162).

The striated appearance on MRI is felt to be characteristic for DCG; however, this may

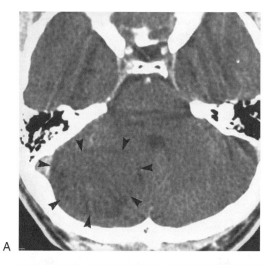

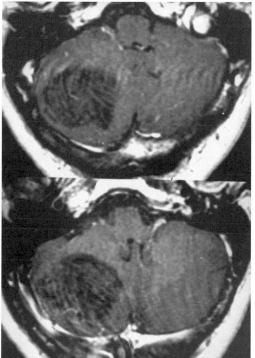

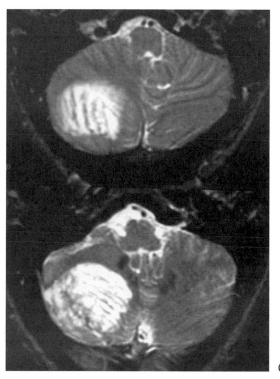

FIG. 14. Dysplastic cerebellar gangliocytoma (Lhermitte-Duclos). **A:** Contrast-enhanced CT reveals a nonenhancing low-density mass (*arrowheads*) with minimal mass effect on the fourth ventricle. **B:** Axial T1 and T2 **(C)** MR demonstrates the typical striated appearance of this lesion due to thickened cerebellar folia.

be confused with acute or subacute cerebellar infarcts. An infarct is differentiated from DCG based on clinical history and the typical evolution of infarcts over time (77,100). The unique striated appearance of DCG helps distinguish this lesion from other tumors.

DESMOPLASTIC INFANTILE GANGLIOGLIOMA

Desmoplastic infantile ganglioglioma (DIG) is a recently described mixed ganglion and glial cell tumor with extensive desmoplasia and large cysts. It is considered a benign tumor despite its high mitotic activity, rapid growth, and aggressive appearance both on imaging and on microscopy. DIGs usually are large and involve more than one lobe. The most common location includes the frontal and parietal lobes, although it has also been observed to involve the temporal and occipital lobes. The tumor is superficially located, and growth into the subarachnoid space and adjacent meninges is uniformly present. A good deal of the desmoplastic component is associated with the meningeal extension (107,155). Extension into the lateral ventricles has been reported (152). Almost all cases occur under 18 months of age, although isolated cases in adults have been reported (76,144,147,155). DIG has significant similarities to other recently described desmoplastic tumors of childhood, including gliofibroma, pleomorphic xanthoastrocytoma, and desmoplastic astrocytoma. Although the lack of ganglion cells in these other desmoplastic tumors provides a distinction for DIG, these tumors may actually represent varying expressions of a single desmoplastic tumor type (29,36,75,122).

The most striking imaging feature of this tumor is its large size. CT reveals a large tumor with formation of a large hypodense cyst and a hyperdense solid component that enhances intensely. This hyperdensity on non-contrast CT can be accounted for by dense collagen deposition. On MRI the cystic component, as expected, is low on T1 and high on T2 images. The signal characteristics of the solid component in this tumor have been variably reported as hypo-, hyper-, or isointense relative to gray matter. The solid component markedly enhances and typically is adjacent to the meninges. A ringlike pattern of enhancement has been described but is uncommon (19,96,144,147). The variable signal characteristics of the solid component as well as its enhancement pattern can be explained by the intermixing of desmoplasia and cellular elements found in these tumors (96). Angiography typically demonstrates a large avascular mass with a small tumor stain (144, 152).

Differential considerations include primitive neuroectodermal tumor, ependymoma, and astrocytoma. DIG should be considered in infants presenting with a large superficial cerebral mass with large cystic components and an enhancing solid component adjacent to meninges (96,147). Its identification is important because it has a significantly better prognosis and different management considerations relative to many other infantile brain tumors.

NEUROCYTOMA

Neurocytomas are composed of small, neoplastic, granular-type neuronal cells resembling oligodendroglioma cells on light microscopy. They are almost exclusively intraventricular and have thus been termed *central neurocytoma* (21,69,135,161). Recently, intracerebral neurocytomas have been described and designated cerebral neurocytomas (108,123). Neurocytomas comprise 0.1% to 0.5% of all brain tumors (69,161). The age range for these tumors is 7–53 years (21,116,121) with a mean age of 25–30 years, with no gender predilection (21,69,161). Patients usually present with symptoms of hydrocephalus, although cerebral neurocytomas can also present with seizures (21,69,108,123, 161). There are case reports of tumors presenting with hemorrhage (96,109,143).

CT of central neurocytoma demonstrates a hyperdense, well-circumscribed intraventricular tumor that enhances homogeneously. Calcifications are present in 52% to 75% of cases, and tiny cystic components are often present (21,47,69,71,123,135,161).

MRI demonstrates a large intraventricular tumor with frequent extension into the third ventricle through the foramen of Monro. Surgically demonstrated points of attachment more commonly include the septum pellucidum and lateral wall of the lateral ventricle, although they have also been reported to be attached to the roof and inferomedial wall of the lateral ventricle and third ventricle (21,47,69,109,161). Extension into or origin from the adjacent brain parenchyma has been reported and has been associated with anaplastic varieties of central neurocytoma (21,136,161). Central neurocytomas are typically isointense to gray matter on T1-weighted MRI, although they may be hyperin-tense, hypointense, or mixed (Fig. 15). T2 imaging may be isointense, mixed isointensity with hyperintensity, or generally hyperintense relative to gray matter. Proton density sequences demonstrate isointense, hyperin-

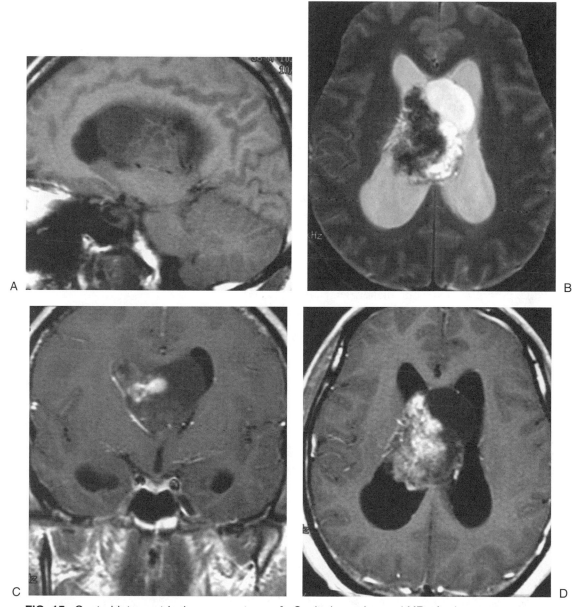

FIG. 15. Central intraventricular neurocytoma. **A:** Sagittal unenhanced MR of a large, complex-appearing intraventricular mass. **B:** Axial T2 MR reveals the typical hyperintense cystic portion of the mass anteriorly, with the mixed high- and low-signal solid portion posteriorly. Coronal (**C**) and axial (**D**) T1-enhanced images demonstrate irregular enhancement of the solid mass, the nonenhancing cyst, and hydrocephalus.

tense, or mixed signal relative to gray matter (21,69,71,161). Serpiginous and punctate signal voids from prominent intratumoral vessels or calcifications frequently can be identified within the tumor (69). In addition, a dilated thalamostriate vein or internal cerebral vein often may be identified (161). The tumor almost always enhances homogeneously. On angiography a vascular stain is shown in 71% of cases. When demonstrated, feeding arteries are typically choroidal or lenticulostriate. Prominent draining veins are less frequently identified (69).

Recurrence of central neurocytomas has been recorded as early as 8 months and as late as 6 years after treatment (39,71,130,164), which suggests that appropriate follow-up imaging is necessary. Isolated cases of intraventricular and spinal dissemination following resection have also been reported and identified on follow-up imaging despite this tumor's benign histology (39).

The few reported cases of cerebral neurocytomas indicate that these tumors have occurred in the frontal and temporal lobes and involve both gray and white matter. They are hypodense and sometimes cystic in appearance on CT, and are without calcifications. MRI demonstrates a tumor that is hyperintense on T2 and hypointense on T1 relative to gray matter (108,123) (Fig. 16).

Differential considerations for central neurocytoma include intraventricular tumors centered around the frontal horn, foramen of Monro, and body of the lateral ventricle, including ependymoma, astrocytoma, oligodendroglioma, metastasis, and lymphoma. Intraventricular meningiomas in older adults and choroid plexus papillomas typically in children tend to occur in the trigone of the lateral ventricles. Subependymomas may look similar to central neurocytoma on nonenhanced studies, but their lack of enhancement and older age distribution tend to differentiate them. Neuroblastoma and glioblastoma multiforme often have a more aggressive appearance, although on occasion they may present a diagnostic difficulty. Many of these tumors have imaging characteristics similar to those described for central neurocytomas, thus making absolute differentiation difficult (37, 58,135).

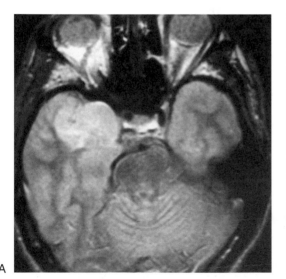 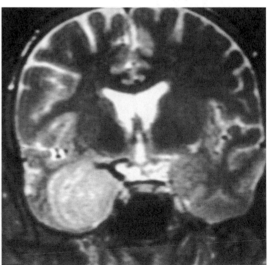

A   B

FIG. 16. Cerebral neurocytoma. **A:** Axial proton density MR reveals a well-defined hyperintense left temporal mass involving gray and white matter. **B:** Coronal T2 MR redemonstrates the hyperintense medial temporal lobe mass. A cyst was not identified.

REFERENCES

1. Abe M, Tabuchi K, Tsuji T, et al. Dysembryoplastic neuro-epithelial tumor: report of three cases. *Surg Neurol* 1995;43:240–245.
2. Altman NR. MR and CT characteristics of gangliocytoma: a rare cause of epilepsy in children. *AJNR* 1982;9:917–921.
3. Altman NR, Purser RK, Post MJ. Tuberous sclerosis: characteristics at CT and MR imaging. *Radiology* 1988;167:527–532.
4. Araki T, Inouye T, Suzuki H, Machida T, Iio M. Magnetic resonance imaging of brain tumors: measurement of T1. *Radiology* 1984;150:95–98.
5. Aronen HJ, Glass J, Pardo FS, et al. Echo-planar MR cerebral blood volume mapping of gliomas. *Acta Radiol* 1995;36:520–528.
6. Asari S, Makabe T, Katayama S, Itoh T, Tsuchida S, Ohmoto T. Assessment of the pathological grade of astrocytic gliomas using an MRI score. *Neuroradiology* 1994;36:308–310.
7. Atlas SW, Grossman RI, Hackney DB. Calcified intracranial lesions: detection with gradient-echo-acquisition rapid MR imaging. *AJNR* 1988;9:253–259.
8. Atlas SW, Lavi E. Intraaxial brain tumors. In: Atals SW, ed. *Magnetic resonance imaging of the brain and spine,* 2nd ed. Philadelphia: Lippincott-Raven, 1996: 423–488.
9. Awwad EE, Levy E, Martin DS, Merenda GO. Atypical MR appearance of Lhermitte-Duclos disease with contrast enhancement. *AJNR* 1995;16:1719–1720.
10. Bagley LJ, Grossman RI, Judy KD, et al. Gliomas: correlation of magnetic susceptibility artifact with histologic grade. *Radiology* 1997;202:511–516.
11. Batltuch GH, Farmer JP, Meagher-Villemure K, et al. Ganglioglioma presenting as a vascular lesion in a 10 year old boy. *J Neurosurg* 1993;79:920–923.
12. Bender JR, Yunis EJ. The pathology of tuberous sclerosis. *Pathol Annu* 1982;17:339–382.
13. Brant-Zawadzki M, Badami JP, Mills CM, Norman D, Newton TH. Primary intracranial tumor imaging: a comparison of magnetic resonance and CT. *Radiology* 1984;150:435–440.
14. Bruner JM. Oligodendroglioma: Diagnosis and prognosis. *Semin Diagn Pathol* 1987;4:251–261.
15. Buchpiguel CA, Alavi JB, Alavi A, Kenyon LC. PET versus SPECT in distinguishing radiation necrosis from tumor recurrence in the brain [clinical conference]. *J Nucl Med* 1995;36(1):159–164.
16. Burger PC, Rawling CE, Cox ER, et al. Clinicopathologic correlation in the oligodendroglioma. *Cancer* 1987;59:1345–1352.
17. Butler AR, Horij SC, Kricheff II, Shannon MB, Budzilovich GN. Computed tomography in astrocytomas: a statistical analysis of the parameters of malignancy and the positive contrast-enhanced CT scan. *Radiology* 1978;129:433–439.
18. Castillo M, Davis PC, Takei Y, Hoffman JCJ. Intracranial ganglioglioma: MR, CT, and clinical findings in 18 patients. *AJNR* 1990;11:109–114.
19. Cerda-Nicolas M, Kepes JJ. Gliofibromas including malignant forms and gliosarcomas: a comparative study and review of the literature. *Acta Neuropathol* 1993;85:349–361.
20. Chamberlain MC, Murovic JA, Levin VA. Absence of contrast enhancement on CT brain scans of patients with supratentorial malignant gliomas. *Neurology* 1988;38:1371–1374.
21. Chang KH, Han MH, Kim DG, Chi JG, et al. MR appearance of central neurocytoma. *Acta Radiol* 1993; 34:520–526.
22. Chiechi MV, Smirniatopoulos JG, Jones RV. Intracranial subependymomas: CT and MR imaging features in 24 cases. *Am J Roentgenol* 1995;165:1245–1250.
23. Chintagumpala MM, Armstrong D, Miki S, et al. Mixed neuronal-glial tumors (gangliogliomas) in children. *Pediatr Neurosurg* 1996;24:306–331.
24. Christoforidis GA, Mehta BA, Agrawal R, Georganos SA, Patel SC. Imaging of oligodendrogliomas. *ASNR Proceedings* 1997; 361.
25. Coates TL, Hinshaw DB, Peckman N, et al. Pediatric choroid plexus neoplasms: MR, CT and pathologic correlation. *Radiology* 1989;173:81–88.
26. Coleman RE, Hoffman JM, Hanson MW, Sostman HD, Schold SC. Clinical application of PET for the evaluation of brain tumors. *J Nucl Med* 1991;32: 616–622.
27. Da Silva AAD, Banerjee T, Coimbra RLM. Lhermitte-Duclos disease (cerebellar gangliocytoma). *South Med J* 1996;89:1208–1212.
28. Daumas-Dupont C, Scheithauer BW, Chodkiewicz JP, et al. Dysembryoplastic neuroepithelial tumor: a surgically curable tumor of young patients with intractable partial seizures: report of thirty-nine cases. *Neurosurgery* 1988;23:545–556.
29. De Chadarevian JP, Pattisapu JV, Faerber EN. Desmoplastic cerebral astrocytoma of infancy: light microscopy, immunohistochemistry and ultrastructure. *Cancer* 1990;66:173–179.
30. Demierre B, Stichnoth FA, Hori A, Spoerri O. Intracerebral ganglioglioma. *J Neurosurg* 1986;65:177–182.
31. Derlon JM, Petit-Taboué MC, Chapon F, et al. The *in vivo* metabolic pattern of low-grade brain gliomas: a positron emission tomographic study using ^{18}F-fluorodeoxyglucose and ^{11}C-L-methylmethionine. *Neurosurgery* 1997;40:276–288.
32. DiChiro G. Positron emission tomography using [^{18}F] fluorodeoxyglucose in brain tumors: a powerful diagnostic and prognostic tool. *Invest Radiol* 1986;22: 360–371.
33. DiChiro G, Oldfield E, Wright DC, et al. Cerebral necrosis after radiotherapy and/or intraarterial chemotherapy for brain tumors: PET and neuropathologic studies. *Am J Roentgenol* 1988;150:189–197.
34. Donliskas CA, Simeone FA. CT characteristics of intraventricular oligodendrogliomas. *AJNR* 1987;8: 1077–1082.
35. Dorne HL, O Gorman AM, Melanson D. Computed tomography of intracranial gangliogliomas. *AJNR* 1986;7:281–285.
36. Duffner PK, Burger PC, Cohen ME, et al. Desmoplastic infantile gangliogliomas: an approach to therapy. *Neurosurgery* 1994;34:583–589.
37. Duong H, Sarazin L, Bourgouin P, Vezina JL. Magnetic resonance imaging of lateral ventricular tumors. *J Assoc Can Radiol* 1995;46:434–442.
38. Earnest IVF, Kelly PJ, Scheithauer BW, et al. Cerebral astrocytomas: histopathologic correlation of MR and CT contrast enhancement with stereotactic biopsy. *Radiology* 1988;166:823–827.

39. Eng DY, Demonte F, Ginsberg L, et al. Craniospinal dissemination of central neurocytoma: report of two cases. *J Neurosurg* 1997;86:547–552.

40. Englund E, Brun A, Larsson EM, Györffy-Wagner Z, Persson B. Tumours of the central nervous system: proton magnetic resonance relaxation times T1 and T2 and histopathologic correlates. *Acta Radiol Diagn* 1986;27(Fasc. 6):653–659.

41. Frerebeau P, Benezech J, Harbi H. Intraventricular tumors in tuberous sclerosis. *Childs Nerv Syst* 1985;1: 45–48.

42. Furie DM, Felsberg GJ, Tien RD, Friedman HS, et al. MRI of gangliocytoma of cerebellum and spinal cord. *JCAT* 1993;17:488–491.

43. Furie DM, Provenzale JM. Supratentorial ependymomas and subependymomas: CT and MR appearance. *JCAT* 1995;19:518–526.

44. Furuta A, Takahashi H, Ikuta F, Onda K, Takeda N, Tanaka R. Temporal lobe tumor demonstrating ganglioglioma and pleomorphic xanthoastrocytoma components. *J Neurosurg* 1992;77:143–147.

45. Gardeur D, Palmieri A, Mashaly R. Cranial computed tomography in the phakomatoses. *Neuroradiology* 1983;25:293–304.

46. Go KG, Kamman RL, Mooyaart EL, et al. Localized proton spectroscopy and spectroscopic imaging in cerebral gliomas, with comparison to positron emission tomography. *Neuroradiology* 1995;37:198–206.

47. Goergen SK, Gonzales MF, McLean CA. Intraventricular neurocytoma: radiologic features and review of the literature. *Radiology* 1992;182:787–792.

48. Goldman S, Levivier M, Pirotte B, et al. Regional glucose metabolism and histopathology of gliomas. *Cancer* 1996;78:1098–1106.

49. Gomez JG, Garcia JH, Colon LE. A variant of cerebral glioma called pleomorphic xanthoastrocytoma: case report. *Neurosurgery* 1985;16:703–706.

50. Hagberg G, Burlina AP, Mader I, Roser W, Radue EW, Seelig J. *In vivo* proton MR spectroscopy of human gliomas: definition of metabolic coordinates for multidimensional classification. *MRM* 1995;34:242–252.

51. Hashimoto M, Fujimoto K, Shinoda S, Masuzawa T. Magnetic resonance imaging of ganglion cell tumours. *Neuroradiology* 1993;35:181–184.

52. Heesters MAAM, Kamman RL, Mooyaart EL, Go KG. Localized proton spectroscopy of inoperable brain gliomas: response to radiation therapy. *J Neurooncol* 1993;17:27–35.

53. Hirose T, Scheithauer BW, Lopes MBS, et al. Ganglioglioma: an ultrastructural and immunohistochemical study. *Cancer* 1997;79:989–1003.

54. Hoeffel C, Boukobza M, Polivka M, et al. MR manifestations of subependymomas. *AJNR* 1995;16: 2121–2129.

55. Holland BA, Kucharcyzk W, Brant-Zawadzki M, et al. MR imaging of calcified intracranial lesions. *Radiology* 1985;157:353–356.

56. Houser OW, Shepherd CW, Gomez MR. Imaging of intracranial tuberous sclerosis. *Ann NY Acad Sci* 1991; 615:81–93.

57. Izukawa D, Lach B, Benoit B. Gangliocytoma of the cerebellum: ultrastructure and immunohistochemistry. *Neurosurgery* 1988;22:576–581.

58. Jelinek J, Smirniatopoulos JG, Parisi JE, Kanzer M. Lateral ventricular neoplasms of the brain: differential

59. Johannsson JH, Rekate HL, Roessmann U. Gangliogliomas: pathological and clinical correlation. *J Neurosurg* 1981;54:58–63.

60. Jooma R, Torrens MJ, Bradshaw J, Brownwell B. Subependymomas of the fourth ventricle: surgical treatment in 12 cases. *J Neurosurg* 1985;62:508–512.

61. Just M, Higer HP, Schwarz M, et al. Tissue characterization of benign brain tumors: use of NMR-tissue parameters. *Magn Reson Imaging* 1988;6:463–472.

62. Kameyama M, Ishiwata K, Tsurumi Y, et al. Clinical application of ^{18}F-FUdR in glioma patients: PET study of nucleic acid metabolism. *J Neurooncol* 1995;23: 53–61.

63. Kawamoto K, Yamanouchi Y, Suwa J, et al. Ultrastructural study of a cerebral gangliocytoma. *Surg Neurol* 1985;24:541–549.

64. Kelly PJ, Daumas-Duport C, Scheithauer BW, Kall BA, Kispert DB. Stereotactic histologic correlations of computed tomography- and magnetic resonance imaging-defined abnormalities in patients with glial neoplasms. *Mayo Clin Proc* 1987;62:450–459.

65. Kendall BE, Jakubowski J, Pullicino P, Symon L. Difficulties in diagnosis of supratentorial gliomas by CAT scan. *J Neurol Neurosurg Psychiatry* 1979;42: 485–492.

66. Kendall B, Reider-Grosswasser I, Valentine A. Diagnosis of masses presenting within the ventricles on computed tomography. *Neuroradiology* 1983;25: 11–22.

67. Kepes JJ, Rubinstein LJ, Eng LF. Pleomorphic xanthoastrocytoma: a distinctive meningocerebral glioma of young subjects with relatively favorable prognosis. A study of 12 cases. *Cancer* 1979;44:1839–1852.

68. Kernohan JW, Mabon RF, Svien HJ, Adson AW. Simplified classification of gliomas. *Mayo Clin Proc* 1949;24:71–75.

69. Kim DG, Chi JG, Park SH, et al. Intraventricular neurocytoma: clinicopathological analysis of seven cases. *J Neurosurg* 1992;76:759–765.

70. Kim DG, Han MH, Lee SH, et al. MRI of intracranial subependymoma: report of a case. *Neuroradiology* 1993;35:185–186.

71. Kim DG, Kim JS, Chi JG, et al. Central neurocytoma: proliferative potential and biological behavior. *J Neurosurg* 1996;84:742–747.

72. Koeller KK, Dillon WP. Dysembryoplastic neuroepithelial tumors: MR appearance. *AJNR* 1992;13: 1319–1325.

73. Komiyama M, Yagura H, Baba M, et al. MR imaging: possibility of tissue characterization of brain tumors using T1 and T2 values. *Am J Neuroradiol* 1987;8: 65–70.

74. Kondziolka D, Lunsford LD, Martinez AJ. Unreliability of contemporary neurodiagnostic imaging in evaluating suspected adult supratentorial (low-grade) astrocytoma. *J Neurosurg* 1993;79:533–536.

75. Kordek R, Biernat W, Alwasiak J, Liberski PP. Pleomorphic xanthoastrocytoma and desmoplastic infantile ganglioglioma: Have these neoplasms a common origin? *Folia Neuropathol* 1994;32:237–239.

76. Kuchelmeister K, Bergmann M, von Wild K, et al. Desmoplastic ganglioglioma: report of two non-infantile cases. *Acta Neuropathol* 1993;85:199–204.

diagnosis based on clinical, CT, and MR findings. *AJNR* 1990;11:567–574.

77. Kulkhantrakorn K, Awwad EE, Levy B, et al. MRI in Lhermitte-Duclos disease. *Neurology* 1997;48: 725–731.

78. Kuroiwa T, Bergey GK, Rothman MI, et al. Radiologic appearance of the dysembryoplastic neuroepithelial tumor. *Radiology* 1995;197:233–238.

79. Kuroiwa T, Kishikawa T, Kato A, et al. Dysembryoplastic neuroepithelial tumors: MR findings. *JCAT* 1994;18:352–356.

80. Labato RD, Sarabia M, Castro S, et al. Symptomatic subependymoma: report of four new cases studied with computed tomography and review of the literature. *Neurosurgery* 1986;19:594–598.

81. Lach B, Duggal N, DaSilva VF, Benoit BG. Association of pleomorphic xanthoastrocytoma with cortical dysplasia and neuronal tumors: a report of three cases. *Cancer* 1996;78:2551–2563.

82. Lang FF, Epstein FJ, Ransohoff J, et al. Central nervous system hanglioglomas part 2: clinical outcome. *J Neurosurg* 1993;79:867–873.

83. Lee YY, Tassel PV. Intracranial oligodendrogliomas: imaging findings in 35 untreated cases. *AJNR* 1989; 10:119–127.

84. Lemsle M, Borsotti JP, Justrabo E, et al. Dysembryoplastic neuroepithelial tumors: a benign tumor cause of partial cpilepsy in young adults. *Rev Neurol* 1996; 152:451–457.

85. Leung SY, Gwi E, Ng HK, et al. Dysembryoplastic neuroepithelial tumor: a tumor with small neuronal cells resembling oligodendroglioma. *Am J Surg Pathol* 1994;18:604–614.

86. Lindbowe CF, Helseth E, Myhr G. Lhermitte-Duclos disease and giant meningiomas as manifestations of Cowden's disease. *Clin Neuropathol* 1995;14: 327–330.

87. Lipper MH, Eberhard DA, Phillips CD, Vezina LG, Cail WS. Pleomorphic xanthoastrocytoma, a distinctive astroglial tumor: neuroradiologic and pathologic features. *AJNR* 1993;14:1397–1404.

88. Liu GT, Galetta SL, Rorkr LB, et al. Gangliogliomas involving the optic chiasm. *Neurology* 1996;46: 1669–1673.

89. Lombardi D, Scheithauer BW, Meyer FB, et al. Symptomatic subependymoma: a clinicopathological and flow cytometric study. *J Neurosurg* 1991;75:585–588.

90. Lu WY, Goldman M, Young B, Davis DG. Optic nerve ganglioglioma. *J Neurosurg* 1993;78:979–982.

91. Lunsford LD, Martinez AJ, Latchaw RE. Magnetic resonance imaging does not define tumor boundaries. *Acta Radiol Suppl* 1986;369:154–156.

92. Luyken C, Hildebrandt G, Scheidhauer K, Krisch B, Schicha H, Klug N. [111]Indium (DTPA-Octreotide) scintigraphy in patients with cerebral gliomas. *Acta Neurochir (Wien)* 1994;127:60–64.

93. Macdonald DR, Brien RA, Gilbert JJ, et al. Metastatic oligodendroglioma. *Neurology* 1989;39:1593–1596.

94. Marano SR, Johnson PC, Spetzler RF. Recurrent Lhermitte-Duclos disease in a child: case report. *J Neurosurg* 1988;69:599–603.

95. Marcus CD, Galeon M, Peruzzi P, et al. Lhermitte-Duclos disease associated with syringomyelia. *Neuroradiology* 1996;38:529–531.

96. Martin DS, Levy B, Awwad EE, Pittman T. Desmoplastic infantile gaglioglioma: CT and MR features. *AJNR* 1991;12:1195–1197.

97. Mattay VS, Frank JA, Santha AKS, et al. Whole-brain functional mapping with isotropic MR imaging. *Radiology* 1996;201:399–404.

98. McConachie NS, Worthington BS, Cornford EJ, et al. Computed tomography and magnetic resonance in the diagnosis of intraventricular cerebral masses. *Br J Radiol* 1994;67:223–243.

99. McLaurin RL, Towbin RB. Tuberous sclerosis: diagnostic and surgical considerations. *Pediatric Neurosci* 1985;12:43–48.

100. Meltzer CC, Smirniatopoulos JG, Jones RV. The striated cerebellum: an MR imaging sign in Lhermitte-Duclos disease (dysplastic gangliocytoma). *Radiology* 1995;194:699–703.

101. Miller DC, Lang FF, Epstein FJ. Central nervous system Gangliogliomas. Part 1: Pathology. J Neurosurg 1993;79:859–866.

102. Moran V, O Keeffe F. Giant cell astrocytoma in tuberous sclerosis: computed tomographic findings. *Clin Radiol* 1986;37:543–545.

103. Mork SJ, Halvorsen TB, Lindegaard KF, et al. Oligodendroglioma: histologic evaluation and prognosis. *J Neuropathol Exp Neurol* 1986;45:65–78.

104. Mork SJ, Lindegaard KF, Halvorsen TB, et al. Oligodendroglioma: incidence and biologic behavior in a defined population. *J Neurosurg* 1985;63:881–889.

105. Morris HH, Estes MI., Gilmore R, et al. Chronic intractable epilepsy as the only symptom of primary brain tumor. *Epilepsia* 1993;34:1038–1043.

106. Morrison G, Sobel DF, Kelley W, et al. Intraventricular mass lesions. *Radiology* 1984;153:435–442.

107. Ng THK, Fung CF, Ma LT. The pathological spectrum of desmoplastic infantile ganglioglimas. *Histopathology* 1990;16:235–241.

108. Nishio S, Takeshita I, Kaneko Y, Fukui M. Cerebral neurocytoma: a new subset of benign neuronal tumors of the cerebrum. *Cancer* 1992;70:529–537.

109. Okamura A, Goto S, Sato K, Ushio Y. Central neurocytoma with hemorhagic onset. *Surg Neurol* 1995;43: 252–255.

110. Oriuchi N, Tamura M, Shibazaki T, et al. Clinical evaluation of thallium-201 SPECT in supratentorial gliomas: relationship to histologic grade, prognosis and proliferative activities. *J Nucl Med* 1993;34: 2085–2089.

111. Ormson MJ, Kispert DB, Sharbrough FW, et al. Cryptic structural lesions in refractory partial epilepsy: MR imaging and CT studies. *Radiology* 1985;160: 215–219.

112. Osawara H, Kiya K, Uozumi T, et al. Multiple oligodendrogliomas: case report. *Neurol Med Chir* 1990;30: 127–131.

113. Ott D, Hennig J, Ernst T. Human brain tumors: assessment with *in vivo* proton MR spectroscopy. *Radiology* 1993;186:745–752.

114. Packer RJ, Sutton LN, Rorke LB, et al. Oligodendroglioma of the posterior fossa in childhood. *Cancer* 1985;56:195–199.

115. Pahapill PA, Ramsay DA, Del Maestro RF. Pleomorphic xanthoastrocytoma: case report and analysis of the literature concerning the efficacy of resection and the significance of necrosis. *Neurosurgery* 1996;38: 822–828.

116. Parker DR. Neuroradiology case of the day: central neurocytoma. *AJR* 1991;156:1311.

117. Perry A, Giannini C, Scheithauer BW, et al. Composite pleomorphic xanthoastrocytoma and ganglioglioma: report of four cases and review of the literature. *Am J Surg Pathol* 1997;21:763–771.

118. Pierpaoli C, Jezzard P, Basser PJ, Barnett A, DiChiro, G. Diffusion tensor MR imaging of the human brain. *Radiology* 1996;201:637–648.

119. Pirotte B, Goldman S, Bidaut LM, et al. Use of positron emission tomography (PET) in stereotactic conditions for brain biopsy. *Acta Neurochir (Wien)* 1995;134:79–82.

120. Poptani H, Gupta RK, Jain VK, Roy R, Pandey R. Cystic intracranial mass lesions: possible role of *in vivo* MR spectroscopy in its differential diagnosis. *Magn Reson Imaging* 1995;13:1019–1029.

121. Porter-Grenn LM, Silbergleit R, Stern HJ, et al. Intraventricular primary neuronal neoplasms: CT, MR, and angiographic findings. *JCAT* 1991;15:365–368.

122. Prayson RA. Gliofibroma: A distinct entity or a subtype of desmoplastic astrocytoma? *Hum Pathol* 1996;24:610–613.

123. Rabinowicz AL, Abrey LE, Hinton DR, Couldwell WT. Cerebral neurocytoma: an unusual cause of refractory epilepsy: case report and review of the literature. *Epilepsia* 1995;36:1237–1240.

124. Rainov NG, Holzhausen HJ, Winfried B. Dysplastic gangliocytoma of the cerebellum (Lhermitte-Duclos disease). *Clin Neurol Neurosurg* 1995;97:175–180.

125. Rand SD, Prost R, Haughton V, et al. Accuracy of single-voxel proton MR spectroscopy in distinguishing neoplastic from nonneoplastic brain lesions. *Am J Neuroradiol* 1997;18:1695–1704.

126. Raymond AA, Halpin SFS, Alsanjari N, et al. Dysembryoplastic neuroepithelial tumour: features in 16 patients. *Brain* 1994;117:461–475.

127. Reiche W, Kolles H, Eymann R, Feiden W. Dysembryoplastic neuroepithelial tumor (DNT): pattern of neuroradiology findings. *Radiologe* 1996;36:884–889.

128. Richieri-Costa A, Frederigue U, Guion-Almelda ML. Holoprosencephaly, hamartomatous growth of the cerebrum, dysplastic gangliocytoma of the cerebellum, unique brain anomalies, and renal agenesis in a Brazilian infant born to a diabetic mother: a clinical and pathologic study. *Birth Defects* 1993;29:389–394.

129. Rimbau J, Isamat F. Dysplastic gangliocytoma of the cerebellum (Lhermitte-Duclos disease) and its relation to the multiple hamartoma syndrome (Cowden disease). *J Neurooncol* 1994;18:191–197.

130. Robbins P, Segal A, Narula B, et al. Central neurocytoma: a clinicopathological, immunohistochemical and ultrastructural study of 7 cases. *Pathol Res Pract* 1995;191:100–111.

131. Rubenstein LJ. Tumors of the central nervous system. *Atlas of tumor pathology*, 2nd series, fascicle 6. Washington, DC: Armed Forces Institute of Pathology, 1972.

132. Rushing EJ, Rorke LB, Sutton L. Problems in the nosology of desmoplastic tumors of childhood. *Pediatr Neurosurg* 1993;19:54–62.

133. Russell DS, Rubinstein LJ. *Pathology of tumors of the nervous system,* 5th ed. Baltimore: Williams & Wilkins, 1989:83–350, 395, 402, 403.

134. Schorner W, Meencke HJ, Felix R. Temporal Lobe epilepsy: comparison of CT and MR imaging. *AJNR* 1987;8:773–781.

135. Schweitzer JB, Davies KG. Differentiating central neurocytoma. *J Neurosurg* 1997;86:543–546.

136. Sgouros S, Walsh AR, Barber P. Central neurocytoma of thalamic origin. *Br J Neurosurg* 1994;8:373–376.

137. Shaw EG, Scheithauer BW, O Fallon JR, et al. Oligodendrogliomas: the Mayo Clinic experience. *J Neurosurg* 1992;76:428–434.

138. Shibamoto Y, Kitakabu Y, Takahashi M, et al. Supratentorial low-grade astrocytoma. *Cancer* 1993;72:190–195.

139. Sjöholm H, Elmqvist D, Rehncrona S, Rosén I, Salford LG. SPECT imaging of gliomas with Thallium-201 and Technetium-99m-HMPAO. *Acta Neurol Scand* 1995;91:66–70.

140. Smith MT, Ludwig CL, Godfrey AD, Armbrustmacher VW. Grading of oligodendrogliomas. *Cancer* 1983;52:2107–2114.

141. Smith NM, Carli MM, Hanieh A, et al. Gangliogliomas in childhood. *Childs Nerv Syst* 1992;8:238–242.

142. Smith RR, Grossman RI, Goldberg HI, et al. MR imaging of Lhermitte-Duclos disease: a case report. *AJNR* 1987;10:187–189.

143. Smoker WRK, Townsend JJ, Reichman MV. Neurocytoma accompanied by intraventricular hemorrhage: case report and literature review. *AJNR* 1991;12:755–770.

144. Sperner J, Gottschalk J, Neumann, et al. Clinical, radiological and histological findings in desmoplastic infantile ganglioglioma. *Childs Nerv Syst* 1994;10:458–463.

145. Tampieri D, Moumdjian R, Melanson D, Ethier R. Intracerebral gangliogliomas in patients with partial complex seizures: CT and MR imaging findings. *AJNR* 1991;12:749–755.

146. Taratuto AL, Pomata H, Sevlever G, et al. Dysembryoplastic neuroepithelial tumor: morphological, immunocytochemical, and deoxyribonucleic acid analyses in a pediatric series. *Neurosurgery* 1995;36:474–481.

147. Tenreico-Picon OR, Kamath SV, Knorr JR, et al. Desmoplastic infantile ganglioglioma: CT and MRI features. *Pediatr Radiol* 1995;25:540–543.

148. Thomas DW, Lewis MA. Lhermitte-Duclos disease associated with Cowden's disease. *Int J Oral Maxillofac Surg* 1995;24:369–371.

149. Tice H, Barnes PD, Gounerova L, et al. Pediatric and adolescent oligodendrogliomas. *AJNR* 1993;14:1293–1300.

150. Tien RO. Intraventricular mass lesions of the brain: CT and MR findings. *Am J Roentgenol* 1991;157:1283–1290.

151. Tonn JC, Paulus W, Warmuth-Metz M, Schachenmayr W, Sorensen N, Roosen K. Pleomorphic xanthoastrocytoma: report of six cases with special consideration of diagnostic and therapeutic pitfalls. *Surg Neurol* 1997;47:162–169.

152. Toshimitsu A, Hiroshi A, Terufumi I, et al. Desmoplastic infantile ganglioglioma. *Neurol Med Chir* 1993;33:463–466.

153. Tovi M. MR imaging in cerebral gliomas: analysis of tumour tissue components. *Acta Radiol* 1993;384 (Suppl):1–24.

154. Van Roost D, Kristof R, Zentner J, Wolf HK, Schramm J. Clinical, radiological, and therapeutic features of pleomorphic xanthoastrocytoma: report of three pa-

tients and review of the literature. *J Neurol Neurosurg Psychiatry* 1996;60:690–692.

155. Vandenberg SR, May EE, Rubinstein LJ, et al. Desmoplastic supratentorial neuroepithelial tumors of infancy with divergent differentiation potential (desmoplastic infantile gangliogliomas): report on 11 cases of a distinctive embryonal tumor with favorable prognosis. *J Neurosurg* 1987;66:58–71.

156. Vonofakos D, Marcu H, Hacker H. Oligodendrogliomas: CT patterns with emphasis on features indicating malignancy. *JCAT* 1979;3:783–789.

157. Wacker MR, Cogen PH, Etzell JE, et al. Diffuse leptomeningeal involvement by a ganglioglioma in a child. *J Neurosurg* 1992;77:302–306.

158. Watanabe M, Tanaka R, Takeda N. Magnetic resonance imaging and histopathology of cerebral gliomas. *Neuroradiology* 1992;34:463–469.

159. Wenz F, Rempp K, Heb T, et al. Effect of radiation on blood volume in low-grade astrocytomas and normal brain tissue: quantification with dynamic susceptibility contrast MR imaging. *AJR* 1996;166:187–193.

160. Whittle IR, Gordon A, Misra BK, Dip MC, Shaw JF, Steers JW. Pleomorphic xanthoastrocytoma. Report of four cases. J Neurosurg 1989;70:463–468.

161. Wichman N, Schubiger O, Von Deimling A, et al. Neuroradiology of central neurocytoma. *Neuroradiology* 1991;33:143–148.

162. Williams DW III, Elster AD, Ginsberg LE, Stanton C. Recurrent Lhermitte-Duclos disease: report of two cases and association with Cowden's disease. *AJNR* 1992;13:287–290.

163. World Health Organization. *Classification of brain tumors.* Zurich: WHO, 1990.

164. Yasargil MG, von Ammos K, von Deimling A, et al. Central neurocytoma: histopathologic variants and therapeutic approaches. *J Neurosurg* 1992;78:32–37.

165. Yoshino MT, Lucio R. Pleomorphic xanthoastrocytoma. *AJNR* 1992;13:1330–1332.

166. Zentner J, Wolf HK, Ostertum B, et al. Gangliogliomas: clinical, radiological, and histopathological findings in 51 patients. *J Neurol Neurosurg Psychiatry* 1994;57: 1497–1502.

167. Zulch KJ. *Brain tumors: their biology and pathology,* 3rd ed. Berlin: Springer-Verlag, 1986:210–341.

The Practical Management of Low-Grade Primary Brain Tumors, edited by Jack P. Rock, Mark L. Rosenblum, Edward G. Shaw, and J. Gregory Cairncross.
Lippincott Williams & Wilkins, Philadelphia, © 1999

3

Classification and Pathobiology of Low-Grade Glial and Glioneuronal Neoplasms

Jorge A. Gutierrez

Department of Pathology (Neuropathology), Henry Ford Hospital, Detroit, Michigan 48202

The principal aim of classifying tumors is to provide attending physicians with a base with which to make therapeutic decisions and predict outcomes. Central nervous system (CNS) tumors are grouped according to their cell of origin (astrocytic, oligodendroglial, etc.) and are graded subsequently in an attempt to predict their behavior from their degree of anaplasia.

The classifications have traditionally been centered on the morphologic appearance of tumors by light microscopy and histochemistry. These techniques have been improved first by the widespread availability of electron microscopy and later by immunohistology. More recently, the advent of new imaging technology has allowed the routine observation *in vivo* of the macroscopic appearance of these tumors and the functional integrity of their vasculature, which may provide a reliable indicator of their outcome (1,31). In the past decade the explosion in cytogenetic and molecular genetic technology has made it possible to delve into the most intricate mechanisms by which these nucleopathies transform a normal cell into a neoplastic one. Morphology, however, remains the gold standard, and the new technology thus far contributes to refine or complement the current morphology-based classifications. In the future it may be possible that the new methodologies will contribute more objective and reproducible parameters for better accuracy and precision in classifying these neoplasms.

The nature of the specimen and the correctness (accuracy) and reproducibility (precision) of the diagnosis are important factors to consider when classifying brain tumors. Tumors of neuroectodermal origin, including gliomas, are well known for their morphologic heterogeneity. A tumor may display a well-differentiated low-grade appearance (phenotype) in one area, appear undifferentiated and of higher grade a few millimeters away, or be mixed with more than one cellular component. Thus sampling from several areas may be necessary to classify the tumor accurately. A technological advance that has greatly affected the approach to brain tumors, as well as the classification of an individual tumor, is stereotactic biopsy. This procedure, by subjecting the patient to a less complicated surgical procedure and allowing for sampling of lesions formerly considered not amenable to biopsy, necessarily provides small samples for morphologic examination. Because of the morphologic heterogeneity of gliomas, these samples may not represent the lesion or may underestimate the grade of the neoplasm (167). In fact, in a study comparing diagnoses made on stereotactically obtained biopsies with the diagnosis rendered on the resection specimens, the correlation was perfect in 63% of cases, imperfect in 30%, and inaccurate in 7% (17). Also of great importance in managing individual cases classified on stereotactic biopsies is the recognition of the ample variability in grading astrocytomas in these small samples when examined not only by different observers but also by the same observer on different occasions. Intraobserver agreement in two readings of 64% and interobserver agreement ranging from 35% for anaplastic astrocytomas to 62% for glioblastomas multiforme have been reported (134). Furthermore, accuracy and precision may be more difficult to achieve when classifying low-grade gliomas, as suggested by a previous report on objective grading of astrocytomas indicating that reproducibility of grading between two observers was lower (81%) for low-grade than for high-grade (96%) astrocytomas (30).

The classification of CNS tumors is a constantly changing, complex process in which the concerted cooperation and educated judgment of the surgeon, radiologist, and pathologist are essential. In this chapter a profile of only the low histologic-grade neoplasms of neuroectodermal origin is sketched, with emphasis on their pathologic characteristics and biologic factors that may predict their behavior. The first section discusses tumors derived from the macroglia (astrocytes, oligodendrocytes, and ependymal cells), and the second and third sections emphasize the neuronal and mixed neuronal/glial neoplasms, respectively.

TUMORS OF GLIAL ORIGIN

Astrocytomas

Astrocytomas are primary neoplasms of the CNS derived from astrocytes. These are the most common tumors of the brain and comprise a broad spectrum of morphologic and clinicopathologic entities with different prognostic implications. A group of astrocytomas infiltrates the brain diffusely and contains the tumors observed more frequently in clinical practice. These usually affect the adult population. Morphologically, these astrocytomas range from tumors of low histologic grade devoid of anaplastic features (grades I and II) to high histologic-grade neoplasms with variable degrees of anaplasia (grades III and IV)

and a significantly worse prognosis. In contrast, other astrocytomas are rather well-circumscribed, present usually during childhood, have a generally characteristic clinicopathologic profile, and usually have a favorable prognosis.

Diffuse Astrocytoma

Diffuse, low-grade, or well-differentiated astrocytoma corresponds to grade II astrocytomas of the World Health Organization (WHO) classification of brain tumors (92), to grade I and II astrocytomas of the St. Anne–Mayo Clinic grading system (30), and to the astrocytoma category of the three-tiered system of Ringertz as used in the Armed Forces Institute of Pathology atlas (13). These tumors may account for as many as 19% of all intracranial gliomas, and usually occur during the third and fourth decades of life (1,66,189). Diffuse, low-grade astrocytomas involve primarily the cerebral hemispheres; they present in the cerebellum less frequently, and there is a rather well-defined subset developing in the brain stem in children. In the spinal cord they appear as a fusiform, diffuse enlargement that can be associated with a syrinx. As implied by their name, diffuse astrocytomas are poorly circumscribed lesions that involve gray and white matter with obliteration of the anatomic landmarks. They may have cystic areas, infrequently have calcification, and most characteristically are devoid of gadolinium enhancement, to the point of making the diagnosis of low-grade astrocytoma highly questionable when enhancement is observed in the imaging studies.

Macroscopically, the tumor may manifest only by increased firmness and grayish discoloration of the brain tissue, with haziness of the gray/white matter interface. Or the tumor may be an obvious tannish-gray mass with firmer fibrillary zones and/or soft gelatinous areas. Typically, the neoplasm is devoid of necrosis or hemorrhage.

Microscopically, three types of normal astrocytes and their neoplastic counterparts are recognized: (a) fibrillary, (b) protoplasmic, and (c) gemistocytic. Usually one cell type predominates in a given tumor, but a variable component of the other cell types is almost always present.

1. *Fibrillary.* In the early, diffusely infiltrating tumors only an increased cellularity of the cerebral parenchyma is detectable. The tumor cells have a round, somewhat vesicular nucleus that appears devoid of cytoplasm (naked nucleus) and are disposed in a fine, almost imperceptible, fibrillary background. These features are better observed on smears of fresh tumor tissue. The lesion may be subtle and difficult to distinguish from a reactive process and even from normal tissue, a task made more difficult by the scant amount of tissue provided by stereotactic biopsies. In many cases, however, there also are areas of the tumor where the nuclei are elongated and atypical, are more closely packed, and have a readily apparent prominent fibrillary background.

2. *Protoplasmic.* Neoplastic protoplasmic astrocytes display a round, vesicular nucleus surrounded by a scant cytoplasm that projects short processes; the processes surround small extracellular cystic spaces (microcysts) that contain proteinaceous/mucinous fluid. This microcystic/mucinous change is frequently observed when the tumor grows in the cerebral cortex.

3. *Gemistocytic.* The neoplastic gemistocytic astrocytes are similar to their reactive nonneoplastic counterparts in that they have a round eccentric nucleus, with possibly a small nucleolus, and an expanded eosinophilic cytoplasm thrown into several processes.

Ultrastructurally, neoplastic astrocytes are no different from nonneoplastic ones and can be recognized as astrocytic by the presence of the distinctive intermediate filaments, which are much more abundant in gemistocytic forms. The filaments may be demonstrated to be glial by immunohistochemistry using an antiserum against glial fibrillary acidic protein (GFAP). These filaments are also immunoreactive with antivimentin serum and may cross-react with other intermediate filament markers (69).

Several systems are used to grade diffuse astrocytomas (13,30,86,92), and their criteria for different grades vary. However, all agree that in low-grade diffuse astrocytomas there is an absence of mitotic figures, microvascular cellular proliferation, or tumor necrosis. The presence of any of these changes, usually associated with prominent nuclear atypia and hypercellularity, indicates a higher histologic grade (III or IV) astrocytoma. A problem arises when in a small biopsy devoid of hypercellularity and nuclear anaplasia a single mitotic figure, proliferated microvessel, or area of necrosis is present; in these cases, correlation with clinical data and imaging findings may help resolve the matter.

In evaluating astrocytomas, histologic grade, age at tumor diagnosis, and vascularity are important factors in predicting tumor behavior. Low histologic grade (grade II) is a most consistent predictor of prolonged survival of patients with astrocytic tumors, under both univariate and multivariate analyses (30,89). Low-grade astrocytomas tend to develop in the third and fourth decades of life, at a younger age than high-grade ones. Age alone (independent of tumor grade) is a most significant predictor of outcome in gliomas (52,89,180). A statistical model has given the best possible survival score to a 16-year-old patient with a low-grade astrocytoma (180). Microvascular cellular proliferation is a manifestation of anaplasia and, by definition, should not be present in low-grade astrocytomas. However, quantifying the density of single-layered microvessels may be a predictor of survival in low-grade astrocytomas. In a recent series, those tumors with seven or fewer microvessels (400× high power field) had a mean survival of 11.2 years, compared with 3.8 years for those with more than seven microvessels (1).

The proliferative activity of these astrocytomas has been investigated and correlated with tumor behavior using different antibodies against the Ki-67 antigen, which is present in the cell nucleus during all phases of the mitotic cycle except for the G0 phase. The results have been somewhat contradictory. Although it is widely accepted that these proliferation indices are more precise than mitotic counts and that high labeling indices (LI) are associated with high-grade astrocytomas and a worse prognosis, the critical values and their predictive potential vary widely. Grade IV astrocytomas have an LI greater than 6%, which is associated with statistically significant shortened survival times (120, 136). In contrast, low-grade gliomas generally have an LI of 3% or less (75,120,136). Accordingly, Ki-67 indices ≥3% (136) or ≥5% (81), or a MIB-1 index >1.5% (75) are reliable predictors of shortened survivals. In one series, the indices are related to survival more significantly than histologic grade and are more accurate than morphology in assigning biologically more aggressive gliomas to a higher histologic grade (75). Another study, using area-related proliferation indices, found that MIB-1 LIs are significantly lower in grade II (median = 6%) than in grade III (median = 12%) astrocytomas. The best discrimination was obtained at 8%, and an index of 15.3% separated the survivors from the nonsurvivors (177). In some studies the prognostic significance of the proliferation indices has been maintained even after multivariate analysis (81,177). However, in a group of 105 astrocytomas, although MIB-1 indices were found to be inversely related to survival, under multivariate analysis the MIB-1 indices did not reach significance, and it was recommended that these indices be used cautiously, if at all (28).

The molecular genetic alterations occurring in gliomas have been investigated as possible predictors of tumor aggressiveness. The natural evolution of astrocytomas is to transform within several years into a higher histologic grade and biologically more aggressive glioma, a phenomenon that occurs in about three-fourths of astrocytomas. This fact is currently attributed to the progressive multistep development of genetic alterations dur-

ing the process of tumorigenesis. Initially, it was thought that the expression of the p53 protein increased with the progression from astrocytoma to anaplastic astrocytoma to glioblastoma multiforme (81). It is now generally accepted that p53 alterations—with or without p53 increased expression, gene mutation, and/or loss of heterozygosity (LOH) of one chromosome 17p (allele) (122)—occur in about two-thirds of low-grade (grade II) astrocytomas and that p53 alterations are an early step in the neoplastic transformation and progression of a large proportion of astrocytic tumors (110,147). Other genetic alterations have been observed in grade II astrocytomas, but the genetic abnormalities characteristic of grade III and IV astrocytomas (LOH of chromosome 19q, LOH of chromosome 10, deletion of pl6, and amplification of EGF-R or CDK4) are rarely observed in low-grade astrocytomas (147,216). Because of the even distribution of p53 alterations throughout the spectrum of astrocytic neoplasm, p53 expression/mutation cannot be used as a marker of anaplasia, and no correlation with survival has been found.

Median survival for patients with supratentorial low-grade astrocytomas has ranged from 23 months to 8.2 years (1,128,210), with the longer survivals in the more recent series attributed in part to an earlier diagnosis of patients presenting with seizures. Patients usually succumb to progressive disease with increasing anaplasia.

Protoplasmic Astrocytoma

Protoplasmic astrocytes are characterized by a paucity of glial filaments and are found in normal gray matter in association with neurons. Certain sparsely fibrillary gliomas arising in the cerebral cortex have been referred to as protoplasmic astrocytomas. Although their existence as a separate histologic entity is debatable, pure protoplasmic astrocytomas may account for about 5% of all low-grade astrocytomas (160). The tumors frequently affect the frontal and temporal lobes, involve the cerebral cortex, and appear gelatinous with possible formation of macroscopic cysts.

Histologically, the neoplastic cells have round or ovoid nuclei set up in a microcystic mucinous background where only sparse, short, fibrillary processes are observed. The GFAP immunoreactivity is focal and sparse. The tumors are low histologic grade (I or II), although microvascular cellular proliferation or a rare mitotic figure may be observed occasionally. The MIB-1 proliferation indices are low (mean = 0.7%), and the p53 protein is expressed in only a few tumors (159). Prognostically, the tumors behave like low-grade gliomas with prolonged survival periods. The differential diagnosis of protoplasmic astrocytoma from other tumors with prominent microcystic changes (oligodendroglioma, pilocytic astrocytoma, dysembryoplastic neuroepithelial tumor), particularly in younger patients, may be difficult and perhaps subjective.

Gemistocytic Astrocytoma

Gemistocytes are plump astrocytes filled with glial filaments. They are observed as reactive astrocytes in pathologic processes of certain duration. Gemistocytes are also an integral component of many gliomas, astrocytic and oligodendroglial, low and high grade, and of other neoplasms, where they may be reacting to the presence of the infiltrating tumor. However, astrocytomas in which most cells, probably more than one-half, have a gemistocytic phenotype are designated as gemistocytic. The exact role of these plump astrocytes in these astrocytomas is uncertain. Most gemistocytes are considered postmitotic: they do not immunoreact with the MIB-1 antibody (100) and have a higher rate of bcl-2 expression than the other cells (217), suggesting that they are not mitosing cells and that they are escaping the apoptotic process. Prognostically, although WHO classifies gemistocytic astrocytomas as low-grade tumors (grade II), it is generally accepted that they have a great proclivity to undergo malignant transformation. Furthermore, it has been observed that gliomas

containing more than 20% gemistocytes have median survival times of about 2.5 years (106). This outcome is more akin to that of anaplastic astrocytomas, thus prompting the suggestion that for therapeutic purposes, gemistocytic astrocytomas should be considered anaplastic astrocytomas (grade III). This assertion is further supported by the observation that WHO grade II astrocytomas containing more than 5% gemistocytes evolved into grade III and IV tumors almost twice as fast (35 months) as those with less than 5% (64 months) (217). Gemistocytic astrocytomas, in addition to the gemistocytes, have a variable population of fibrillary astrocytes frequently displaying atypical nuclei and cycling activity. A consistent change in gemistocytic astrocytomas is a perivascular infiltrate of lymphocytes. In the past, and before it was recognized that oligodendrogliomas may have cells resembling gemistocytes (gliofibrillary oligodendrocytes and minigemistocytes), gemistocytic astrocytomas may have been overdiagnosed (see the section entitled "Oligodendroglioma" later).

Circumscribed Astrocytomas

Pleomorphic Xanthoastrocytoma (PXA)

PXA is one of the superficial cerebral desmoplastic astrocytomas with a characteristic histology that, because of its pleomorphic appearance, may be misinterpreted as a high-grade neoplasm, although it usually has a favorable prognosis. The tumor was described by Kepes (85) while studying xanthomatous lesions of the CNS. The tumor presents in children, although it also occurs in adults.

Typically, the lesion involves the surface of the frontotemporal lobe in close contact with the leptomeninges and dura. The outline of the tumor tends to circumscription. The cut surface may be tannish-yellow or orangish because of the high lipid content. The tumor tissue is focally dense and firm, and frequently contains cysts, occasionally with a dominant cyst and a mural nodule.

Microscopically, the morphology may be atypical because of the prominent cellular pleomorphism manifested by bizarre, giant, or multinucleated tumor cells. A characteristic feature is the presence of large lipidized cells with foamy, finely vesicular cytoplasm resembling histiocytes. A third distinctive finding is the abundant deposition of reticulin fibers around nests of individual tumor cells, which imparts a desmoplastic character to the tumor. Commonly, the tumors are diffusely or focally infiltrated by lymphocytes.

A few mitotic figures are sometimes observed, and scant microvascular cellular proliferation may be present. The tumor cells are to a variable degree immunoreactive with GFAP. This fact allowed Kepes to characterize these masses resembling xanthomatous lesions as astrocytic neoplasms (85). The positive GFAP reaction is also useful to rule out a morphologically close mimic, the malignant fibrous histiocytoma (56). The PXA tumor cells may also be immunoreactive with vimentin, S100, and some histiocyte markers (104).

The coexistence of PXA and ganglioglioma (GG) as separate tumors has been reported (95). Another occurrence is the presence of clusters of neoplastic neurons, immunoreactive with the neuronal markers NFP and SYN, in otherwise characteristic PXAs (104). In addition, coexpression of GFAP, SYN, and NFP has been demonstrated in some of the characteristic PXA's pleomorphic cells (157). These findings suggest a possible relationship of PXA with other neuroectodermal tumors, demonstrating a glioneuronal phenotype, and possibly even with subependymal giant cell astrocytoma (see later) (157).

The prognosis of PXAs is favorable with prolonged disease-free survival (85), but more recent reports indicate that a minority of cases recur rapidly and may evolve into anaplastic astrocytoma or glioblastoma multiforme. The presence of tumor necrosis is accepted as an indicator that the lesion is a high-grade astrocytoma (grade IV); otherwise, there are no reliable clinicopathologic criteria to predict malignant transformation (220). However, it has been suggested that promi-

nent mitotic activity (4/10 hpf) may predict anaplastic progression (125), although the patient reported was alive and free of disease 6 years after the recurrence despite a glioblastoma multiforme morphology.

Mutations in the p53 gene and epidermal growth factor (EGF) amplification have been described in PXAs, but the unusual location of the mutations and the appearance of the changes only after tumor recurrence suggest that the genetic events in PXA tumorigenesis are different from those in diffuse astrocytomas (153).

Subependymal Giant Cell Astrocytoma (SEGA)

SEGAs are WHO grade I intraventricular tumors that occur in patients with tuberous sclerosis (TS). The cell of origin of these tumors, despite their denomination as astrocytomas, is uncertain. SEGAs are almost exclusively observed in patients with TS and occur in about 6% of TS subjects with symptomatic tumors (192). Tumors usually become symptomatic during the first and second decades of life and are occasionally the presenting feature of the disorder.

The classical location of these intraventricular tumors is the lateral ventricles in the vicinity of the orifice of Monro. The lesion is well-circumscribed, is firm, and may have secondary changes, such as cyst formation, hemorrhage, necrosis, and/or calcification. Microscopically, the tumor is moderately cellular with a prominent fibrillary background and an admixture of spindle, plump, and neuronlike cells. In the diagnostic areas, the tumor cells are similar to gemistocytes, with an eccentric nucleus containing a prominent nucleolus and a single tapering or straplike cytoplasmic process extending opposite the nucleus. A perivascular pseudorosette pattern is most distinctive, although it is not usually as well-defined or as frequent as in ependymomas. Mitotic figures, microvascular cellular proliferation, and/or areas of necrosis may be present, but these features of atypia do not indicate malignant transformation (192), as they do in classical astrocytomas. In accord with their low aggressive potential, the MIB-1 proliferation index tends to be low, with a mean of 1.1% (57), and most (12 of 13 tumors tested) are diploid (192).

Most neoplastic cells are immunoreactive with astrocytic markers, including GFAP, vimentin, and S100. Some of the large polygonal and ganglion-like cells react with antibodies against neurofilament, tubulin, and microtubule-associated protein, all of which are neuronal cytoskeletal proteins (119). Furthermore, some cells have also reacted with antibodies to neuropeptides, and an occasional cell has coexpressed both glial and neuronal epitopes. The tumor cells in SEGAs have not shown reactivity with an HMB-45 antiserum (57), a feature observed in some extramural tissues of patients with TS.

The presence of glial, neuronal, and neuropeptide proteins in the neoplastic cells suggests that the lesions probably arise from subependymal cells with potential to undergo glioneuronal and neuroendocrine differentiation (119). The morphology of the SEGAs is similar to the smaller intraventricular hamartomatous lesions of TS patients, the candle guttering. By convention the lesions that by their larger size become symptomatic are classified as tumors.

The prognosis of SEGAs is most favorable, with no known cases of malignant transformation or dissemination. The fatal cases are most likely secondary to treatment complications (192). Thus their distinction from intraventricular ependymomas and astrocytomas is most important.

Pilocytic Astrocytoma

Pilocytic astrocytoma (PA) is a low-grade (WHO grade I), well-circumscribed astrocytic neoplasm that occurs more frequently in children and young adults, and has a favorable prognosis. These neoplasms have also been designated as juvenile pilocytic astrocytomas (JPAs) or cystic astrocytomas, or names have been assigned according to their locations (e.g., cerebellar astrocytomas, optic nerve gliomas, chiasmatic/hypothalamic gliomas).

PAs usually manifest clinically during the first three decades of life and are the most common glioma in children. In the cerebellum only 11% of PAs occur in adults older than 30 years (183). PA has a characteristic topographic distribution with an overall tendency to develop in midline periventricular zones. In the infratentorial compartment they are the most common cerebellar astrocytoma, where the majority (80%) involve the hemispheres (64). Much less frequently, they develop within the brain stem, in a few cases forming pontomedullary exophytic masses (87). Supratentorially, the optic nerve–optic chiasm/tract/hypothalamus area, and thalamus around the third ventricle are characteristic locations. Less commonly, they develop in the cerebral hemispheres with a predilection for the mesial temporal lobe (84). In the spinal cord a certain proportion of intramedullary gliomas are PAs.

PAs have gross pathologic features that set them apart from the diffuse fibrillary astrocytomas, the other low-histologic-grade astrocytomas. The PA is a well-circumscribed, solid tumor mass that macroscopically appears well demarcated from the surrounding brain tissue, but microscopically frequently infiltrates surrounding parenchyma (20,64). With the exception of the optic pathway tumors, where the neoplasm diffusely infiltrates the anatomic structures and frequently the leptomeninges, the classic PA tumor pushes aside surrounding structures and provides a cleavage plane that allows for possible complete resection. A feature observed in about one-third of cases is the formation of a large cyst that contains amber-colored, clear fluid and sometimes a mural nodule; this finding, although characteristic, is also observed in other low-grade gliomas (GG, oligodendroglioma, etc.). Otherwise the solid tumors may be heterogeneous, with firm, tannish-gray areas; soft, gray, mucinous zones; and orange-yellow areas of remote bleeding. Occasionally, they are vascular to the point of resembling a vascular malformation (50), a feature observed particularly in supratentorial examples (118). The prominent vascularity of PA, both macroscopic and microscopic, is responsible for the almost universal gadolinium enhancement of these tumors; the enhancement characteristically has minimal or no associated edema (20).

Microscopically, the neoplastic cell from which the tumor derives its name is the piloid (hairlike) astrocyte, which is a fibrillary glial cell with a narrow, elongated nucleus and a single thin and long glial process extending from one or both nuclear poles, a morphology better appreciated on smear preparations. The tumors are sparsely or moderately cellular, with the cells arranged in a diagnostic biphasic pattern made of dense and heavily fibrillated areas, frequently perivascular, intermingled with looser areas where the cells are rounder and secrete mucosubstances with formation of microcysts. Presumably, the coalescence of these loose areas gives origin to the dominant macrocyst. Two other features of diagnostic importance are the sausage-shaped, eosinophilic Rosenthal fibers, which are more commonly present in sparsely cellular and heavily fibrillated areas, and the intracellular, granular eosinophilic bodies or inclusions, which are identified more easily in cellular zones with microcystic change. Other features characteristic of PA are nuclear pleomorphism; microvascular proliferation with formation of glomeruloid structures, frequently in the wall of the cyst; and less frequently, congeries of microvessels with thick hyalinized walls. Mitotic figures are occasionally present, and there may be focal necrosis without pseudopalisading. The morphology of the tumor may be heterogeneous, and its diagnosis, particularly its distinction from the diffuse fibrillary astrocytoma, may sometimes be difficult. This problem occurs frequently with small biopsies obtained from eloquent areas such as the spinal cord, brain stem, central gray matter, and optic pathway. Correlation of the characteristic clinicoradiologic features with the morphologic findings is necessary to classify these cases. The more reliable histologic diagnostic findings are the

piloid cellular component, the biphasic distribution of the neoplastic cells, and the presence of Rosenthal fibers. The identification of these diagnostic features in small focal areas of some glial cerebellar tumors allowed for the recognition of the diffuse variant of PA (64). This variant is not uncommon and has been reported in 15% of all PAs (183). Because of its resemblance to fibrillary astrocytomas, this tumor type may have been diagnosed in the past as diffuse fibrillary astrocytoma.

The neoplastic cells in PA are immunoreactive with GFAP and vimentin. Somewhat paradoxically, Rosenthal fibers are not immunoreactive with GFAP, or only a thin outline of the fiber may be positive. The fibers are reactive with sera against α B-crystallin (a lens protein present also in other organs' ground substance) and ubiquitin (a modulator protein of nonlysosomal protein degradation) (206).

PAs are WHO grade I neoplasms, even considered by some as hamartomatous lesions. The presence of nuclear atypia, mitoses, microvascular proliferation, and necrosis—features that in diffuse astrocytomas indicate neoplastic progression—has no prognostic significance in PA (64). Thus PAs are not graded histologically. However, malignant transformation may occur spontaneously or after therapy (surgery and/or radiation) in about 3% of cases (205), with a latency period that ranges between 5 and 52 years. These transformed tumors have zones of clearly recognizable pilocytic morphology, with transition areas to high histologic grade astrocytoma. When the tumors are compared with nonmalignant pilocytic astrocytomas, features highly indicative of malignant transformation are a high mitotic rate of at least 1 mitosis per 250 × microscopy field, and a high percentage of cells in the S-phase (7.6% ± 2.49%) (205); however, these malignant cases have had prolonged survival.

PAs are low-grade, slow-growing, well-circumscribed neoplasms amenable to complete resection and cure. The best predictor of outcome is the extent of resection, with gross total resection being associated with better disease-free survival in both supratentorial (50) and cerebellar tumors (23,64,77).

Chromosomal and molecular genetic analysis of PAs has demonstrated that although about half are diploid, they may also be aneuploid and tetraploid, and no correlation exists between ploidy status and histologic features or prognosis (50,64). LOH of chromosome 17p, a common occurrence in low-grade diffuse astrocytomas, is seldom observed in PA. However, a fraction of supratentorial and infratentorial PAs, which are sporadic and related to neurofibromatosis type 1 (NF1), has allelic loss of 17q chromosome in the NF1 region (214), without any correlation with histologic features. The association of PA with NF1 and the 17q loss in PA suggests the existence of a tumor suppressor gene in the long arm of chromosome 17 involved in PA tumorigenesis. Surprisingly, NF1 gene transcripts, instead of being down-regulated, are found overexpressed in sporadic PA (155). The p53 protein in PA has been found to be high (11,111), intermediate (152), or absent (115). The p53 overexpression has been observed with (152) or without (111) mutation of the p53 gene, an observation that has prompted the suggestion that oncogenesis in childhood astrocytomas may be different from that in adults (115). A high proportion of PAs (one-third) commonly exhibit chromosomal gains of chromosomes 7 and 8 (219), gains that are either absent in fibrillary astrocytomas (219) or seldom observed in grade II astrocytomas with good prognosis (178).

Desmoplastic Cerebral Astrocytoma of Infancy

Desmoplastic cerebral astrocytoma of infancy (DCAI) is a WHO grade I rare astrocytic tumor, in which neoplastic astrocytes lay down basal lamina; in contrast with the desmoplastic infantile ganglioglioma, it lacks a neuronal component.

The tumor was described initially as superficial cerebral astrocytoma attached to dura (201), pointing out two gross cardinal features of the lesion. It is a characteristic clinico-pathologic entity affecting children during the first 2 years of life, and consists of a mass located on the surface of the brain that has a favorable prognosis despite its large size and desmoplastic atypical histologic appearance.

In the original report, DCAIs were 1.25% of 483 intracranial tumors in children (201). The tumors frequently manifest during infancy with progressive macrocephaly. The lesion is a large, supratentorial tumor on the surface of the brain, in close relationship with the dura, and usually has a significant cystic component.

At surgery, the tumor may appear plaque-like, attached to the dura and surface of the brain (123,201), commonly involving more than one lobe (frontal, parietal, or temporal). The tumors are large (3–13 cm) and consist of a superficial firm, gray, or white bosselated component, and frequently a deeply located cystic component. Histologically, DCAIs are spindle-celled neoplasms that focally may be cellular and have atypical nuclear features, thus resembling a malignant tumor. Focal storiform zones may suggest a fibrous histiocytic lesion. However, the neoplastic cells are astrocytes as demonstrated by their positive immunoreactivity for GFAP, and the ultrastructural observation of intracytoplasmic intermediate filaments (34,123,201). The firmness of the tumor is provided by the extensive deposition of basal lamina material and collagen fibers in between the tumor cells. This feature may be observed ultrastructurally (6) or may be demonstrated with a reticulum stain as a rich reticulin network, frequently surrounding individual cells. The basal lamina, like other basal laminae, contains collagens I and IV but is devoid of fibronectin (123). In contrast with desmoplastic infantile GGs, which clinically and pathologically are similar to DCAIs, there is no neuronal component. DCAIs may have plump astrocytes and nuclear pleomorphism, which may suggest the possibility of the tumor being a PXA, another superficial tumor of the brain with extensive desmoplasia; however, PXAs occur at an older age, and their diagnostic lipidization of astrocytes is not present in DCAIs.

Mitoses, microvascular cellular proliferation, and necrosis are not features of DCAIs. A single case, however, has been reported with mitotic activity, an elevated proliferating cell nuclear antigen (PCNA) labeling index, and aneuploidy (6). The outcome is good in DCAIs after adequate surgical resection, but the follow-up periods have been short. It is thought that the neoplastic process involves the subpial astrocyte, because of the tumor's extensive deposition of basal lamina and superficial location. In contrast with other astrocytomas, LOH of chromosomes 17 or 10 and alterations in the p53 gene were not observed in two DCAIs (123).

Regional Astrocytomas

In evaluating low-grade astrocytomas, and after excluding the other circumscribed astrocytomas, the differential diagnosis between PA and diffuse astrocytoma is crucial because of the expected better outcome of PA. These two astrocytomas involve specific structures, resulting in characteristic clinicopathologic syndromes (i.e., optic nerve gliomas, brain stem gliomas, etc.), and their relative distribution, age of onset, and morphology are different, depending on the particular region of the brain involved. Thus the location of the tumor in the neuraxis poses different diagnostic problems. The better outcome of PA, however, may not apply to all PAs. In a series of low-grade astrocytomas in children that controlled statistically for site of tumor and age of patient, the histology of PA versus diffuse astrocytoma had no impact on survival; and in a series of midline tumors in children the rates of recurrence and death were higher for the PAs than for fibrillary astrocytomas (74).

Cerebellar Astrocytomas

The average age for the occurrence of all cerebellar astrocytomas is 14.5 years. Half of them occur during the first 5 years of life, and 71% are seen in children (77). About 80% of

cerebellar astrocytomas are PAs, and at presentation their mean age is 12 years, vastly different from the mean age of 52 years in diffuse astrocytomas (64). No differences have been reported in outcome between pilocytic and diffuse tumors in the cerebellum (77). However, a more recent series has observed a statistically significant difference in 5-, 10-, and 20-year disease-free survival between PA (85%, 81%, and 78%, respectively) and diffuse astrocytoma (10%, 5%, and 5%) (64). A similar favorable outcome for cerebellar PA has been observed with the Wiston-Gilles classification in which the glioma A category, which encompasses the PA, had better overall and progression-free survival than the glioma B that contains other gliomas (23).

Supratentorial Astrocytomas

The median age of presentation for supratentorial PA is the middle second decade, in sharp contrast with the median age of 34 years for diffuse astrocytoma (189). The incidence of supratentorial PA not involving the optic pathway is about equal in the temporal lobe (51%) and in the basal ganglia, thalamus, and hypothalamus together (50%) (50). The survival rate of these PAs is as high as 82% at 20 years (50), which is significantly better than the 7% survival rate of diffuse astrocytomas in a similar location (189).

Spinal Cord Astrocytomas

Intramedullary spinal cord tumors are most frequently gliomas, both astrocytomas and ependymomas, and about one-fourth to one-half are PAs (133,173). Most spinal cord astrocytomas are low grade (WHO grade I or II), usually involve several cervicothoracic segments (166), and only rarely become holocord tumors. The survival for PA and diffuse astrocytoma together at 10 years ranges between 50% and 82% (133,166,173) but is significantly better for PAs alone (81%) than for diffuse alone (15%) (133), and shortens with higher histologic grades (166). Surprisingly, in a series of spinal cord tumors in children under 3 years, considered as congenital tumors, there were no PAs, and most (89%) were low-grade neoplasms that had an overall 5-year progression-free survival of 76.2% (22).

Optic Pathway Gliomas

Gliomas of the optic pathway involve the optic chiasm and hypothalamus more frequently than the intraorbital optic nerve (2,3). Most gliomas in patients with NF-1 occur in the optic-hypothalamic region (74). The tumors involving the optic nerve expand the nerve, spread into the leptomeningeal space, and may extend backward into the chiasm. Primary chiasmatic tumors frequently also involve the hypothalamus and are considered as a separate subset of optic pathway gliomas (2). Most tumors are low-grade astrocytomas, with the malignant variants occurring in older patients. The gliomas in the optic nerve have better survival than the chiasmatic ones, as they are more frequently completely excised (3,74). In the chiasmatic/hypothalamic group, 60% are PAs and 40% are fibrillary. Patients overall have prolonged survivals, but those younger than 5 years and older than 20 years frequently have tumors with aggressive behavior, which cannot be predicted histologically (2). Furthermore, hypothalamic tumors have a high incidence of multicentric dissemination, particularly when incompletely resected (127).

Brain Stem Gliomas

Astrocytomas occurring in the brain stem tend to affect children and young adults. The tumors have been associated with a dismal survival measured in months, but recently their outcome has greatly improved, probably as a result of earlier diagnosis. The tumors frequently infiltrate the brain stem diffusely, with their external appearance having been described as pontine/brain stem hypertrophy. The characteristic tumor is a fibrillary astrocytoma infiltrating the pons diffusely, with the tumor cells extending along and in between fiber tracts and appearing somewhat piloid. These diffuse astrocytomas have a tendency for malignant transformation, most of them eventuating into high-grade tumors (9). There is, however, a subset of tumors—23.5% in a series of 51 patients with brain stem gliomas (87)—at the cervicomedullary junction that form exophytic masses projecting into the fourth ventricle, cerebellopontine angle, or upper cervical spinal cord. These neoplasms generally occur in young patients, are almost always low-grade astrocytomas amenable to total/subtotal resection, and result in survival periods that are longer than those of other brain stem gliomas (21,73,87, 171). About 4% of individuals with NF-1 have brain stem astrocytomas. These tumors are mostly medullary. Close to one-half are exophytic and appear to be less aggressive than their spontaneous pontine counterparts (135).

Oligodendroglioma

Oligodendrogliomas are neoplasms originating from oligodendrocytes that, like astrocytomas, have different degrees of anaplasia but generally have a better prognosis. The accurate classification of oligodendrogliomas is difficult because of the absence of a reliable immunohistologic marker for neoplastic oligodendrocytes. Contributing to the problem are the frequent occurrence of both GFAP-positive elements in oligodendrogliomas and naked nuclei with perinuclear haloes in other gliomas.

Oligodendrogliomas comprise about 4% to 8% of all intracranial tumors (66) and from 0.8% to 4.7% of spinal cord and filum tumors (51). These figures, however, may underestimate the true incidence of oligodendrogliomas. With the recognition that neoplastic oligodendrocytes may develop an astrocyte phenotype, which frequently resembles a plump gemistocyte, many tumors formerly classified as mixed oligoastrocytomas or gemistocytic astrocytomas would currently be classified as oligodendrogliomas. Moreover, a sizable proportion of diffuse fibrillary astrocytomas may really be oligodendrogliomas (32). It is expected that in future series, oligodendrogliomas will become a more frequent glioma, probably second only to the glioblastoma multiforme. In fact, in a recent series (32) pure oligodendrogliomas accounted for 33% of supratentorial gliomas in adults.

Like low-grade astrocytomas, oligodendrogliomas peak in the fourth decade of life (32, 66,189). In children, oligodendroglial neoplasms are uncommon. Most oligodendrogliomas are sporadic and unassociated with any phakomatosis, although familial cases have been reported (99).

Oligodendrogliomas are more common in the frontal and temporal lobes (32,204), frequently manifest clinically by seizures, and characteristically involve cerebral cortex and adjacent white matter. They also affect deeper structures and occasionally are inside the ventricles (113). Spinal oligodendrogliomas constitute only 1.6% of all oligodendrogliomas (51), where they develop more frequently in cervical segments, although they can involve the cord throughout.

Spinal tumors have a greater tendency (60%) than their cerebral counterparts (20%) to disseminate into the leptomeninges, with seeding throughout the spinal or cerebral fluid, the so-called oligodendromatosis (51).

Oligodendrogliomas may infiltrate the brain diffusely or may form masses of solid tumor. In the diffuse form the brain tissue is firm and tannish-gray, with partial or total obliteration of gray and white matter. When a mass is present, it has ill-defined borders. Sparsely or moderately cellular tumors with prominent fibrillary background are firm and tan, whereas cellular tumors have gray-semifirm or translucent-gelatinous tissue, frequently with cystic change. There is calcification in approximately half of the tumors (12,191). Calcification may be fine and involve the tumor diffusely, providing a gritty cut surface, or it may be focal, usually in sparsely cellular and highly vascularized areas of the tumor. Sometimes the calcification is in the adjacent cerebral cortex.

Some oligodendrogliomas have an angiomatoid component of small vessels with thick, hyalinized walls, tumors that may be referred to as angiogliomas. Hemorrhage, sometimes massive, may complicate low- and high-grade tumors; it has been related to the tumor's rich vascular network. Large zones of necrosis are a feature of malignant oligodendrogliomas.

The distinctive histologic pattern of oligodendroglioma is that of a cellular proliferation of cells with uniformly round, centrally located nuclei surrounded by a clear, hydropic perinuclear halo, which is delimited by a cytoplasmic membrane. This appearance has been likened to a fried egg, and the back-to-back arrangement of the cells is referred to as a honeycomb. The tumor cells are separated into pseudolobules by a rich network of thin, branching, and interanastomozing capillary-type vessels, a pattern described as chicken wire. The morphologic features that identify a cell as an oligodendrocyte, neoplastic or otherwise, are the round nuclear outline and the high chromatin density with a few chromocenters or small nucleolus. The perinuclear haloes, although characteristic of oligodendroglial cells, are an artifact not present in optimally fixed specimens.

There is a morphologic spectrum that ranges from low- to high-histologic-grade tumors. At one end there are sparsely cellular neoplasms growing as isolated tumor cells devoid of atypia that infiltrate diffusely relatively well-preserved gray and white matter, probably grade I tumors. At the other end there are cellular tumors that replace the brain tissue and have features of anaplasia such as nuclear pleomorphism and hyperchromasia, frequent mitoses, microvascular cellular proliferation, and extensive necrosis. These tumors are malignant oligodendrogliomas (grade III) and merge imperceptibly with the glioblastoma multiforme (grade IV).

Ultrastructurally, oligodendroglioma cells have a paucity of cytoplasmic organelles and may have short, microtubule-containing processes or cytoplasmic membrane folds stacked around the cell's periphery (132).

The accurate diagnosis of oligodendroglioma rests almost exclusively on nuclear morphology and architectural features. This is due to the absence of an immunohistochemical marker for neoplastic oligodendrocytes that can be used in paraffin-embedded tissue and has high sensitivity and specificity. Several antisera for antigens present in normal, developing, and adult oligodendrocytes have been tested. Some are myelin proteins such as MBP, MAG, and PLP; others include carbonic anhydrase, Leu-7 (a leukocyte marker that immunoreacts also with myelin), and galactocerebroside. The results have been inconsistent or difficult to interpret, or have low specificity (140). Galactocerebroside appears promising, but results have been also inconsistent.

GFAP-positive cells occur frequently in oligodendrogliomas (27). These astrocyte-like cells may be the predominant cell type in a given tumor, consequently making the recognition and typing of these tumors as oligodendrogliomas a difficult and controversial task. Despite their GFAP positivity, these cells have been classified as neoplastic oligodendrocytes because they occur in areas of solid oligodendroglial tumor growths and have the characteristic densely chromatic round nuclei of oligodendroglial cells. These cells have been classified morphologically as minigemistocytes or signet ring cells (12) and gliofibrillary oligodendrocytes (GFOCs). Minigemistocytes and GFOCs are believed to be transitional forms between oligodendrocytes and astrocytes. The presence of these cells may vary from just a few cells to the predominant cell. The tumors have been referred to as transitional oligodendrogliomas, either minigemistocytoma or gliofibrillary oligodendrogliomas. The distinction between a minigemistocytoma and a true gemistocytic astrocytoma may be difficult and subjective, particularly in small samples that do not contain areas of typical oligodendroglioma.

Attempts have been made to sort out the prognostic significance of these GFAP-positive cells in oligodendrogliomas. Interestingly, minigemistocytes and true gemisto-

cytes do not react with MIB-1, which indicates that they are noncycling, postmitotic cells (100). Their presence, however, may signal tumor progression. A retrospective study of 111 oligodendrogliomas that compared the survival rates of different grade oligodendrogliomas with and without GFAP-positive cells found no significant difference; however, the survival time was reduced by one-half in those tumors containing true gemistocytes (102). In another study, the presence of signet ring cells did not appear to influence the prognosis of the tumors, but these cells seemed to occur more frequently in neoplasms with high cellularity and necrosis or vascular proliferation (12).

In the last few years, neuronal markers have been observed in cerebral oligodendrogliomas. This finding further complicates the differential diagnosis with other neoplasms characterized by round, hyperchromatic nuclei, and perinuclear haloes (e.g., central neurocytoma, cerebral neurocytoma, and dysembryoplastic neuroepithelial tumor [DNET]) or with neoplasms containing glial and neuronal elements (i.e, the GGs). Neoplastic cells in supratentorial oligodendrogliomas have been reported as immunoreactive with the neuronal markers synaptophysin, NSE, PGP 9.5, and MAP 2. In addition, some cells in these tumors have organelles and membrane specializations interpreted as neuronal synaptic vesicles or membranes (144). Synaptophysin and PGP have also been demonstrated in glial neoplasms containing oligodendroglial areas (59). These immunophenotypic and ultrastructural features are characteristic of DNETs and neurocytomas, both of which are considered to be of neuronal derivation. The presence of neuronal features in oligodendroglial neoplasms suggests that tumorigenesis is occurring in a bipotential precursor cell. Such cells have been demonstrated in the rat. The N-O cell is capable of differentiation into neurons and oligodendrocytes (221). Furthermore, in ethylnitrosourea-induced murine oligodendrogliomas, the tumor cells express both neuronal and glial markers (209).

Although most patients eventually die of tumor recurrence, the overall prognosis of oligodendrogliomas is better than that of astrocytomas (188). The median survival has ranged between 5.1 and 7.5 years (12,15,31, 191).

Histologic grading of oligodendrogliomas is less well-defined than that for astrocytomas. It is recognized that there are short-, intermediate-, and long-term survivors, but the histologic features that define these groups remain unclear. The systems used are based on features of anaplasia and include the four-tiered ones of Kernohan, Smith (195), and WHO, and the three-tiered one of Kros (101). A recent system divides oligodendrogliomas in two groups of long- and short-term survivors by evaluating the microvasculature by combined histologic and radiologic methods (31). However, histologic features do have a strong predictive value. In a series of 81 pure supratentorial oligodendrogliomas, low-grade tumors (grades I and II of Kernohan and St. Anne Mayo systems) had a median survival time of 9.8 years and 5- and 10-year survival rates of 75% and 46%, respectively, versus 3.9 years and 41% and 20% rates for the high-grade tumors (grades III and IV) (191). In a morphologic study of 71 oligodendrogliomas to determine the predictive value of histologically detected nuclear atypia, microvascular proliferation, mitoses, and necrosis, the parameters more commonly used to assign tumor grade—necrosis and mitoses—were most important, and necrosis was the only independently significant variable (12). In a recently proposed classification of oligodendrogliomas (31), tumors are divided based on the presence (group B) or absence (group A) of endothelial proliferation and/or gadolinium enhancement. The difference in the median survival time of 3.5 years for grade B and 11 years for grade A was highly significant, whereas nuclear atypia, mitoses, and necrosis did not have significant predictive value.

Age of the patient and presence of neurologic deficit at time of diagnosis are important prognostic factors in oligodendrogliomas.

The age of the patient, as in astrocytomas, is strongly related to survival. It has been observed that patients younger than 20 years of age have a 5-year survival rate of about 80%, whereas those older than 60 years have a median survival of 1.8 years and 5- and 10-year survival rates of 14% and 0, respectively. Patients between age 20 and 60 years have intermediate survival rates (191). These data agree with others' observations of a significantly worse prognosis in patients older than 50 or 60 years (25,98). However, in a study of 79 pure oligodendrogliomas, a significantly worse prognosis was observed in patients younger than 20 years (probably related to the deep location of the tumors), and although shortened survival in patients older than 51 years was noted, the difference was not statistically significant (31). The presence of neurologic deficit at the time of diagnosis, probably secondary to the destructive effect of the tumor mass, is also a strong predictor of outcome. In a study of pure oligodendrogliomas, there was a median survival time of 2.5 years in patients with neurologic deficit at diagnosis and 11 years for patients without deficit (31). Similarly, patients with low-grade oligodendrogliomas who present clinically with seizures and have no neurologic deficits have a significantly better outcome than those with raised intracranial pressure or neurologic deficits (15). Other positive predictive clinical factors include gross total or subtotal removal, frontal location (98), and absent computed tomography (CT) enhancement (15, 191).

The proliferative activity of oligodendrogliomas is also an important predictive tool. Coons and Johnson observed in oligodendrogliomas and oligoastrocytomas that a MIB-1 LI below 5 predicted survival more than three times longer than neoplasms with indices greater than 5 (24). Similarly, in a large group of pure oligodendrogliomas, a significant difference in survival was detected between tumors with a MIB-1 LI of less than 0.1 and greater than 0.2 (98). It has also been observed that high LI may predict more aggressive behavior in low-grade tumors, and low LI suggests a more indolent course in high-grade neoplasms (24).

Evaluation of proliferative activity by chromatin ploidy analysis by flow cytometry has been found to have no predictive value, with a tendency for better survival in tetraploid or aneuploid tumors than in diploid tumors (52,103). Although ploidy has no predictive value, the S-phase fraction may have strong prognostic significance. It may allow for discrimination of survival between grade II and III tumors, in which prediction of survival is more uncertain, thus possibly being a better predictor of behavior than tumor grade (25).

The expression of molecular markers of neoplasia has also been investigated in oligodendrogliomas as a possible predictor of tumor behavior. In contrast with astrocytomas, TP53 mutations are infrequent in oligodendrogliomas (126). The mutation is a late phenomenon in oligodendroglia tumorigenesis, as it is only the high-grade oligodendrogliomas that demonstrate frequent positivity for p53 (7,154). In a study of pure oligodendrogliomas, there was no correlation between tumor grade and p53 LI, but patients with neoplasms with greater than 75% positive cells had a survival of about 1 year only (97), thus suggesting that p53 positivity in low-grade oligodendrogliomas may herald a more aggressive behavior (59). Similarly, the expression of telomerase, a DNA polymerase that maintains telomere length after mitosis and may immortalize cells, is confined to high-grade oligodendrogliomas (36).

During the process of tumorigenesis of oligodendrogliomas, LOH of chromosomes 1p and 19q is a characteristic early genetic event (8,165,215). Detecting abnormalities in the 1p 36.3 locus by ISH in paraffin sections (174) may become an objective tool to separate neoplasms of oligodendroglial lineage from those of astrocytic origin. Telomerase may also be a factor in oligodendroglial tumorigenesis, as it has been found in 100% of 19 oligodendrogliomas examined (112).

There are several hypotheses to explain the origin and mechanism of tumorigenesis of oligodendrogliomas. The hypothesis needs to explain the wide morphologic spectrum of oligodendrogliomas that ranges from almost pure oligodendrocytic tumors to tumors with an extensive astrocytic phenotype, and in between a large majority of cases that have various proportions of both elements. The current, more popular hypothesis is that the neoplastic process involves a bipotential precursor cell that may differentiate into oligodendrocyte or astrocyte lineages. This theory is supported by the demonstration in developing rat optic nerve of two precursor cells with different reactivity to two oligodendroglia markers—A2B5 and galactocerebroside (162). The O-2A cell is A2B5 positive and develops further into galactocerebroside-positive oligodendrocytes and type 2 astrocytes. The other cell is A2B5 negative and gives origin to type 1 astrocytes. The neoplastic transformation would involve the O-2A bipotential cell and manifest in both oligodendrocytic and astrocytic components of the tumor.

The origin of oligodendroglioma from the O-2A progenitor cell is supported by observations made on clinical material. In a group of tumors containing various mixtures of oligodendroglioma and astrocytoma, oligodendroglioma tumor cells are usually galactocerebroside (GC) and/or A2B5 immunoreactive, and GFAP-positive neoplastic cells are frequently positive with GC and/or A2B5 antibodies; these findings suggest that oligodendrogliomas with or without an astrocytoma component are derived from O-2A progenitor cells (35). Indirect support for the bipotential precursor cell theory is provided by the molecular genetic disorders observed in gliomas.

A characteristic pattern in oligodendrogliomas during early stages of neoplastic evolution, and most atypical for astrocytomas, is the deletion of genetic material in chromosomes 19q and 1p (8,165). In examining separate areas of pure oligodendroglioma and pure astrocytoma from three mixed oligoastrocytomas, von Deimling's group (96) found the characteristic LOH of 19q and 1p in both areas, astrocytic and oligodendroglial. Through a different approach, mixed gliomas have been examined by computer-assisted microscopy analysis of Feulgen-stained nuclei, a method that by quantitating 30 different variables can differentiate the nuclear morphology of oligodendrogliomas from that of astrocytomas. It was observed that the nuclear morphology of the great majority of mixed gliomas is more similar to oligodendrogliomas than to astrocytomas (33). The host's local factors and stage of development may determine the neoplasm's phenotype: protoplasmic astrocytoma in gray matter, classical oligodendroglioma in mature tumor, and low-grade glioma at very early stages of development. This field is the object of intense research and will probably provide for more accurate classification of tumors.

Ependymomas

Ependymomas are gliomas that develop in close proximity to the ventricular system, central canal, or filum terminale and are derived from ependymal or subependymal cells. The tumors occur frequently in children in an infratentorial location and intraspinally in adults, and have a behavior less closely related to their histologic grade than other gliomas.

Overall, ependymomas are infrequent neoplasms, accounting for only 1.2% of all primary intracranial tumors (137) and 2.9% of intracranial gliomas (66). Their incidence in the spinal cord is much higher, where they comprise more than half of all the neoplasms and about one-third of all intraspinal glial tumors (137). Ependymomas have a characteristic age-related distribution. They develop more frequently during childhood when ependymomas are 15% of intracranial gliomas, and most are infratentorial (48,137, 184). This age-related distribution is also evident in the spinal cord tumors, where more than 85% of ependymomas occur after age 15 years, whereas close to two-thirds of the intracranial ones develop in children (137,184).

Morphologically, three major types of ependymoma are recognized: diffuse, myxopapillary, and subependymoma; each has a characteristic location. The diffuse type, and its papillary variant, may occur throughout

the neuraxis; the myxopapillary ependymomas are observed almost exclusively in the lumbosacral spine, and the subependymomas are almost all intraventricular.

Topographically, ependymomas have a well-defined distribution. Of all the ventricular ependymomas, 31% are lateral, 8% involve the third ventricle (148), and the remaining 61% arise from the floor of the fourth ventricle. The supratentorial tumors are in close relationship with the lateral wall of the ventricles, with a tendency for a paraventricular rather than an intraventricular location. The fourth ventricular tumors have been divided according to their microanatomic location. The *midfloor type* arises in the caudal half of the ventricle and has a tendency to extend into the dorsal upper cervical spinal cord through the orifice of Magendie. The *lateral type* develops in the vestibular area and frequently grows into the cerebellomedullary cystern through the foramen of Luschka; and the *roof type* extends from the inferior medullary velum (76). Ependymomas, usually cystic, may also develop in the cerebral hemispheres away from the ventricles, a variant that has been referred to as ectopic.

The intraspinal ependymomas may be intramedullary in relationship with the central canal or may develop in the region of the cauda equina. The intramedullary ependymomas develop all along the cord but have a predilection for the cervical and cervicothoracic segments (129) and are usually low-grade cellular tumors that occur in young and middle-aged adults. In the lumbosacral area the tumors develop in middle-aged adults at the conus medullaris or along the filum terminale. In about equal proportions the tumors are either cellular ependymomas or myxopapillary ependymomas; however, most myxopapillary tumors occur in this area (196).

On rare occasions, primary ependymomas may develop in the pelvic/abdominal cavity or subcutaneous sacrococcygeal tissue. In the latter location, the mass lesion is usually diagnosed in a young adult as a pilonidal cyst or sinus (67) and is rarely associated with a spinal defect. These tumors are presumed to originate from the coccygeal medullary vestige at the end of the coccyx.

Ependymomas tend to be better circumscribed than other gliomas. The cut surface of the tumors is usually heterogeneous with pinkish-gray areas intermingled with hemorrhagic zones, is frequently gritty due to calcification, and may have areas of necrosis. The intracerebral tumors may be solid or papillary and frequently contain cysts. Infratentorially, the tumor may fill the ventricular cavity and appear solid or papillary. The spinal intra-axial lesions are nonencapsulated but characteristically are well-circumscribed, elongated lesions. There is frequently a proximal syringomyelic cavity and focal attachment to the central canal. At the cauda equina, the tumor may be intra-axial and growing in the conus medullaris or extra-axial attached to the filum terminale, and may present as a circumscribed mass or wrap around the region's anatomic structures.

Microscopically, the neoplastic ependymal cells grow in a fine, fibrillary background and have a predominantly ovoid nucleus with heavy, fine, and uniformly distributed chromatin. The hallmark of ependymomas that allows for their immediate recognition is the ependymal pseudorosette. This structure is formed by carrot-shaped cells aligned circumferentially around a vessel, with their fibrillary processes directed perpendicularly to the vessel wall, thus forming a perivascular rim of tissue devoid of nuclei. Although this feature may be observed in other tumors, the diagnosis of ependymoma in its absence is somewhat doubtful. True ependymal rosettes and canals are also diagnostic but occur rarely, as is the case with blepharoplasts and cilia. The spectrum of the neoplasms extends from cellular and sparsely fibrillary tumors, the cellular ependymomas, to sparsely cellular and heavily fibrillary ones. Some of the latter tumors have been recognized as the tanicytic variant of ependymoma. The subependymoma, another heavily fibrillary variant, and the myxopapillary ependymoma have characteristic microscopy features (see later). Papillary structures, where the central core

vessel is surrounded by an ependymofibrillary frond, may occur focally in otherwise typical cellular ependymomas. When papillae formation is the predominant feature, the tumors resemble choroid plexus papillomas and are referred to as papillary ependymomas. A clear cell variant, with tumor cells having perinuclear halos and resembling oligodendrocytes, is also recognized. This variant can be misdiagnosed as oligodendroglioma or central neurocytoma.

Immunoperoxidase staining with GFAP may be helpful in diagnosing questionable cases, as it demonstrates the tapering fibrillary processes of the perivascular neoplastic ependymal cells forming the pseudorosettes. The tumors are also immunoreactive with vimentin, the reaction being stronger in the high-grade tumors (26) and allowing for a differential diagnosis with choroid plexus papillomas, which are GFAP and vimentin negative. Tumor cells may also be positive with the epithelial markers cytokeratin and epithelial membrane antigen. Ultrastructural studies are not usually necessary to diagnose ependymomas, but the cells do have characteristic intermediate filaments, intercellular junctions, and blepharoplasts.

In contrast with astrocytomas and oligodendrogliomas, there is no well-defined grading system for ependymomas. The WHO (92) describes a low-grade (grade II) tumor and an anaplastic ependymoma (grade III). The anaplastic neoplasm is cellular, is rather undifferentiated, and has frequent mitoses and prominent vascular proliferation. In ependymomas the presence of necrosis does not have the ominous implications that it has in astrocytic tumors (65,156).

It is generally accepted that in ependymomas there is no close correlation between histologic grade and prognosis (48,49,65,124, 184,218). However, a median survival without recurrence of 15.5 years, and 1.5 years for low- and high-grade ependymomas, respectively, has been reported (43). Tumor recurrence almost always develops at the primary site, with recurrent low-grade tumors and first relapses having a less aggressive progression (54).

Being in close relationship with the ventricular system, ependymomas have direct access to the cerebrospinal fluid (CSF), but dissemination of ependymomas through the CSF pathway is uncommon (141,218). When it does occur, it has been reported to not influence prognosis (156). However, in a recently reported series, 11.4% of tumors disseminated, and dissemination significantly worsened prognosis. The younger age of patients, biopsy or subtotal resection, myxopapillary phenotype, and high proliferative indices (13% compared with 2% for the nondisseminated ones) characterized the cases undergoing dissemination (168).

Metastases outside of the CNS are exceptional with low-grade gliomas. In ependymomas they appear in as many as 6% of the cases and develop without any relationship with degree of anaplasia (143). The metastases involve chest and abdominal structures, the latter in association with peritoneal shunts.

Ependymomas, despite their usually low histologic grade, may behave aggressively, particularly in children, in whom ependymomas may have worse outcomes than medulloblastomas (66), especially in the long term (198). The median survival rate for ependymomas ranges between an overall 5.4 years for intracranial childhood tumors (156) to 15.5 years for supratentorial low-grade ependymomas (43). The 5-year survival rates are between 45% and 61% (65,141,156), and the 10-year survival rates are about 45% (65,156).

In ependymomas young age is an unfavorable prognostic factor. Anaplastic ependymomas tend to occur at a young age (218), in sharp contrast with astrocytomas, and to a certain degree with oligodendrogliomas, where advancing age is associated with higher histologic grade and worse prognosis. Median survival times of 28.5 months for patients younger than age 15 years and of 52 months for those older than age 15 have been reported (218). Children younger than 6 years (124,141,156) have shortened survival, and the 5-year survival is close to 0 in children 24 months or younger (65,156).

A factor predictive of improved survival time is complete surgical removal without residual disease or infiltration (124,141,156). As expected, the location of the tumor very much determines the extent of resection. There does not appear to be a difference in outcome between supratentorial and infratentorial ependymomas (156). There is, however, a significantly lower mean survival time and lower 5-year cumulative survival rate for lateral (i.e., vestibular [40 months and 21%]) than for midfloor (i.e., caudal [170 months and 73%]) fourth ventricular ependymomas (76). Spinal cord and cauda equina tumors have better outcomes than intracranial ones (184).

Histologically, high cellularity and mitotic indices have not correlated with survival in some reports (65,156), whereas in other studies tumor cellularity (49) and number of mitoses (141,184) have had significant predictive value. The immunoperoxidase demonstration of increased expression of vimentin in the neoplastic cells, with a GFAP/vimentin ratio of less than 1, is associated with a 5.4 times higher risk of death (46).

The proliferative activity of intracranial malignant and intracranial/intraspinal low-grade ependymomas, determined by bromodeoxyuridine labeling, is not significantly different (5); however, in this series, all cases with an index greater than 1% recurred within 24 months after diagnosis. MIB-1 LIs with a median of 3.8% (186) or mean around 2.0% (83,175) are characteristic of low-grade ependymomas. High-grade tumors have a median of 9.5% (186) or means between 6.7% and 34% (83,175). However, individual cases may not conform (175), and overlapping indices are frequent. Similarly, as with other CNS tumors, DNA ploidy in ependymomas is not useful at the individual tumor level in segregating low- from high-grade neoplasms (179). Another possible objective marker of heightened aggressiveness of tumors is the activity of telomerase, an enzyme up-regulated during neoplastic transformation. The enzyme is overexpressed in high-grade ependymoma and demonstrates a close correlation with elevated MIB-1 LI (175).

Abnormalities in chromosome 22 appear to be important in tumorigenesis of ependymomas, which is different from other gliomas. Full or partial deletions of chromosome 22 have been described commonly in sporadic ependymomas (163,172), and monosomy of chromosome 22 occurs in familial ependymomas. Furthermore, ependymomas are one of the CNS neoplasms that develop in neurofibromatosis II (NF2), the gene of which is located on chromosome 22. However, by examining intracranial ependymomas it has been suggested that a gene other than the NF2 gene may be involved in sporadic and familial ependymoma tumorigenesis (194). Also, in a *de novo* constitutional translocation the breakpoint occurred away from the NF2 gene (151). Since NF2-associated ependymomas usually develop in the spinal cord, it is possible that the NF2 mutation is distinctive of intramedullary ependymomas. Other chromosomal abnormalities have also been described, but less consistently. Frequently in ependymomas (199) there are abnormalities of chromosome 17, the seat of the p53 gene. However, p53 mutations are unusual in ependymomas (146). A viral agent may also be a factor in the process of neoplastic transformation of ependymomas. In 10 of 11 ependymomas, a segment of the papova virus SV40 T-antigen has been demonstrated (10). This protein, and other viral proteins, may inactivate p53 with consequential effects on the regulation of the cell cycle.

Myxopapillary Ependymoma

Myxopapillary ependymomas are a morphologically distinct type of ependymoma that develops almost exclusively in the lumbosacral area. They are believed to originate from ependymal cells at the level of the filum terminale. Rarely, they may present in other segments of spinal cord, in the cerebrum, or in the sacrococcygeal subcutaneous region (67). These tumors constitute from one-fourth to one-third of all spinal ependymomas (137,184,196). Most myxopapillary ependymomas occur after age 16 years (184),

with a central distribution in the fourth decade (158,196).

The tumors characteristically originate from the filum terminale and may extend upward into the conus medullaris. They may present as a discrete encapsulated mass or surround neighboring nerve roots.

The formation of papillae and the production of mucin are the distinctive microscopy features. The neoplastic ependymal cells have round or ovoid nuclei with fine chromatin and an appreciable amount of cytoplasm. The perivascular space forming the typical ependymal pseudorosette accumulates abundant mucin around the core vessel, and the zone may eventually hyalinize. The ependymovascular units become discohesive and form papillae. In the more solid areas, the cells grow in sheets and appear more epithelial-like, with occasional intracellular mucin. Nuclear atypia may be focal, but cellular anaplasia is not usually present. The immunophenotype of the myxopapillary ependymal cells is similar to that of the other ependymomas. Ultrastructurally, the myxopapillary cells are different in that they demonstrate prominent basal lamina.

Myxopapillary ependymomas are low histologic-grade tumors (WHO grade I). Mitotic activity is low, as is the MIB-1 LI, around 1% (158,175,186). The LI, however, tends to be higher in the tumors that disseminate (168).

Myxopapillary ependymomas are slowly growing neoplasms that have high rates of dissemination (33%) (168) and recurrence (43%) (158), which, as expected, are greater when the tumors have been piecemeal or incompletely resected (196). In this large series, the mean survival time of completely resected tumors was 19 years.

As in other ependymomas, p53 expression is not a feature of tumorigenesis in myxopapillary tumors (158). A rearrangement of chromosome 1p has been described (181).

Subependymomas

Subependymomas are low-grade, abundantly fibrillated ependymal neoplasms that occur during adulthood and are usually amenable to complete resection. Because of their rich gliofibrillary matrix and their presumed origin from subependymal glial cells, they also have been described as subependymal glomerate astrocytomas.

The prototypical subependymoma is a small, lobular tumor in the fourth or lateral ventricle found incidentally in an elderly individual. In many cases, however, tumors become symptomatic. The symptomatic tumors characteristically present in patients older than 15 years (117) and tend to be diagnosed at an earlier age (39 years) than asymptomatic ones (59 years) (182). These symptomatic lesions are usually large, with diameters of 4–5 cm and are located in eloquent areas, close to the orifice of Monroe, cerebral aqueduct, fourth ventricle, or spinal cord (182).

Subependymomas occur throughout the ventricular system (78), seldom in the third ventricle (72) and in the spinal cord, usually close to the central canal. Most tumors are almost totally intraventricular (117), but cases have been reported intracerebrally (94) and on the surface of the spinal cord (72).

Classical subependymomas are firm, lobulated, tannish-white tumors projecting from the surface of the ventricle. Microscopically, they are sparsely cellular lesions, with the tumor cells arranged in lobules and disposed in a paucicellular dense fibrillary background that forms the main part of the tumor. The tumor cells have the finely powdery chromatin characteristic of ependymal cells, and the cytoplasm may appear vacuolated. The fibrillary matrix may be immunoreactive with GFAP, and the tumor cells may be positive with epithelial markers. Ultrastructurally, the cells have features of ependymal cells, such as microvilli, lumina, and intercellular attachments (94). Areas of subependymoma may be found in otherwise characteristic ependymomas. These mixed tumors should probably be diagnosed as ependymomas, and the subependymoma designation should be reserved only for those cases where the great bulk of the tumor has the distinctive sybependymoma morphology (13).

Because of their superficial location and circumscribed character, subependymomas are amenable to complete excision. A large size, however, predicts a negative outcome (182). In this series, collected before microscopy neurosurgery became available, a majority of the fatal cases were mixed tumors with a cellular ependymoma component, and many of the patients died soon after surgery.

Mixed Gliomas

Mixed gliomas are those tumors with more than one neoplastic glial cell phenotype. Most of these gliomas are oligoastrocytomas, a minor fraction may be oligoependymomas, and a few could be ependymoastrocytomas. Recognizing that gliomas are morphologically heterogeneous tumors and that pure tumors are rare, the concept of mixed gliomas, their histogenesis, and the criteria for their diagnosis have been widely debated.

The incidence of mixed gliomas varies according to the criteria used for their diagnosis. In a large series of gliomas, 9.2% were classified as mixed (66). They occur more frequently during the fourth decade of life. The most frequent presenting symptom is seizures, followed by headaches. About 50% develop in the frontal lobe. Calcification ranges between 14% when detected by CT and 60% when detected microscopically (61, 190).

According to the distribution of the neoplastic glial components, the tumors are considered compact when discrete zones of each tumor are present and diffuse when the two cellular elements are intermingled (61). The grading of these neoplasms remains controversial, but probably the presence of frequent mitoses, microvascular cellular proliferation, and necrosis separates the low- from the high-grade tumors (190). Considering that pure gliomas comprised exclusively of a single type of macroglial cell are uncommon, an important question is when to call a tumor a mixed glioma. Originally, Hart et al. (61) proposed that neoplasms be classified as mixed when the proportion of the two cellular components was about equal or when both components were present as separate zones. More recently, it has been arbitrarily suggested that the presence of 30% of a second glial phenotype suffices for a mixed designation.

The importance of separating mixed gliomas from pure oligodendrogliomas or astrocytomas is more than academic if their respective prognoses were different. The median survival of mixed gliomas has ranged between 3 years, placing them prognostically closer to astrocytomas (61), and 5.8 years, a survival intermediate between astrocytomas and oligodendrogliomas (190). In both series, tumor grade is a predictor of survival, with low grades (Kernohan's 1 and 2) having a significantly better prognosis. However, whether the predominant component was astrogial or oligodendroglial, or the mixture was compact or diffuse, had no differential predictive value. Mixed gliomas, like other gliomas, usually progress into histologically high-grade neoplasms indistinguishable from glioblastomas, a tendency attributed primarily to their astrocytic component.

The origin of these neoplasms is probably from oligodendroglia, possibly through a process of neoplastic transformation more akin to the misdifferentiation model (see Chapter 13 in this volume). Quantitative comparison by computerized image analysis of Feulgen-stained nuclei of mixed oligoastrocytomas with those of typical oligodendrogliomas and astrocytomas demonstrates that most cell phenotypes are closer to grade II oligodendrogliomas than to astrocytomas and that a remaining smaller population resembles oligodendroglioma grade III (33). Furthermore, the characteristic allelic deletions in chromosomes 19q and lp observed during early oncogenesis of oligodendrogliomas are also present in oligoastrocytomas (96), although oligoastrocytomas may have more heterogeneous patterns. Experimentally, most N-nitrosomethylurea-induced murine gliomas are either mixed oligoastrocytomas (>54%) or oligodendrogliomas (23%), and the p53 mutation, a characteristic event in early tumorigenesis of astrocytomas, does not occur in these

tumors (93). The existence of a glial neoplasm phenotypically composed of astrocytes and oligodendrocytes has been proposed to be the result of a neoplastic process involving the O2-A progenitor cell capable of differentiating into an oligodendrocyte and/or a type 2A astrocyte (see the preceding section entitled "Oligodendroglioma"). The proliferative advantage would involve this bipotential cell, and other factors would determine phenotypic expression.

TUMORS OF NEURONAL ORIGIN

The presence of neoplastic neurons is the essential element in neuronal cell tumors. Neuronal proliferation may be the only element of the neoplasm, as is the case in pure neuronal tumors, or there may be a concomitant neoplastic glial proliferation (i.e., the glioneuronal neoplasms). The neoplastic neurons that resemble large pyramidal neurons are referred to as ganglion cells, and the small ones that resemble internuncial neurons are called neurocytes. The pure neuronal tumors are rare and include the gangliocytoma; a special form confined to the cerebellum, the cerebellar dysplastic gangliocytoma; and the central neurocytoma.

Gangliocytomas

Gangliocytomas (GC) are WHO grade I neoplasms made of pyramidal-type neurons proliferating in a nonneoplastic glial background. The tumors are rare, tend to manifest in young adults, and occur more frequently in the cerebrum, cerebellum (45), and spinal cord. The neoplastic neurons may be functional and produce hormones or releasing factors, with development of acromegaly and Cushing's disease (4,176). In these functional cases, the GC is usually associated with a pituitary adenoma, and both tumors may be intrasellar.

GCs are usually well-circumscribed masses that may mimic gray matter or may be firm and grayish when they have an abundant reticulin content. Microscopically, the ganglion cells have well-defined neuronal features with large nucleolus, ample perikaryon, Nissl substance, and multipolar processes. The neurons may have bizarre shapes, may be bi- or multinucleated, and may be distributed haphazardly or form clusters. The background is neuropil-like with a neurofibrillar mesh, sparse glial cells, and various amounts of reticulin fibers. Ultrastructurally and immunohistochemically, the cells have a neuronal phenotype. In addition, the ganglion cells may immunoreact with peptide hormones and/or amines (45). The neoplastic neurons may also contain different types of electron-dense membranous structures, which resemble lipid inclusions of abnormal storage disorders (79) and are probably of a degenerative nature.

Cerebellar Dysplastic Gangliocytoma

Cerebellar dysplastic gangliocytoma (CDG) is a hamartomatous, perhaps neoplastic, neuronal lesion of the cerebellum that has a characteristic morphology and may be associated with Cowden's disease. The lesion is also known as Lhermitte-Duclos disease or Purkinjeoma.

CDG may present at all ages, but a mean age of 33.7 years has been determined from published cases (211). The lesion is rare, and the more recent reports refer to either its characteristic imaging appearance or its association with Cowden's disease. Cowden's disease is an autosomal-dominant inherited disorder characterized by multiple hamartomas of the skin and oral mucosa, and increased incidence of tumors of thyroid, breast, ovary, and gastrointestinal tract. The abnormal gene has been localized to chromosome 10q22–23 (142). More recently recognized features of the syndrome are megalocephaly and CDG. CDG is frequently associated with macrocephaly and thinning of the occipital bone (44), and with malformations of fingers, leontiasis ossea, syringomyelia, and astrocytoma (169). Although it appears that CDG can be an isolated lesion, its association with Cowden's disease is being advocated as a new

phakomatosis (149), but how often this association occurs is unknown. The relationship between a CDG treated by total resection alone and the presentation 17 years later of a gemistocytic astrocytoma in the contralateral parieto-occipital lobe (38) is also uncertain. The clinical presentation of CDG is usually secondary to increased intracranial pressure, the result of hydrocephalus.

CDG is a single or multifocal lesion of the cerebellum that may involve the vermis or the hemispheres. It is characterized by expansion of the cerebellar tissue with broadening of the folia, but with preservation of the folial architecture. The lesional tissue is pale. Microscopically, the broadened folia have a bilayered cortex with a superficial layer (molecular) occupied by dense bundles of thick, myelinated axons, and a deeper hypercellular layer (granular). Some of the cells in the granular layer have the appearance of pyramidal neurons, but the majority are round cells resembling hypertrophied granular neurons. Purkinje cells and normal granular neurons may be inconspicuous, and the white matter in the core of the folium may be thin or absent. Ultrastructurally, both types of proliferated cells have neuronal features with characteristic microtubules, clear and dense core vesicles, and synaptic junctions (169). The molecular layer axons are thinly myelinated. Immunohistochemically, the proliferated cells react with neuronal markers. The axons from the enlarged, granular-like neurons have shown a normal pattern of neurofilament phosphorylation (225). The MIB-1 labeling index of the lesion is low, and the p53 protein is not expressed.

The prognosis of CDG is good, particularly in the more recently reported cases; however, recurrent cases have been described in long-term survivors (211), even after gross total removal.

It is commonly believed that CDG involves primarily the granular neurons, because the orientation of the superficial, large, myelinated fibers is similar to the axonal distribution of normal granular neurons. However, the demonstration in the abnormal cells of immunophenotypic patterns characteristic of both Purkinje and granular neurons suggests that both cell types are involved in the dysplastic process (193). The physiologic phosphorylation pattern of the lesional axonal neurofilament proteins suggests that the cells are hypertrophic/hyperplastic rather than neoplastic.

Central Neurocytomas

Central neurocytomas (CNs) are low-histologic-grade (WHO grade I) neoplasms with neuronal differentiation that occur intraventricularly in the supratentorial compartment and have a favorable outcome. The tumors are currently a well-characterized clinicopathologic entity, but formerly they were diagnosed as oligodendrogliomas, ependymomas, or neuroblastomas because of their microscopy appearance or location.

CNs represent less than 0.5% of all CNS tumors (63,212) and may account for about one-half of all supratentorial intraventricular tumors in adults (63). The tumors occur in young adults, with a mean age of 29 years; almost half are diagnosed during the third decade; and two out of three cases become clinically apparent between 20 and 40 years of age (63). Clinical manifestations of raised intracranial pressure due to hydrocephalus are a characteristic presentation of CNs. The tumors develop in the lateral and third ventricles in the neighborhood of the orifice of Monro, where they are frequently described as attached to the septum pellucidum, lateral ventricle, or corpus callosum. Many of the tumors occupy the anterior half of the lateral ventricle (63) and may straddle the midline. The tumors may involve both lateral and third ventricles, and a unique case even extended into the fourth ventricle (226). CNs have been described in other sites such as thalamus (187), cerebellum (41), and spinal cord (121, 203).

CNs are grossly well-circumscribed tumors. They have various degrees of calcification that range from a finely gritty cut surface to a calcified mass, such as the one present in one of the two initial cases of CN reported by Hassoun (62).

The microscopic appearance of CNs is characteristic, although it may be easily misinterpreted as other neoplasms. The tumor is moderately cellular and made of uniform round cells growing in sheets with a very fine fibrillary background that has a delicate capillary-type vascular network. The nuclei have a stippled chromatin, and the cytoplasm may be clear and form a perinuclear halo, giving a honeycomb appearance to the solid tumor growth; these features are reminiscent of clear cell ependymoma or the classical pattern of oligodendroglioma. The background of CNs is finely fibrillary, neuropil-like. This background may occupy sizable areas where the tumor is devoid of nuclei, forming the so-called pineocytoma-like rosettes, which are a most distinctive feature of the CN and are absent in oligodendrogliomas. In perivascular areas the background fibrillary processes may produce small ependymoma-like rosettes that, unlike the pseudo-rosettes in ependymomas, are GFAP negative. In some cases, prominent ectatic, focally hyalinized vascularity is present (170). Although there may be slight nuclear atypia, uniform cellularity is observed throughout, and mitotic figures or areas of necrosis are unusual findings. This is in contrast with the neuroblastomas, another one of the look-alikes, in which the tumor cells are blastic in type, with prominent nuclear atypia, individual cell necrosis, and prominent mitotic figures.

The classical CN can be readily recognized with hematoxylin and eosin stain preparations, but confirmation of its neuronal nature requires immunohistochemistry, and perhaps electron microscopy examination in some questionable cases. The tumors are uniformly immunoreactive for the glycolytic enzyme neuron-specific enolase (NSE), which lacks specificity, because it is present in many other neoplasms. Most CNs, with one exception (107), are immunopositive with antisera against the synaptic vesicle protein synaptophysin (47,55,68,90,170,185,212,213), with the few negative cases attributed to prolonged formaldehyde fixation (47,55,68), which presumably denatures the protein. The antisynaptophysin reaction may be tenuous and focal, but it is consistently positive in the neuropil-like background and is readily identified in the pineocytic rosettes and in perivascular zones. Other neuronal markers such as calcineurin (55), MAP2 (55,68), class III P-tubulin (68), and the adhesion molecules Ll and isoform 180 of nerve cell adhesion molecule (N.CAM) (47) are also consistently present in CN. Results with neurofilament proteins have been inconsistent (47,68,212). The neuroendocrine marker chromogranin (47) has not been detected immunohistologically. Reactive GFAP-positive astrocytes may be present in perivascular areas and at the periphery of the tumor. However, focal GFAP expression by tumor cells has been reported (197), and von Deimling has described in three of four CNs perikaryal expression of GFAP in many tumor cells with frequent coexpression of synaptophysin (213). Furthermore, CN cells in culture have also coexpressed synaptophysin and GFAP (207).

The ultrastructural distinctive features of CNs are neuronal cytoskeletal and synaptic structures in the perikaryon of cells, but more prominent in the processes-rich interperikaryal neuropil. The structures are microtubules, light and dense core secretory vesicles, and well formed to rudimentary synapses (47,62, 68,88,107,170,212).

CNs have a good prognosis (90,107,185). An overall actuarial 5-year survival of 81% (185) has been reported; even patients with subtotal removal may remain free of recurrence or progression of disease (90). However, gross total resection may have a better local control rate (100%) than subtotal resections (70%) (185). Occasional patients, probably less than 7% (42), have recurrences (88, 90,107,170,187,207) or craniospinal dissemination (42). Some tumors have either *de novo* (212,226) or after recurrence (187) histologic features of anaplasia (i.e., anaplastic or malignant CN), raising the possibility of aggressive behavior or malignant transformation. Overall, however, there is no correlation between aggressive behavior and histologic atypia (42,88,170,207), and the final outcome of these atypical variants is unknown. CNs occurring after age 50 have a poor prognosis (197).

The proliferation indices of CNs have been reported as less than 1% (88,170). A study exploring the correlation among MIB-1 LI, histologic findings, and outcome observed that a MIB-1 LI of more than 2% correlates closely with vascular proliferation and has a 63% chance of relapse (versus 22% for CNs with less than 2% MIB-1 LI). The authors propose that these tumors should be classified as atypical CN (WHO grade II) (197).

The protooncogene N-*myc* is not overexpressed in CNs (213) as it usually is in neuroblastomas, nor has overexpression of p53 been observed (42). Cytogenetically, loss of chromosome 17 has been reported in one CN (16). The tumor cells in CNs have been found to be diploid (88), with a mean cytometrically determined proliferation index of 7.8%.

The nature and origin of CNs remain a subject of debate. In view of their positive immunoreactivity with neuronal markers and their ultrastructurally observed neuronal elements, it is widely accepted that CNs are neuronal neoplasms made up of fairly well-differentiated cells. The absence of protein pp60+, normally present in postmitotic neurons, suggests that CN cells have not completed the process of neurogenesis (213). The absence of large ganglion cells and the paucity or absence of neurofilaments suggest that CN cells are small, mature neurons similar to striatal and thalamic granular interneurons (68). It is postulated that the tumors arise from the subependymal plate, a structure that contains cells with neurogenic potential (68, 213) and is present in the lateral and third ventricles, but not in the fourth ventricle, of adult mammals. Alternatively, the cell of origin may be a pluripotential cell with a strong commitment for neuronal differentiation, but with a potential for glial development (207, 213). This theory is based on the questionable phenotypic glial differentiation and on the coexpression of synaptophysin and GFAP in histology sections (213) and in cells cultured from two neurocytomas (207).

A nosology problem has arisen recently by the report of intraparenchymal CNS neoplasms with a neurocytoma appearance with or without an astrocytic component (53), or of histologically malignant intracerebral neoplasms with ultrastructural and immunoreactive features of neurocytoma (i.e., malignant neurocytoma [139]), or of oligodendrogliomas (144) in which neuronal markers and/or ultrastructural features indicate a neuronal nature.

Also, neoplasms that are described as cerebral neurocytomas but that probably are DNETs have been reported (145). Whether these tumors are bona fide neurocytomas or oligodendrogliomas that may express neuronal features remains to be established.

MIXED NEURONAL AND GLIAL TUMORS

The glioneuronal tumors are not as rare as the pure neuronal tumors and comprise the following: GGs, which present usually in young adults; a special form observed in infants, the desmoplastic infantile GG; and the dysembryoplastic neuroepithelial tumor, which characteristically becomes symptomatic in young adults.

Ganglioglioma

Ganglioglioma is a low-histologic-grade tumor (WHO grade I or II) with a neuronal and a glial component. A high-grade anaplastic variant is also recognized (WHO grade III). In the spectrum of neuroepithelial neoplasms, GGs have a mixture of neuronal and glial cells, the neurons being large with a prominent perikaryon, thus resembling pyramidal neurons (i.e., ganglion cells).

GGs are tumors of children and young adults, with a tendency for those in the midline to manifest at an earlier age than cerebral hemispheric ones (58,109). Most supratentorial GGs present with seizures, and GGs may be the tumors most frequently resected surgically for treatment of epilepsy (161,222).

GGs are uncommon tumors, with an incidence of 0.4% to 1.3% of all intracranial tumors. In a large series of CNS tumors, GGs were 1.4% of all gliomas and 5.8% of all low-grade astrocytomas excluding PAs (105).

GGs occur more frequently in the cerebral hemispheres, where the temporal lobe is a most common and characteristic location. A frontal lobe involvement is also common, and a few develop in the midline around the third ventricle. Another frequent site is the spinal cord, where they may be even more common than in the cerebrum (109), and usually involve several segments. Brain stem and cerebellar involvement is also observed. Primary tumors in the anterior optic pathway, where normally there are no neurons, are unusual (18), but the chiasm may be involved secondarily (116). GGs have been reported in patients with neurofibromatosis, tuberous sclerosis, and congenital malformations (58).

GGs appear grossly as circumscribed lesions, but at surgery and microscopy examination the margins are usually not well defined. Cystic areas are frequent, with the formation occasionally of a mural nodule. The tumors develop in areas rich in neurons, with a preferential involvement of the cerebral cortex. The tumors are usually solid masses of firm, variably cystic, tannish-gray tissue with frequent calcium deposition.

Microscopically, the tumor has a neuronal and a glioma component. The large ganglion cells are distinctive and set the lesion apart from the neurocytomas, where the neuronal element is small and tends to resemble granular neurons. Similarly, the glioma component is essential, as it separates GGs from gangliocytoma, where the nongangliocytic element is glial but not of a neoplastic nature. The ganglion cells have a large nucleus with a prominent nucleolus, and the cytoplasm or perikaryon is ample, occasionally with Nissl substance. With the electron microscope (EM), the ganglion cells have numerous cellular processes and contain distinctive neuronal cytoskeleton, including microtubules and neurofilaments, and diagnostic membrane-bound dense core vesicles (200). Dendrosomatic synapses may occasionally be detected on the surface of the ganglion cells. The ganglion cells may be differentiated from normal native neurons, in the vicinity of or being overrun by the expanding tumor, by their abnormally large size, shape, and/or distribution/orientation. The glioma component of GGs is most commonly a fibrillary astrocytoma, but not infrequently it is a pilocytic astrocytoma (71,223). The glial phenotype has also been described as oligodendroglial (19), and exceptionally as ependymal. In most GGs, the glioma is of low histologic grade, but in some cases features of anaplasia such as dysplastic nuclei, microvascular cellular proliferation, and multifocal necrosis (105,131,223) indicate a high histologic grade or anaplastic ganglioglioma (AGG). In a report of malignant transformation of a GG 3 years after radiotherapy, the anaplastic features involved both neurons and astrocytes (82). Other characteristic but not constant features of GGs are binucleated neurons, a prominent fibrous stroma, focal mineralization, and a lymphocytic infiltrate. In a few tumors the fibrous stroma may be prominent and provide the mass with a desmoplastic character. The presence of collagen and inflammatory cells in GGs has been associated with their indolent course (80). Glioneuronal hamartias, cortical dysplasia, neuronal heterotopias, and other migrational disorders frequently occur in the neighborhood of GGs (161,223,227).

The mix of neuronal and glial elements in GG varies between tumors and within a tumor. Ganglion cells may be the predominant component, raising the possible diagnosis of gangliocytoma, or the tumor may be predominantly astrocytic with only scant neuronal elements, which may require immunostains for their demonstration. Antibodies to neurofilament and microtubule proteins are immunoreactive with neoplastic ganglion cells. Antibodies against synaptophysin provide a most sensitive marker for ganglion cells (37,71,130). The dense perikaryal surface pattern of synaptophysin staining of the ganglion cells has been described as diagnostic of neoplastic ganglion cells (131). This criterion,

however, needs to be applied carefully because a similar pattern of staining has been observed in nonneoplastic neurons of the spinal cord (228). Chromogranin A, a component of the soluble protein fraction of dense core granules in neuroendocrine cells, is not as sensitive a ganglion cell marker as is synaptophysin (37,71), but its uniform staining of the perikaryon provides for a less controversial detection and interpretation of neoplastic neurons. Neuronal enzymes and polypeptides have also been used as ganglion cell markers with various results (200).

GGs, considered by some as hamartomatous growths, are slow-growing neoplasms, particularly those in the temporal lobes (105), with a favorable prognosis (109) and potential for cure when completely resected. Gross total resection is the best predictor of prolonged overall and event-free survival (19,37,58,105, 227). Total resection has a better overall outcome than subtotal (19), but subtotal resection may still have a good prognosis (14) and recurrence-free survival (37). Attributed to easier access for total removal, tumor location in the cerebral hemisphere has been found to be the single factor predictive of better outcome (109), as tumors in the midline, brain stem, and spinal cord have a greater risk of recurrence or death (58,109).

Histologic grading of GGs is not a good predictor of behavior (109). Anaplastic features, however, may predict unfavorable outcomes (60) and may influence the prognosis in incompletely resected tumors (58). Furthermore, there is a tendency for higher-grade neoplasms to have a shorter time to recurrence (109). GGs frequently have infiltration of the adjacent subarachnoid space, but this feature does not seem to adversely affect prognosis (19,161,223). The Ki-67 and MIB-1 LI of GGs have ranged between 1.1% and 2.7% (71,161), with most tumors being below 10.5% (71,161,223) and high indices being related with recurrences (71). Similarly, a BrDU index of less than 1% has been determined in eight nonrecurring GGs, and of 1.3% in one case that recurred twice (105). The astrocytic component is the cycling cell population in

GGs, the one responsible for the anaplastic transformation. That the neurons are also neoplastic is suggested by the presence in a tumor that was cultured of large, ganglion-like cells that were actively dividing (131), and by tumors that have been reported to have PCNA-positive neuronal elements (223), presumably in the mitotic phase. Expression of the p53 protein has ranged from totally negative (223) to a mean labeling index of 15.6%, suggesting that the expression of the protein may be related with recurrence (71).

Desmoplastic Infantile Ganglioglioma

Desmoplastic infantile ganglioglioma (DIGG), one of the superficial desmoplastic tumors of the cerebrum, is a WHO grade I supratentorial glioneuronal neoplasm that distinctively occurs in infants and, despite an immature cellular component, has a favorable prognosis.

DIGGs are uncommon CNS neoplasms that amounted to only 0.4% in a series of more than 6,500 brain tumors (208), although they have been reported to comprise up to 2% of malignant brain tumors in infants (39). Most cases present during the first year of life, frequently as progressive megalocephaly.

DIGGs are superficial tumors that involve frontal, parietal, temporal, and rarely occipital lobes, frequently extending beyond one lobe, because they are usually large (several centimeters). A deep-seated location is unusual (150). The tumors may be attached to the dura matter and usually have a cystic and a solid component.

Microscopically, DIGGs have neuronal and astrocytic elements in variable densities and proportions, with the tumor cells being disposed either diffusely in a densely desmoplastic background or in focal zones surrounded by loosely arranged collagenous strands. The neuronal cells may be atypical ganglion cells or smaller round neurons in a fine fibrillary background. The glial component is of variable cellular density and primarily astrocytic; it is more prominent in the desmoplastic zones, where it may be associated with a dense reticulin network. Characteristically, DIGGs have a third cellular element of small, undifferentiated cells where areas of necrosis, mitotic figures, and microvascular cellular proliferation may be present. These high-histologic-grade zones may be extensive and, if the more diagnostic glioneuronal areas are not observed, may lead to an inaccurate malignant diagnosis. The neuronal and glial tumor cells are readily identified with immunohistochemistry or ultrastructural methods. The astrocytes are characteristically associated with basal lamina (208) and collagen. The nature of the small cell component is uncertain (208).

DIGGs are probably a variant of GGs that occur during the neonatal period. In contrast with the classical GG, a tumor that usually develops in older individuals, DIGGs are extensively desmoplastic, have an undifferentiated cellular component, and are devoid of an inflammatory infiltrate. The nosology of desmoplastic GGs with inflammatory cells, probably more akin to classical GG (108), is uncertain. Similarly, the relationship of DIGG with DCAI (see earlier), a tumor that has similar clinical and macroscopic features but lacks the neuronal and undifferentiated elements, has yet to be defined. It has been suggested that they are probably the same tumor but that in DCAI the neuronal cells have escaped detection.

The prognosis of DIGGs is overall favorable (40,208), with complete resection predicting a prolonged survival. Incomplete resection, particularly when residual tumor is deeply situated, may be most unfavorable (150). Because of the undifferentiated cellular component, DIGGs may be misdiagnosed as malignant cerebral tumors such as desmoplastic neuroblastomas, malignant gliomas, or malignant meningiomas (40). A thorough sampling of an infantile superficial cerebral tumor will decrease the possibility of missing diagnostic glioneuronal areas.

Dysembryoplastic Neuroepithelial Tumor

Dysembryoplastic neuroepithelial tumor (DNET) is a low-histologic-grade glioneuronal lesion (WHO grade I) of the cerebral cortex that is probably hamartomatous and is associated with chronic intractable epilepsy.

DNET is a clinicopathologic entity that manifests during childhood or early adulthood in the form of focal seizures, frequently of temporal localization, that last for many years and are refractory to medical treatment. DNETs constitute about 1.5% of all pediatric intracranial tumors (202). DNETs are an important fraction of all the lesions encountered in surgical resections for intractable epilepsy; their incidence in these specimens ranges from around 6% (29,138) in children, to 14% in adults (164), to a high of 25% in a mixed population (224). The occurrence of DNET in two children with NF1 is probably coincidental (114). The tumors are preferentially located in the temporal lobe, followed in frequency by the frontal lobe, and only occasionally in other lobes. In agreement with their chronicity, associated cranial bone deformities may be present (202).

Macroscopically, DNETs are mostly confined to the cerebral cortex, although they may extend into the adjacent white matter (91,114). Typically, the lesion is small, rather ill defined, and lobular. It may fragment easily; it may be richly vascularized and/or mucinous. Histologically, there is an overall nodularity and the presence of a specific element. In specimens containing neighboring cortex an associated cortical dysgenesis is commonly present. The nodular component is usually made of oligodendroglia-like cells (OLC); only occasionally is it of a predominantly astrocyte phenotype (70). The specific element consists of OLCs distributed within a mucinous matrix, within which normal and dysplastic ganglion-like neurons appear to be floating. The proportion of each component, the nodular and the specific, varies greatly from case to case. Mitotic figures are infrequent, and when present appear to take place in astrocytes (164). Characteristically, the lesion is devoid of anaplastic changes, although increased cellularity and some pleomorphism have been reported (164). A PCNA mean proliferative index of 2.1% has been determined;

however, in the same specimens a MIB-1 antibody labeled only sporadic nuclei (202), and with one exception all DNETs were found to be diploid.

The nature of the glioneuronal elements of DNETs has been explored with immunohistochemistry and electron microscopy. Astrocytes have been demonstrated with GFAP, some of them resembling reactive cells, others having OLC phenotype and appearing like gliofibrillary oligodencrocytes with the presence ultrastructurally of glial filaments and microtubules (70). Most OLCs are immunoreactive with S100, indicating their glial nature, and frequently have structural oligodendrocyte features. However, focally, these OLCs do react with synaptophysin and contain synapses ultrastructurally (70), features that demonstrate their neuronal character. Therefore it appears that the cellular elements of DNETs are heterogeneous and composed of dysmorphic ganglion cells, small neurons, oligodendrocytes, and astrocytes in various proportions. Based on these observations, it has been proposed that DNETs originate from progenitor cells with potential for glial and neuronal differentiation (70).

The outcome of surgery for DNETs is excellent; there are no recurrences, even after incomplete resection (29,202). In view of this clinical behavior, the dysplastic appearance of the tumor and of surrounding cerebral cortex, and the low proliferative indices, the lesion has been interpreted as a hamartoma (70, 202). In contrast, because of the presence of some pleomorphism, few mitotic figures, and increased cellularity, it has been suggested that DNET may actually be a neoplasm (202).

CONCLUSION

Classification of brain tumors is a complex endeavor intended to facilitate patient management and requires the close cooperation of surgeons, radiologists, and pathologists. As may be observed throughout this chapter, morphology is still the mainstay of these tumor classifications, but alone it falls short of accurately predicting patients' outcome, and other factors may be as important in determining the approach to therapy. The quest, of course, continues for more objective and reproducible indicators of tumor biological potential, with great hopes centered on the new technologies, but with the realization that the microscope still has a great deal to contribute.

REFERENCES

1. Abdulrauf SI, Edvardsen K, Ho K-L, Yang XY, Rock JP, Rosenblum ML. Vascular endothelial growth factor expression and vascular density as prognostic markers of survival in patients with low-grade astrocytomas. *J Neurosurg* 1998;88:513–520.
2. Alshail E, Rutka JT, Becker LE, Hoffman HJ. Optic chiasmatic-hypothalamic glioma. *Brain Pathol* 1997; 7:799–806.
3. Alvord EC, Lofton S. Gliomas of the optic nerve or chiasm: outcome by patient's age, tumor site, and treatment. *J Neurosurg* 1988;68:85–98.
4. Asa SL, Scheithauer BW, Bilbao JM, et al. A case for hypothalamic acromegaly: a clinicopathological study of six patients with hypothalamic gangliocytomas producing growth hormone-releasing factor. *J Clin Endocrinol Metab* 1984;58:796–803.
5. Asai A, Hoshino T, Edwards MS, Davis RL. Predicting the recurrence of ependymomas from the bromodeoxyuridine labeling index. *Childs Nerv Syst* 1992;8: 273–278.
6. Aydin F, Ghatak NR, Salvant J, Muizelaar P. Desmoplastic cerebral astrocytoma of infancy: a case report with immunohistochemical, ultrastructural and proliferation studies. *Acta Neuropathol* 1993;86:666–670.
7. Barbareschi M, Iuzzolino P, Pennella A, et al. p53 protein expression in central nervous system neoplasms. *J Clin Pathol* 1992;45:583–586.
8. Bello MJ, Vaquero J, DeCampos JM, et al. Molecular analysis of chromosome 1 abnormalities in human gliomas reveals frequent loss of 1p in oligodendroglial tumors. *Int J Cancer* 1994;57:172–175.
9. Berger MS, Edwards MSB, LaMasters D, Davis RL, Wilson CBD. Pediatric brain stem tumors: radiographic, pathological, and clinical correlations. *Neurosurgery* 1983;12:298–302.
10. Bergsagel DJ, Finegold MJ, Butel JS, Kupsky WJ, Garcea RL. DNA sequences similar to those of simian virus 40 in ependymomas and choroid plexus tumors of childhood. *N Engl J Med* 1992;326:988–993.
11. Bodey B, Groger AM, Bodey B Jr, Siegel S, Kaiser HE. Immunohistochemical detection of p53 protein expression in various childhood astrocytoma subtypes: significance in tumor progression. *Anticancer Res* 1997;17:1187–1194.
12. Burger PC, Rawlings CE, Cox EB, McLendon RE, Schold SC, Bullard DE. Clinicopathologic correlations in the oligodendroglioma. *Cancer* 1987;59: 1345–1352.
13. Burger PC, Scheithauer BW. Atlas of tumor pathology: tumors of the central nervous system. Washington, DC: Armed Forces Institute of Pathology, 1994.
14. Celli P, Scarpinati M, Nardacci B, Cervoni L, Cantore GP. Gangliogliomas of the cerebral hemispheres: report of 14 cases with long-term follow-up and review of the literature. *Acta Neurochir (Wien)* 1993;125: 52–57.
15. Celli, P, Nofrone I, Palma L, Cantore G, Fortuna A. Cerebral oligodendroglioma: prognostic factors and life history. *Neurosurgery* 1994;35:1018–1035.
16. Cerda-Nicolas M, Lopez-Gines C, Peydro-Olaya A, Llombart-Bosch A. Central neurocytoma: a cytogenetic case study. *Cancer Genet Cytogenet* 1993;65: 173–174.
17. Chandrasoma PT, Smith MM, Apuzzo MLJ. Sterotactic biopsy in the diagnosis of brain masses: comparison of results of biopsy and resected surgical specimen. *Neurosurgery* 1989;24(2):160–165.
18. Chilton J, Caughron MR, Kepes JJ. Ganglioglioma of the optic chiasm: case report and review of the literature. *Neurosurgery* 1990;26:1042–1045.
19. Chintagumpala MM, Armstrong D, Miki S, et al. Mixed neuronal-glial tumors (gangliogliomas) in children. *Pediatr Neurosurg* 1996;24:306–313.
20. Coakley KJ, Huston J, Scheithauer BW, Forbes G, Kelly PJ. Pilocytic astrocytomas: well-demarcated magnetic resonance appearance despite frequent infiltration histologically. *Mayo Clin Proc* 1995;70: 747–751.
21. Cohen ME, Duffner PK, Heffner RR, Lacey DJ, Brecher M. Prognostic factors in brainstem gliomas. *Neurology* 1986;36:602–605.
22. Constantini S, Houten J, Miller DC, et al. Intramedullary spinal cord tumors in children under the age of 3 years. *J Neurosurg* 1996;85:1036–1043.
23. Conway PD, Oechler HW, Kun LE, Murray KJ. Importance of histologic condition and treatment of pediatric cerebellar astrocytoma. *Cancer* 1991;67: 2772–2775.
24. Coons SW, Johnson PC. MIB-1/Ki-67 labeling index predicts patient survival for oligodendroglial tumors. *J Neuropathol Exp Neurol* 1995;54:440.
25. Coons SW, Johnson PC, Pearl DK, Olafsen AG. Prognostic significance of flow cytometry deoxyribonucleic acid analysis of human oligodendrogliomas. *Neurosurgery* 1994;34:680–687.
26. Cruz-Sanchez FF, Rossi ML, Hughes JT, Cervos-Navarro J. An immunohistological study of 66 ependymomas. *Histopathology* 1988;13:443–454.
27. Cruz-Sanchez FF, Rossi ML, Buller JR, Carboni P, Fineron PW, Coakham HB. Oligodendrogliomas: a clinical, histological, immunocytochemical and lectin-binding study. *Histopathology* 1991;19:361–367.
28. Cunningham JM, Kimmel DW, Scheithauer BW, O'-Fallon JR, Novotny PJ, Jenkins RB. Analysis of proliferation markers and p53 expression in gliomas of astrocytic origin: relationships and prognostic value. *J Neurosurg* 1997;86:121–130.
29. Daumas-Duport C, Scheithauer BW, Chodkiewicz J-P, Laws ER, Vedrenne C. Dysembryoplastic neuroepithelial tumor: a surgically curable tumor of young patients with intractable partial seizures. *Neurosurgery* 1988; 23:545–556.
30. Daumas-Duport C, Scheithauer B, O'Fallon J, Kelly P. Grading of astrocytomas: a simple and reproducible method. *Cancer* 1988;62:2152–2165.
31. Daumas-Duport C, Tucker M-L, Kolles H, et al. Oli-

godendrogliomas. Part II: A new grading system based on morphological and imaging criteria. *J Neurooncol* 1997;34:61–78.

32. Daumas-Duport C, Varlet P, Tucker M-L, et al. Oligodendrogliomas. Part I: Patterns of growth, histological diagnosis, clinical and imaging correlations: a study of 153 cases. *J Neurooncol* 1997;34:37–59.

33. Decaestecker C, Lopes BS, Gordower L, et al. Quantitative chromatin pattern description in Feulgen-stained nuclei as a diagnostic tool to characterize the oligodendroglia and astroglial components in mixed oligoastrocytomas. *J Neuropathol Exp Neurol* 1997;56:391–402.

34. De Chadarévian J-P, Pattisapu JV, Faerber EN. Desmoplastic cerebral astrocytoma of infancy. Light microscopy, immunocytochemistry, and ultrastructure. *Cancer* 1990;66:173–179.

35. De la Monte, SM. Uniform lineage of oligodendrogliomas. *Am J Pathol* 1989;135:529–540.

36. DeMasters BKK, Markham N, Lillehei KO, Shroyer KR. Differential telomerase expression in human primary intracranial tumors. *Am J Clin Pathol* 1997;107:548–554.

37. Diepholder HM, Schwechheimer K, Mohadjer M, Knoth R, Volk B. A clinicopathologic and immunomorphologic study of 13 cases of ganglioglioma. *Cancer* 1991;68:2192–2201.

38. Domingo Z, Fisher-Jeffes ND, DeVilliers JC. Malignant occipital astrocytoma in a patient with Lhermitte-Duclos disease (cerebellar gangliocytoma). *Br J Neurosurg* 1996;10:99–102.

39. Duffner PK, Horowitz ME, Krischer JP, et al. Postoperative chemotherapy and delayed radiation in children less than 3 years of age with malignant brain tumors. *N Engl J Med* 1993;328:1725–1731.

40. Duffner PK, Burger PC, Cohen ME, et al. Desmoplastic infantile gangliogliomas: an approach to therapy. *Neurosurgery* 1994;34:583–589.

41. Enam SA, Rosenblum ML, Ho K-L. Neurocytoma in the cerebellum: case report. *J Neurosurg* 1997;87:100–102.

42. Eng DY, DeMonte F, Ginsberg L, Fuller GN, Jaeckle, K. Craniospinal dissemination of central neurocytoma: report of two cases. *J Neurosurg* 1997;86:547–552.

43. Ernestus RI, Wilcke O, Schroder R. Supratentorial ependymomas in childhood: clinicopathological findings and prognosis. *Acta Neurochir (Wien)* 1991;111:96–102.

44. Faillot T, Sichez J-P, Brault J-L, et al. Lhermitte-Duclos disease (dysplastic gangliocytoma of the cerebellum). *Acta Neurochir* 1990;105:44–49.

45. Felix I, Bilbao JM, Asa SL, Tyndel F, Kovacs K, Becker LE. Cerebral and cerebellar gangliocytomas: a morphological study of nine cases. *Acta Neuropathol* 1994;88:246–251.

46. Figarella-Branger D, Gambarelli DG, Dollo C, et al. Infratentorial ependymomas of childhood: correlation between histological features, immunohistological phenotype, silver nucleolar organizer region staining values and post-operative survival in 16 cases. *Acta Neuropathol* 1991;82:208–216.

47. Figarella-Branger D, Pellissier JF, Daumas-Duport C, et al. Central neurocytomas: critical evaluation of a small-cell neuronal tumor. *Am J Surg Pathol* 1992;16:97–109.

48. Fokes EC, Earle KM. Ependymomas: clinical and pathological aspects. *J Neurosurg* 1969;30:585–593.

49. Foreman NK, Love S, Thorne R. Intracranial ependymomas: analysis of prognostic factors in a population-based series. *Pediatric Neurosurg* 1996;24:119–125.

50. Forsyth PA, Shaw EG, Scheithauer BW, et al. Supratentorial pilocytic astrocytomas: a clinicopathologic, prognostic and flow cytometric study of 51 patients. *Cancer* 1993;72:1335–1342.

51. Fortuna A, Celli P, Palma L. Oligodendrogliomas of the spinal cord. *Acta Neurochir* 1980;52:305–329.

52. Ganju V, Jenkins RB, O'Fallon JR, et al. Prognostic factors in gliomas: a multivariate analysis of clinical, pathologic, flow cytometric, cytogenetic, and molecular markers. *Cancer* 1994;74:920–927.

53. Giangaspero F, Cenacchi G, Losi L, Cerasoli S, Bisceglia M, Burger PC. Extraventricular neoplasms with neurocytoma features: a clinicopathological study of 11 cases. *Am J Surg Pathol* 1997;21:206–212.

54. Goldwein JW, Glauser TA, Packer RJ, et al. Recurrent intracranial ependymomas in children: survival, patterns of failure, and prognostic factors. *Cancer* 1990;66:557–563.

55. Goto S, Nagahiro S, Ushio Y, Kitaoka M, Nishio S, Fukui M. Immunocytochemical detection of calcineurin and microtubule-associated protein 2 in central neurocytoma. *J Neurooncol* 1993;16:19–24.

56. Grant JW, Gallagher PJ. Pleomorphic xanthoastrocytoma: immunohistochemical methods for differentiation from fibrous histiocytomas with similar morphology. *Am J Surg Pathol* 1986;10:336–341.

57. Gyure KA, Prayson RA. Subependymal giant cell astrocytoma: a clinicopathologic study with HMB45 and MIB-1 immunohistochemical analysis. *Mod Pathol* 1997;10:313–317.

58. Haddad SF, Moore SA, Menezes AH, Van Gilder JC. Ganglioglioma: 13 years of experience. *Neurosurgery* 1992;31:171–178.

59. Hague K, Kotsianti A, Morgello S. Heterogeneity of oligodendrogliomas. *J Neuropathol Exp Neurol* 1997;56:585.

60. Hakim R, Loeffler JS, Anthony DC, Black PM. Gangliogliomas in adults. *Cancer* 1997;79:127–131.

61. Hart MN, Petito CK, Earle KM. Mixed gliomas. *Cancer* 1974;33:134–140.

62. Hassoun J, Gambarelli D, Grisoli F, et al. Central neurocytoma: an electron-microscopic study of two cases. *Acta Neuropathol (Berl)* 1982;56:151–156.

63. Hassoun J, Soylemezoglu F, Gambarelli D, Figarella-Branger D, von Ammon K, Kleihues P. Central neurocytoma: a synopsis of clinical and histological features. *Brain Pathol* 1993;3:297–306.

64. Hayostek CJ, Shaw EG, Scheithauer BW, et al. Astrocytomas of the cerebellum: a comparative clinicopathologic study of pilocytic and diffuse astrocytomas. *Cancer* 1993;72:856–869.

65. Healey EA, Barnes PD, Kupsky WJ, et al. The prognostic significance of postoperative residual tumor in ependymoma. *Neurosurgery* 1991;28:666–672.

66. Helseth A, Mork SJ. Neoplasms of the central nervous system in Norway. III. Epidemiological characteristics of intracranial gliomas according to histology. *APMIS* 1989;97:547–555.

67. Helwig EB, Stern JB. Subcutaneous sacrococcygeal

myxopapillary ependymoma: a clinicopathologic study of 32 cases. *Am J Clin Pathol* 1984;81:156–161.

68. Hessler, RB, Lopes MBS, Frankfurter A, Reidy J, Vandenberg SR. Cytoskeletal immunohistochemistry of central neurocytomas. *Am J Surg Pathol* 1992;16:1031–1038.

69. Hirato J, Nakazato Y, Ogawa A. Expression of nonglial intermediate filament proteins in gliomas. *Clin Neuropathol* 1994;13:1–11.

70. Hirose T, Scheithauer BW, Lopes BS, Vandenberg SR. Dysembryoplastic neuroepithelial tumor (DNT): an immunohistochemical and ultrastructural study. *J Neuropathol Exp Neurol* 1994;53:184–195.

71. Hirose T, Scheithauer B, Lopes M, et al. Ganglioglioma: an ultrastructural and immunochemical study. *Mod Pathol* 1996;9:140A, 819.

72. Hoeffel C, Boukobza M, Polivka M, et al. MR manifestations of subependymomas. *AJNR* 1995;16:2121–2129.

73. Hoffman HJ, Becker L, Craven MA. A clinically and pathologically distinct group of benign brain stem gliomas. *Neurosurgery* 1980;7:243–248.

74. Hoffman HJ, Soloniuk DS, Humphreys RP, et al. Management and outcome of low-grade astrocytomas of the midline in children: a retrospective review. *Neurosurgery* 1993;33:964–971.

75. Hsu DW, Louis DN, Efird JT, Hedley-Whyte ET. Use of MIB-1 (Ki-67) immunoreactivity in differentiating grade II and grade III gliomas. *J Neuropathol Exp Neurol* 1997;56:857–865.

76. Ikezaki K, Matsushima T, Inoue T, Yokoyama N, Kaneko Y, Fukui M. Correlation of microanatomical localization with postoperative survival in posterior fossa ependymomas. *Neurosurgery* 1993;32:38–44.

77. Ilgren EB, Stiller CA. Cerebellar astrocytomas: clinical characteristics and prognostic indices. *J Neurooncol* 1987;4:293–308.

78. Iqbal Z, Sutcliffe JC. Subependymoma of the lateral ventricle: case report and literature review. *Br J Neurosurg* 1994;8:83–85.

79. Itoh Y, Yagishita S, Chiba Y. Cerebral gangliocytoma: an ultrastructural study. *Acta Neuropathol (Berl)* 1987;74:169–178.

80. Jaffey PB, Mundt AJ, Baunoch DA, et al. The clinical significance of extracellular matrix in gangliogliomas. *J Neuropathol Exp Neurol* 1996;55:1246–1252.

81. Jaros E, Perry RH, Adam L, et al. Prognostic implications of p53 protein, epidermal growth factor receptor, and Ki-67 labelling in brain tumours. *Br J Cancer* 1992;66:373–385.

82. Jay V, Squire J, Becker LE, Humphreys R. Malignant transformation in a ganglioglioma with anaplastic neuronal and astrocytic components. *Cancer* 1994;73:2862–2868.

83. Karamitopoulou E, Perentes E, Diamantis I, Maraziotis T. Ki-67 immunoreactivity in human central nervous system tumors: a study with MIB 1 monoclonal antibody on archival material. *Acta Neuropathol* 1994;87:47–54.

84. Katsetos CD, Krishna L. Lobar pilocytic astrocytomas of the cerebral hemispheres. I: Diagnosis and nosology. *Clin Neuropathol* 1994;13:295–305.

85. Kepes JJ, Rubinstein LJ, Eng LF. Pleomorphic xanthoastrocytoma: a distinctive meningocerebral glioma of young subjects with relatively favorable prognosis: a study of 12 cases. *Cancer* 1979;44:1839–1852.

86. Kernohan JW, Mabon RF, Svien HJ, Adson AW. A simplified classification of gliomas. *Proc Staff Meet Mayo Clin* 1949;24:71–75.

87. Khatib ZA, Heideman RL, Kovnar EH, et al. Predominance of pilocytic histology in dorsally exophytic brain stem tumors. *Pediatr Neurosurg* 1994;20:2–10.

88. Kim DG, Kim JS, Chi JG, et al. Central neurocytoma: proliferative potential and biological behavior. *J Neurosurg* 1996;84:742–747.

89. Kim TS, Halliday AL, Hedley-Whyte ET, Convery K. Correlates of survival and the Daumas-Duport grading system for astrocytomas. *J Neurosurg* 1991;74:27–37.

90. Kim DG, Chi JG, Park SH, et al. Intraventricular neurocytoma: clinicopathological analysis of seven cases. *J Neurosurg* 1992;76:759–765.

91. Kirkpatrick PJ, Honavar M, Janota I, Polkey CE. Control of temporal lobe epilepsy following en bloc resection of low-grade tumors. *J Neurosurg* 1993;78:19–25.

92. Kleihues P, Burger PC, Scheithauer BW. World Health Organization. International histological classification of tumours. *Histological typing of tumours of the central nervous system,* 2nd ed. Berlin: Springer-Verlag, 1993.

93. Kokkinakis DM, Rushing EJ, Watson ML, Land KJ, Schold SC. Modeling glial tumors in rats: an insight in brain tumorigenesis. *J Neuropathol Exp Neurol* 1997;56:610.

94. Kondziolka D, Bilbao JM. Mixed ependymoma-astrocytoma (subependymoma?) of the cerebral cortex. *Acta Neuropathol* 1988;76:633–637.

95. Kordek R, Biernat W, Sapieja W, Alwasiak J, Liberski PP. Pleomorphic xanthoastrocytoma with a gangliogliomatous component: an immunohistochemical and ultrastructural study. *Acta Neuropathol* 1995;89:194–197.

96. Kraus JA, Koopmann J, Kaskel P, et al. Shared allelic losses on chromosomes 1p and 19q suggest a common origin of oligodendroglioma and oligoastrocytoma. *J Neuropathol Exp Neurol* 1995;54:91–95.

97. Kros JM, Godschalk JJCJ, Krishnadath KK, van Eden CG. Expression of p53 in oligodendrogliomas. *J Pathol* 1993;171:285–290.

98. Kros JM, Hop WCJ, Godschalk JJCJ, Krishnadath KK. Prognostic value of the proliferation-related antigen Ki-67 in oligodendrogliomas. *Cancer* 1996;78:1107–1113.

99. Kros JM, Lie S-T, Stefanko SZ. Familial occurrence of polymorphous oligodendroglioma. *Neurosurgery* 1994;34:732–736.

100. Kros JM, Schouten WCD, Janssen PJA, van der Kwast TH. Proliferation of gemistocytic cells and glial fibrillary acidic protein (GFAP)-positive oligodendroglial cells in gliomas: a MIB-1/GFAP double labeling study. *Acta Neuropathol* 1996;91:99–103.

101. Kros JM, Troost D, van Eden CG, van Der Werf AJM, Uylings HBM. Oligodendroglioma: a comparison of two grading systems. *Cancer* 1988;61:2251–2259.

102. Kros JM, Van Eden CG, Stefanko SZ, Waayer-Van Batenburg M, van der Kwast Th H. Prognostic implications of glial fibrillary acidic protein containing cell types in oligodendrogliomas. *Cancer* 1990;66:1204–1212.

103. Kros JM, van Eden CG, Vissers CJ, Mulder AH, van der

Kwast Th H. Prognostic relevance of DNA flow cytometry in oligodendroglioma. *Cancer* 1992;69:1791–1798.

104. Kros JM, Vecht CJ, Stefanko SZ. The pleomorphic xanthoastrocytoma and its differential diagnosis: a study of five cases. *Hum Pathol* 1991;22:1128–1135.

105. Krouwer HGJ, Davis RL, McDermott MW, Hoshino T, Prados MD. Gangliogliomas: a clinicopathological study of 25 cases and review of the literature. *J Neurooncol* 1993;17:139–154.

106. Krouwer HGJ, Davis RL, Silver P, Prados M. Gemistrocytic astrocytomas: a reappraisal. *J Neurosurg* 1991;74:399–406.

107. Kubota T, Hayashi M, Kawano H, et al. Central neurocytoma: immunohistochemical and ultrastructural study. *Acta Neuropathol* 1991;81:418–427.

108. Kuchelmeister K, Bergmann M, von Wild K, et al. Desmoplastic ganglioglioma: report of two non-infantile cases. *Acta Neuropathol* 1993;85:199–204.

109. Lang FF, Epstein FJ, Ransohoff J, et al. Central nervous system gangliogliomas. Part 2: Clinical outcome. *J Neurosurg* 1993;79:867–873.

110. Lang FF, Miller DC, Koslow M, Newcomb EW. Pathways leading to glioblastoma multiforme: a molecular analysis of genetic alterations in 65 astrocytic tumors. *J Neurosurg* 1994;81:427–436.

111. Lang FF, Miller DC, Pisharody S, Koslow M, Newcomb EW. High frequency of p53 protein accumulation without p53 gene mutation in human juvenile pilocytic, low grade and anaplastic astrocytomas. *Oncogene* 1994;9:949–954.

112. Langford LA, Piatyszek MA, Xu R, Schold SC, Shay JW. Telomerase activity in human brain tumours. *Lancet* 1995;346:1267–1268.

113. Lee KS, Kelly DL. Primary oligodendroglioma of the lateral ventricle. *South Med J* 1990;83:254–255.

114. Lellouch-Tubiana A, Bourgeois M, Vekemans M, Robain O. Dysembryoplastic neuroepithelial tumors in two children with neurofibromatosis type 1. *Acta Neuropathol* 1995;90:319–322.

115. Litofsky NS, Hinton D, Raffel C. The lack of a role for p53 in astrocytomas in pediatric patients. *Neurosurgery* 1994;34:967–973.

116. Liu GT, Galetta SL, Rorke LB, et al. Gangliogliomas involving the optic chiasm. *Neurology* 1996;46:1669–1673.

117. Lobato RD, Sarabia M, Castro S, et al. Symptomatic subependymoma: report of four new cases studied with computed tomography and review of the literature. *Neurosurgery* 1986;19:594–598.

118. Lombardi D, Scheithauer BW, Piepgras D, Meyer FB, Forbes GS. "Angioglioma" and the arteriovenous malformation-glioma association. *J Neurosurg* 1991;75:589–596.

119. Lopes MBS, Altermatt HJ, Scheithauer BW, Shepherd CW, Vandenberg SR. Immunohistochemical characterization of subependymal giant cell astrocytomas. *Acta Neuropathol* 1996;91:368–375.

120. Louis DN, Edgerton S, Thor AD, Hedley-Whyte ET. Proliferating cell nuclear antigen and Ki-67 immunohistochemistry in brain tumors: a comparative study. *Acta Neuropathol* 1991;81:675–679.

121. Louis DN, Swearingen B, Linggood RM, et al. Central nervous system neurocytoma and neuroblastoma in adults: report of eight cases. *J Neurooncol* 1990;9:231–238.

122. Louis DN, von Deimling A, Chung RY, et al. Comparative study of p53 gene and protein alterations in human astrocytic tumors. *J Neuropathol Exp Neurol* 1993;52:31–38.

123. Louis DN, von Deimling A, Dickersin GR, Dooling EC, Seizinger BR. Desmoplastic cerebral astrocytomas of infancy: a histopathologic, immunohistochemical, ultrastructural and molecular genetic study. *Hum Pathol* 1992;23:1402–1409.

124. Lyons MK, Kelly PJ. Posterior fossa ependymomas: report of 30 cases and review of the literature. *Neurosurgery* 1991;28:659–665.

125. Macaulay RJB, Jay V, Hoffman HJ, Becker LE. Increased mitotic activity as a negative prognostic indicator in pleomorphic xanthoastrocytoma: case report. *J Neurosurg* 1993;79:761–768.

126. Maintz D, Fiedler K, Koopmann J, et al. Molecular genetic evidence for subtypes of oligoastrocytomas. *J Neuropathol Exp Neurol* 1997;56:1098–1104.

127. Mamelak AN, Prados MD, Obana WG, Cogen PH, Edwards MSB. Treatment options and prognosis for multicentric juvenile pilocytic astrocytoma. *J Neurosurg* 1994;81:24–30.

128. McCormack BM, Miller DC, Budzilovich GN, Voorhees GJ, Ransohoff J. Treatment and survival of low-grade astrocytoma in adults—1977–1988. *Neurosurgery* 1992;31:636–642.

129. McCormick PC, Torres R, Post KD, Stein BM. Intramedullary ependymoma of the spinal cord. *J Neurosurg* 1990;72:523–532.

130. Miller DC, Koslow M, Budzilovich GN, Burstein DE. Synaptophysin: a sensitive and specific marker for ganglion cells in central nervous system neoplasms. *Hum Pathol* 1990;21:271–276.

131. Miller DC, Lang FF, Epstein FJ. Central nervous system gangliogliomas. Part 1: Pathology. *J Neurosurg* 1993;79:859–866.

132. Min K-W, Scheithauer BW. Oligodendroglioma: the ultrastructural spectrum. *Ultrastructural Pathol* 1994;18:47–60.

133. Minehan KJ, Shaw EG, Scheithauer BW, Davis DL, Onofrio BM. Spinal cord astrocytoma: pathological and treatment considerations. *J Neurosurg* 1995;83:590–595.

134. Mittler MA, Walters BC, Stopa EG. Observer reliability in histological grading of astrocytoma stereotactic biopsies. *J Neurosurg* 1996;85:1091–1094.

135. Molloy PT, Bilaniuk LT, Vaughan SN, Needle MN, et al. Brainstem tumors in patients with neurofibromatosis type 1: a distinct clinical entity. *Neurology* 1995;45:1897–1902.

136. Montine TJ, Vandersteenhoven JJ, Aguzzi A, et al. Prognostic significance of Ki-67 proliferation index in supratentorial fibrillary astrocytic neoplasms. *Neurosurgery* 1994;34:674–679.

137. Mork SJ, Loken AC. Ependymoma: a follow-up study of 101 cases. *Cancer* 1977;40:907–915.

138. Morris HH, Estes ML, Gilmore R, et al. Chronic intractable epilepsy as the only symptom of primary brain tumor. *Epilepsia* 1993;34:1038–1043.

139. Mrak RE. Malignant Neurocytic tumor. *Hum Pathol* 1994;25:747–752.

140. Nakagawa Y, Perentes E, Rubinstein LJ. Immunohistochemical characterization of oligodendrogliomas: an analysis of multiple markers. *Acta Neuropathol (Berl)* 1986;72:15–22.

141. Nazar GB, Hoffman HJ, Becker LE, Jenkin D, Humphreys RP, Hendrick EB. Infratentorial ependymomas in childhood: prognostic factors and treatment. *J Neurosurg* 1990;72:408–417.

142. Nelen MR, Padberg GW, Peeters EAJ, et al. Localization of the gene for Cowden disease to chromosome 10q22–23. *Nat Genet* 1996;13:114–116.

143. Newton HB, Henson J, Walker RW. Extraneural metastases in ependymoma. *J Neurooncol* 1992;14: 135–142.

144. Ng H-K, Ko HCW, Tse CCH. Immunohistochemical and ultrastructural studies of oligodendrogliomas revealed features of neuronal differentiation. *Int J Surg Pathol* 1994;2:47–56.

145. Nishio S, Takeshita I, Kaneko Y, Fukui M. Cerebral neurocytoma: a new subset of benign neuronal tumors of the cerebrum. *Cancer* 1992;70:529–537.

146. Ohgaki H, Eibl RH, Wiestler OD, Gazi Yasargil M, Newcomb EW, Kleihues P. p53 mutations in nonastrocytic human brain tumors. *Cancer Res* 1991;51: 6202–6205.

147. Ohgaki H, Schauble B, zur Hausen A, von Ammon K, Kleihues P. Genetic alterations associated with the evolution and progression of astrocytic brain tumours. *Virchows Arch* 1995:427:113–118.

148. Oppenheim JS, Strauss RC, Mormino J, Sachdev VP, Rothman AS. Ependymomas of the third ventricle. *Neurosurgery* 1994;34:350–353.

149. Padberg GW, Schot JDL, Vielvoye GJ, Bots GThAM, de Beer FC. Lhermitte-Duclos disease and Cowden disease: a single phakomatosis. *Ann Neurol* 1991;29: 517–523.

150. Parisi JE, Scheithauer BW, Priest JR, Okazaki H, Komori T. Desmoplastic infantile ganglioglioma (DIG): a form of gangliogliomatosis? *J Neuropathol Exp Neurol* 1992;51:365.

151. Park JP, Chaffee S, Noll WW, Rhodes CH. Constitutional *de novo* t(1;22)(p22;q11.2) and ependymoma. *Cancer Genet Cytogenet* 1996;86:150–152.

152. Patt S, Gries H, Giraldo M et al. p53 gene mutations in human astrocytic brain tumors including pilocytic astrocytomas. *Hum Pathol* 1996;27:586–589.

153. Paulus W, Lisle DK, Tonn JC, et al. Molecular genetic alterations in pleomorphic xanthoastrocytoma. *Acta Neuropathol* 1996;91:293–297.

154. Pavelic J, Hlavka V, Poljak M, Gale N, Pavelic K. p53 immunoreactivity in oligodendrogliomas. *J Neurooncol* 1994;22:1–6.

155. Platten M, Giodano MJ, Dirven CMF, Gutmann DH, Louis DN. Up-regulation of specific NF1 gene transcripts in sporadic pilocytic astrocytomas. *Am J Pathol* 1996;149:621–627.

156. Pollack IF, Gerszten PC, Martinez AJ, et al. Intracranial ependymomas of childhood: long-term outcome and prognostic factors. *Neurosurgery* 1995;37: 655–667.

157. Powell SZ, Yachnis AT, Rorke LB, Rojiani AM, Eskin TA. Divergent differentiation in pleomorphic xanthoastrocytoma: evidence for a neuronal element and possible relationship to ganglion cell tumors. *Am J Surg Pathol* 1996;20:80–85.

158. Prayson RA. Myxopapillary ependymomas: a clinicopathologic study of 14 cases including MIB-1 and p53 immunoreactivity. *Mod Pathol* 1997;10:304–310.

159. Prayson RA, Estes ML. MIB1 and p53 immunoreactivity in protoplasmic astrocytomas. *Pathol Inter* 1996; 46:862–866.

160. Prayson RA, Estes ML. Protoplasmic astrocytoma: a clinicopathologic study of 16 tumors. *Am J Clin Pathol* 1995;103:705–709.

161. Prayson RA, Khajavi K, Comair YG. Cortical architectural abnormalities and MIB1 immunoreactivity in gangliogliomas: a study of 60 patients with intracranial tumors. *J Neuropathol Exp Neurol* 1995;54: 513–520.

162. Raff MC, Miller RH. Glial cell development in the rat optic nerve. *TINS* 1984;7:469–472.

163. Ransom DT, Ritland SR, Kimmel DW, et al. Cytogenetic and loss of heterozygosity studies in ependymomas, pilocytic astrocytomas, and oligodendrogliomas. *Genes Chrom Cancer* 1992;5:348–356.

164. Raymond AA, Halpin SFS, Alsanjari N, et al. Dysembryoplastic neuroepithelial tumor: features in 16 patients. *Brain* 1994;117:461–475.

165. Reifenberger J, Reifenberger G, Liu L, James CD, Wechsler W, Collins VP. Molecular genetic analysis of oligodendroglial tumors shows preferential allelic deletions on 19q and 1p. *Am J Pathol* 1994;145: 1175–1190.

166. Reimer R, Onofrio BM. Astrocytomas of the spinal cord in children and adolescents. *J Neurosurg* 1985; 63.669–675.

167. Revesz T, Scaravilli F, Coutinho L, Cockburn H, Sacares P, Thomas DGT. Reliability of histological diagnosis including grading in gliomas biopsied by image-guided stereotactic technique. *Brain* 1993;116; 781–793.

168. Rezai AR, Woo HH, Lee M, Cohen H, Zagzag D, Epstein FJ. Disseminated ependymomas of the central nervous system. *J Neurosurg* 1996;85:618–624.

169. Reznik M, Schoenen J. Lhermitte-Duclos disease. *Acta Neuropathol (Berl)* 1983;59:88–94.

170. Robbins P, Segal A, Narula S, et al. Central neurocytoma: a clinicopathological, immunohistochemical and utrastructural study of 7 cases. *Path Res Pract* 1995;191:100–111.

171. Robertson PL, Allen JC, Abbott IR, Miller DC, Fidel J, Epstein FJ. Cervicomedullary tumors in children: a distinct subset of brainstem gliomas. *Neurology* 1994; 44:1798–1803.

172. Rogatto SR, Casartelli C, Rainho CA, Barbieri-Neto J. Chromosomes in the genesis and progression of ependymomas. *Cancer Genet Cytogenet* 1993;69: 146–152.

173. Rossitch E, Zeidman SM, Burger PC, et al. Clinical and pathological analysis of spinal cord astrocytomas in children. *Neurosurgery* 1990;27:193–196.

174. Rosso SM, van Dekken H, Krishnadath KK, Alers JC, Kros JM. Detection of chromosomal changes by interphase cytogenetics in biopsies of recurrent astrocytomas and oligodendrogliomas. *J Neuropathol Exp Neurol* 1997;56:1125–1131.

175. Rushing EJ, Yashima K, Brown DF, et al. Expression of telomerase RNA component correlates with the MIB-1 proliferation index in ependymomas. *J Neuropathol Exp Neurol* 1997;56:1142–1146.

176. Saeger W, Puchner MJA, Lüdecke DK. Combined sellar gangliocytoma and pituitary adenoma in acromegaly or Cushing's disease: a report of 3 cases. *Virchows Archiv* 1994;425:93–99.

177. Sallinen PK, Haapasalo HK, Visakorpi T, et al. Prognostication of astrocytoma patient survival by Ki-67 (MIB-1), PCNA, and S-phase fraction using archival paraffin-embedded samples. *J Pathol* 1994;174: 275–282.

178. Sallinen S-L, Sallinen P, Haapasalo H, et al. Accumulation of genetic changes is associated with poor prognosis in grade II astrocytomas. *Am J Pathol* 1997;151: 1799–1807.

179. Salmon I, Kruczynski A, Camby I, et al. DNA histogram typing in a series of 707 tumors of the central and peripheral nervous system. *Am J Surg Pathol* 1993;17:1020–1028.

180. Salmon I, Dewitte O, Pasteels J-L, et al. Prognostic scoring in adult astrocytic tumors using patient age, histopathological grade, and DNA histogram type. *J Neurosurg* 1994;80:877–883.

181. Sawyer JR, Crowson ML, Roloson GJ, Chadduck WM. Involvement of the short arm of chromosome 1 in a myxopapillary ependymoma. *Cancer Genet Cytogenet* 1991;54:55–60.

182. Scheithauer BW. Symptomatic subependymoma: report of 21 cases with review of the literature. *J Neurosurg* 1978;49:689–696.

183. Scheithauer BW, Hayostek C, Shaw EG, O'Fallon J. Astrocytomas of the cerebellum: parameters and prognosis in 132 cases. *Path Res Pract* 1991;187:763.

184. Schiffer D, Chio A, Giordana MT, et al. Histologic prognostic factors in ependymoma. *Childs Nerv Syst* 1991;7:177–182.

185. Schild SE, Scheithauer BW, Haddock MG, et al. Central neurocytomas. *Cancer* 1997;79:790–795.

186. Schroder R, Ploner C, Ernestus R-I. The growth potential of ependymomas with varying grades of malignancy measured by the Ki-67 labeling index and mitotic index. *Neurosurg Rev* 1993;16:145–150.

187. Sgouros S, Walsh AR, Barber P. Central neurocytoma of thalamic origin. *Br J Neurosurg* 1994;8:373–376.

188. Shaw EG, Scheithauer B, O'Fallon J. Astrocytomas (A), oligo-astrocytomas (OA) and oligodendrogliomas (O): a comparative survival study. *Neurology* 1992; 42(Suppl 3):342.

189. Shaw EG, Scheithauer BW, O'Fallon JR. Supratentorial gliomas: a comparative study by grade and histologic type. *J Neurooncol* 1997;31:273–278.

190. Shaw EG, Scheithauer BW, O'Fallon JR, Davis DH. Mixed oligoastrocytomas: a survival and prognostic factor analysis. *Neurosurgery* 1994;34:577–582.

191. Shaw EG, Scheithauer BW, O'Fallon JR, Tazelaar HD, Davis DH. Oligodendrogliomas: the Mayo Clinic experience. *J Neurosurg* 1992;76:428–434.

192. Shepherd CW, Scheithauer BW, Gomez MR, Altermatt HJ, Katzmann JA. Subependymal giant cell astrocytoma: a clinical, pathological, and flow cytometric study. *Neurosurgery* 1991;28:864–868.

193. Shiurba RA, Gessaga EC, Eng LF, et al. Lhermitte-Duclos disease: an immunohistochemical study of the cerebellar cortex. *Acta Neuropathol (Berl)* 1988;75: 474–480.

194. Slavc I, MacCollin MM, Dunn M, et al. Exon scanning for mutations of the NF2 gene in pediatric ependymomas, rhabdoid tumors and meningiomas. *Int J Cancer (Pred Oncol)* 1995;64:243–247.

195. Smith MT, Ludwig CL, Godfrey AD, Armbrustmacher VW. Grading of oligodendrogliomas. *Cancer* 1983;52: 2107–2114.

196. Sonneland, PRL, Scheithauer BW, Onofrio BM. Myxopapillary ependymoma: a clinicopathologic and immunocytochemical study of 77 cases. *Cancer* 1985;56: 883–893.

197. Soylemezoglu F, Scheithauer BW, Esteve J, Kleihues P. Atypical central neurocytoma. *J Neuropathol Exp Neurol* 1997;56:551–556.

198. Stiller CA, Bunch KJ. Brain and spinal tumours in children aged under two years: incidence and survival in Britain, 1971–85. *Br J Cancer* 1992;66(Suppl 18): S50–S53.

199. Stratton MK, Darling J, Llantos PL, Cooper CS, Reeves BK. Cytogenetic abnormalities in human ependymomas. *Int J Cancer* 1989;44:579–581.

200. Takahashi H, Wakabayashi K, Kawai K, et al. Neuroendocrine markers in central nervous system neuronal tumors (gangliocytoma and ganglioglioma). *Acta Neuropathol* 1989;77:237–243.

201. Taratuto AL, Monges J, Lylyk P, Leiguarda R. Superficial cerebral astrocytoma attached to dura: report of six cases in infants. *Cancer* 1984;54:2505–2512.

202. Taratuto AL, Pomata H, Sevlever G, Gallo G, Monges J. Dysembryoplastic neuroepithelial tumor: morphological, immunocytochemical, and deoxyribonucleic acid analyses in a pediatric series. *Neurosurgery* 1995; 36:474–481.

203. Tatter SB, Borges LF, Louis DN. Central neurocytomas of the cervical spinal cord: report of two cases. *J Neurosurg* 1994;81:288–293.

204. Tice H, Barnes PD, Goumnerova L, Scott M, Tarbell NJ. Pediatric and adolescent oligodendrogliomas. *AJNR* 1993;14:1293–1300.

205. Tomlinson FH, Scheithauer BW, Hayostek CJ, et al. The significance of atypia and histologic malignancy in pilocytic astrocytoma of the cerebellum: a clinicopathologic and flow cytometric study. *J Child Neurol* 1994;9:301–310.

206. Tomokane N, Iwaki T, Tateishi J, Iwaki A, Goldman J. Rosenthal fibers share epitopes with αB-crystallin, glial fibrillary acidic protein, and ubiquitin, but not with vimentin. *Am J Pathol* 1991;138:875–885.

207. Valdueza JM, Westphal M, Vortmeyer A, Muller D, Padberg B, Herrmann H-D. Central neurocytoma: clinical, immunohistologic, and biologic findings of a human neuroglial progenitor tumor. *Surg Neurol* 1996; 45:49–56.

208. Vandenberg SR. Desmoplastic infantile ganglioglioma and desmoplastic cerebral astrocytoma of infancy. *Brain Pathol* 1993;3:275–281.

209. Vaquero J, Coca S, Moreno M, et al. Expression of neuronal and glial markers in so-called oligodendroglial tumors induced by transplacental administration of ethyl-nitrosourea in the rat. *Histol Histopathol* 1992;7:647–651.

210. Vertosick FT, Selker RG, Arena VC. Survival of patients with well-differentiated astrocytomas diagnosed in the era of computed tomography. *Neurosurgery* 1991;28:496–501.

211. Vinchon M, Blond S, Lejeune JP, et al. Association of Lhermitte-Duclos and Cowden disease: report of a new case and review of the literature. *J Neurol Neurosurg Psychiatry* 1994;57:699 704.

212. Von Deimling A, Janzer R, Kleihues P, Wiestler OD. Patterns of differentiation in central neurocytoma: an immunohistochemical study of eleven biopsies. *Acta Neuropathol* 1990;79:473–479.

213. Von Deimling A, Kleihues P, Saremaslani P, et al. Histogenesis and differentiation potential of central neurocytomas. *Lab Invest* 1991;64:585–591.

214. Von Deimling A, Louis DN, Menon AG, et al. Deletions on the long arm of chromosome 17 in pilocytic astrocytoma. *Acta Neuropathol* 1993;86:81–85,

215. Von Deimling A, Louis DN, von Ammon, et al. Evidence for a tumor suppressor gene on chromosome 19q associated with human astrocytomas, oligodendrogliomas, and mixed gliomas. *Cancer Res* 1992;52: 4277–4279.

216. Von Deimling A, Louis DN, Wiestler OD. Molecular pathways in the formation of gliomas. *Glia* 1995;15: 328–338.

217. Watanabe K, Tachibana O, Yonekawa Y, Kleihues P, Ohgaki H. Role of gemistocytes in astrocytoma progression. *Lab Invest* 1997;76:277–284.

218. West CR, Bruse DA, Duffner PK. Ependymomas: factors in clinical and diagnostic staging. *Cancer* 1985; 56:1812–1816.

219. White FV, Anthony DC, Yunis EJ, Tarbell NJ, Scott RM, Schofoeld DE. Nonrandom chromosomal gains in pilocytic astrocytomas of childhood. *Hum Pathol* 1995;26;979–986.

220. Whittle IR, Gordon A, Misra BK, Shaw JF, Steers JW. Pleomorphic xanthoastrocytoma: report of four cases. *J Neurosurg* 1989;70:463–468.

221. Williams BP, Read J, Price J. The generation of neurons and oligodendroctyes from a common precursor cell. *Neuron* 1991;7:685–693.

222. Wolf HK, Campos MG, Zentner J, et al. Surgical pathology of temporal lobe epilepsy: experience with 216 cases. *J Neuropathol Exp Neurol* 1993;52:499–506.

223. Wolf HK, Muller MB, Spanle M, Zentner J, Schramm J, Wiestler OD. Ganglioglioma: a detailed histopathological and immunohistochemical analysis of 61 cases. *Acta Neuropathol* 1994;88:166–173.

224. Wolf HK, Wellmer J, Müller MB, et al. Glioneuronal malformative lesions and dysembryoplastic neuroepithelial tumors in patients with chronic pharmacoresistant epilepsies. *J Neuropathol Exp Neurol* 1995;54: 245–254.

225. Yachnis AT, Trojanowski JQ, Memmo M, Schlaepfer WW. Expression of neurofilament proteins in the hypertrophic granule cells of Lhermitte-Duclos disease: an explanation for the mass effect and the myelination of parallel fibers in the disease state. *J Neuropathol Exp Neurol* 1988;47:206–216.

226. Yasargil MG, von Ammon K, von Deimling A, Valavanis A, Wichmann W, Wiestler OD. Central neurocytoma: histopathological variants and therapeutic approaches. *J Neurosurg* 1992;76:32–37.

227. Zentner J, Wolf HK, Ostertun B, et al. Gangliogliomas: clinical, radiological, and histopathological findings in 51 patients. *J Neurol Neurosurg Psychiatry* 1994;57: 1497–1502.

228. Zhang PJ, Rosenblum MK. Synaptophysin expression in the human spinal cord: diagnostic implications of an immunohistochemical study. *Am J Surg Pathol* 1996; 20:273–276.

SECTION II

Management Alternatives

The Practical Management of Low-Grade Primary Brain Tumors, edited by Jack P. Rock, Mark L. Rosenblum, Edward G. Shaw, and J. Gregory Cairncross. Lippincott Williams & Wilkins, Philadelphia, © 1999

4

Surgery for Adult Low-Grade Primary Brain Tumors

Jack P. Rock, Marianne E. Naftzger, and Mark L. Rosenblum

Department of Neurosurgery, Henry Ford Hospital, Detroit, Michigan 48202

The literature on low-grade glioma does not allow for dogmatic recommendations for patient care (also see Chapter 9 in this volume). All treatment recommendations will naturally be subject to physician bias even though such bias may be based on extensive experience (Fig. 1). Unfortunately, well-designed studies capable of indicating best practice are lacking, largely owing to the low incidence of low-grade brain tumors at any one medical center. However, there are several practical and other, more theoretical rationales for brain tumor surgery. Surgery will provide a tissue diagnosis, may improve symptoms and delay the onset of new symptoms, and may improve long-term survival and at least buy time for adjunctive therapies to work against a more limited tumor burden. Theoretically, surgical resection can remove poorly oxygenated and radiation-resistant tumor cells, poorly vascularized regions within the tumor that are sequestered from intravenous therapies, and tumor cells that are resistant to various therapies. In addition, decreasing the number of neoplastic cells may alter cell kinetics to allow for greater chemosensitivity and reduce the statistical chances of malignant transformation within a population of cells.

Currently, radiographic imaging cannot definitively diagnose a primary brain tumor. The radiographic differential diagnosis of a lesion typically considered to be a low-grade brain tumor may include neoplasms of varying types (which may be managed differently), infection, granuloma, demyelinating disease, infarct, radiation necrosis, and hemorrhage. Certain of these lesions can be diagnosed after waiting a few weeks to see what changes occur on the magnetic resonance imaging (MRI) scan. For those patients in whom the lesion remains suggestive of a low-grade brain tumor, one may then choose to follow the patient without tissue diagnosis as long as the lesion remains stable. Presently, the literature does not provide unbiased information supporting the option to surgically intervene or the wait-and-see policy. Assuming, however, that the physician and patient agree that tissue diagnosis and possibly surgical resection are indicated, several management scenarios are available. The surgical strategies for the patient with a presumed low-grade glioma consist of two arms: biopsy alone for diagnosis or biopsy for diagnosis followed by varying degrees of resection.

BIOPSY FOR DIAGNOSIS

Various methods for tumor biopsy have been reported and vary from burr-hole-based hand-guided biopsy to computer-assisted stereotactic biopsy. Although the risks of the stereotactic biopsy procedure include hemorrhage, infection, and increased neurologic deficit, the reported incidence of such compli-

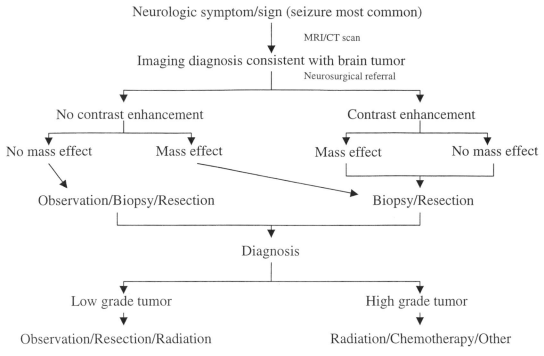

FIG. 1. Approach to the patient with low-grade brain tumor.

cations is under 5% (3). Stereotactic biopsy using computed tomography (CT) or MRI-assisted tomography is the preferred method to obtain pathologic tissue, although biopsies using frameless stereotactic methods are becoming more prevalent. The stereotactic head frame is placed on the patient, using local anesthesia, immediately prior to the neuroimaging procedure. The patient is directly transferred to the CT or MRI suite for imaging and localization of target coordinates, and subsequently returned to the operating room. Utilizing awake local anesthetic technique, with intravenous sedation as necessary, a small hole is placed with a cranial perforator or twist drill at an appropriate location on the skull and the stereotactic needle is guided to the tumor target. After histologic confirmation, the skin incision is closed and the frame is removed. The patient is transferred to the general practice unit, followed overnight in hospital, and discharged the following morning. Sutures are generally removed 7 days later, and radiation

therapy, if indicated, can begin 1–2 weeks after the surgical procedure. Alternatively, craniotomy for resection can follow any time after the stereotactic procedure.

RESECTION AFTER BIOPSY

As opposed to biopsy alone, the initial surgical procedure for a patient with a presumed low-grade glioma can be a standard craniotomy. This is based on the intention to immediately follow the biopsy with resection, because, presumably, overall patient management will benefit from surgical resection of the lesion. It is well-known that certain primary brain tumors can be surgically removed, providing the patient with an excellent prognosis and, in some cases, cure (Table 1). In general, these lesions have well-demarcated boundaries and can be cleanly dissected from normal brain, although such dissection can be performed with lowest morbidity only in specific areas of the brain.

TABLE 1. *Tumors potentially curable with surgery*

Pilocytic astrocytoma
Ependymoma and subependymoma
Oligodendroglioma type A
Neurocytoma
Ganglioglioma
Pleomorphic xanthoastrocytoma
Subependymal giant cell astrocytoma

Regions of the brain in which radical resection of tumor is possible without the likely development of neurologic deficit include the frontal lobes of both hemispheres (the posterior aspect of the frontal lobe [i.e., motor cortex, bilaterally] and speech regions in the inferior frontal gyrus such as Broca's area in the left hemisphere, will require additional attention and monitoring) and the temporal lobes (the middle temporal gyrus and the superior temporal gyrus on the left must be either functionally mapped during the operation or avoided) (Table 2). The posterior frontal and anterior parietal lobes contain the motor and sensory strips, respectively. Intraoperative mapping should be conducted when operating in these regions. The occipital lobes contain the optic radiations and the calcarine cortex; these anatomic projections can be spared despite removal of significant portions of these lobes. Based on the preceding anatomic considerations, lesions in the right frontal and temporal lobes can generally be radically removed with minimal risk, whereas lesions in the remaining regions of the brain are less amenable to radical removal, but with careful use of intraoperative cortical and subcortical mapping they frequently can be removed radically, depending on the histology.

Unfortunately, the most common lesions encountered in adults—including fibrillary astrocytoma, most oligodendrogliomas, and mixed gliomas—do not have well-defined boundaries and are characterized by the presence of neoplastic cells within areas of histologically normal and functional brain parenchyma. Although a considerable portion of these lesions can usually be removed, it remains unclear whether radical removal will positively impact the patient's prognosis. Kelly et al. (6) have proposed a classification system based on biopsy materials. In this system, type 1 tumor biopsies are composed of tumor tissue only, and complete surgical resection should be considered. The common lesions in this group include gangliogliomas, pilocytic astrocytomas, xantho-astrocytomas, protoplasmic astrocytomas, and some oligodendrogliomas. Type 2 tumor biopsies demonstrate regions of tumor tissue surrounded by normal brain parenchyma infiltrated by isolated tumor cells. Surgical resection may improve symptoms in these patients, but survival benefit is uncertain because significant amounts of tumor tissue will remain. Type 3 biopsies demonstrate normal brain parenchyma infiltrated with tumor cells and no islands of pure tumor tissue. Like patients with type 2 tumors, the survival benefit of surgical resection for patients with type 3 tumors is unclear. Although intuitively attractive, the lack of long-term patient follow-up makes definite conclusions on the utility of this classification system impossible to judge.

Generally undisputed indications for surgical intervention are to treat tumors that are potentially curable, tumors with potential for ventricular obstruction and resultant hydrocephalus (e.g., subependymal giant cell astrocytoma as part of the hereditary syndrome of tuberous sclerosis, fourth ventricular ependymoma), and large lesions causing neurologic impairment for which debulking can lead to

TABLE 2. *Operable brain regions*

	Right	Left
Frontal lobes	Anterior two-thirds operable Posterior third requires mapping	
Parietal lobes	Operable but intraoperative mapping preferred	
Occipital lobes	Operable but medial inferior region should be avoided (calcarine cortex)	
Temporal lobes	Operable	Operable with mapping for speech in middle and superior gyri*

*If patient is left-hand dominant, preoperative hemispheric dominance testing (i.e., Wada test) should be performed.

improvement in symptoms and frequently improved quality of life. More controversial indications for surgical intervention include the radical but clearly subtotal removal of diffuse tumors that are not causing neurologic deficits. These lesions account for the majority of surgical procedures. Arguments, although unproved, for operating on this latter group usually invoke the theories of multistep malignant progression and immune surveillance. Respectively, these theories imply that the overall reduction in the number of tumor cells will lead to a decrease in the potential for malignant degeneration and presumed greater efficacy of adjuvant treatments and natural immune mechanisms. However, despite significant advances in anesthetic, microsurgical, and brain-mapping techniques as well as postoperative treatment strategies, complications of surgical intervention still occur.

The major causes of surgical morbidity include inadequate exposure (e.g., imprecise surface localization and restricted brain surface exposure), improper tissue handling, imprecise knowledge of and implications of the extent and histologic character of the lesion, and the relationship of the lesion to the surrounding functional brain. Additional morbidity can be caused by improper attention to the scalp flap design and care because many of these patients will eventually require radiation therapy, chemotherapy, and reoperation. These flaps will be devitalized to a certain extent, and careful attention to preservation of maximal blood supply with meticulous attention to tissue handling at the time of scalp closure is imperative.

Preoperatively, lesion location and size, and surrounding infiltrated and/or edematous parenchyma are assessed. The local parenchymal brain pressure surrounding a tumor with extensive edema may be decreased considerably by preoperative treatment with high-dose steroids for 48–72 hours which facilitates the surgical procedure even when preoperative neurologic deficit is not significant. An edematous brain will make the intraoperative dissection more difficult because of swelling into the operative field that will compromise the surgeon's appreciation of tumor boundaries and impede tissue handling. This difficulty will be compounded if exposure is limited. It is generally a safe practice to make larger cranial openings when extensive edema is present.

Surface landmarks (e.g., pterion, coronal suture, external auditory meatus) can help guide tumor localization, but frame-based and more recently, frameless stereotactic advances have led to reliable three-dimensional imaging guidance from the cranial surface to the tumor and subsequent dissection. We use the viewing wand technology (ISG Technologies, Toronto, Canada), which is based on preoperative MRI with fiducial placement and patient registration the following day in the operating room. This technology provides for accuracy ranging from 2 to 4 mm and guides accurate placement of the skin incision, tailored craniotomy when appropriate, and placement of the lesion in the center of the bony opening.

The relationship of the tumor to the surrounding brain and the functionality of that surrounding brain are critical. Eloquent areas are considered to be the motor and sensory gyri (i.e., pre- and postcentral gyri, respectively) in both hemispheres, speech centers in Broca's and Wernicke's areas (i.e., posterior region of the inferior frontal and supramarginal and angular gyri, respectively), superior and middle temporal gyri on the dominant hemisphere, visual radiations and calcarine cortex, and the internal capsule as it courses through the deep gray matter of the basal ganglia. The location of the motor strip can be estimated and is denoted by a line passing from the bony vertex 2 inches posterior to the coronal suture and extending on a 45-degree angle to the orbitomeatal baseline with origin at the pterion (Fig. 2) (10). Using intraoperative surface mapping to correlate with preoperative MRI, Berger et al. (2) recently demonstrated the motor strip to be predictably located at the posterior end of the superior frontal sulcus, where this sulcus runs perpendicular into the precentral sulcus. The precentral

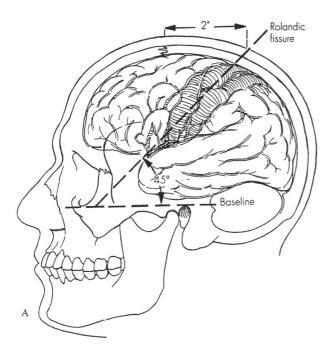

FIG. 2. Taylor-Haughton lines. (From Salcman M. Intrinsic cerebral neoplasms. In: Apuzzo MLJ, ed. *Brain surgery: complication avoidance and management.* New York: Churchill Livingstone, 1993:379–390. Reprinted with permission.)

sulcus serves as the anterior bank of the motor strip. In addition, the central sulcus, best noted on the T2 images as the posterior bank to the motor strip and the anterior bank of the sensory strip, is generally the sulcus, which extends closest to the midline in a transverse plane (Fig. 3). Broca's and Wernicke's areas are best located in relation to the Sylvian fissure at the posterior end of the inferior frontal gyrus and inferior parietal lobule, respectively. The speech center in the superior temporal gyrus is located immediately inferior to the Sylvian fissure. The middle temporal gyrus (located immediately inferior to the superior temporal gyrus) may also contain speech function. However, the surgeon must exercise great caution in basing dissection on surface landmarks when language function is of concern because these regions vary between individuals. Ojemann et al. (9) and Haglund et al. (4) have presented important data demonstrating that language function can be located in the temporal lobe even as far anterior as the temporal tip and as far inferior as the middle temporal gyrus. Based on this in-

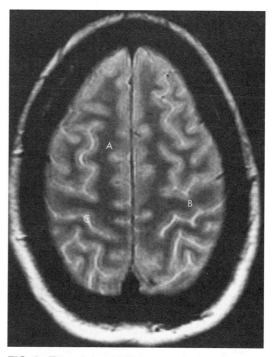

FIG. 3. T2-weighted MR image depicting the superior frontal gyrus (**A**), motor strip (**B**), and central sulcus (**C**).

formation, operations in the dominant hemisphere that involve language function usually require the patient to be awake during the procedure to reliably limit morbidity.

Although many surgeons may choose to avoid operation altogether when lesions are located in close proximity to eloquent regions, techniques have been developed to decrease the morbidity of radical resection even when lesions abut, displace, or undercut these regions. The localization of the motor strip can be estimated reliably in an anesthetized patient by cortical motor mapping. This technique involves neurophysiologic methods to stimulate the cortex, causing the patient's face, tongue, and limbs to move and thereby indicating the precise location of functional brain. Similar technology is employed in the awake patient to localize the speech areas. Speech will halt or become garbled when the eloquent cortex is stimulated.

In general, a bipolar electrode with 5-mm spacing is used to stimulate the cortex. A constant current generator produces biphasic waves at a frequency of 50 Hz. For the anesthetized patient, a minimum alveolar concentration of anesthetic agent is maintained at approximately 0.5, and stimulatory currents range from 2 to 20 mA; for the awake patient the cortex will frequently stimulate with less than 6 mA. When the visible cortex does not stimulate, strip electrodes can be placed under the edge of the bone flap to determine whether the eloquent cortex is nearby and what is its relation to the exposed surface. Focal seizures resulting from cortical stimulation can be controlled by short-acting barbiturates but, in some cases, will interfere with mapping information. In these situations, electrocoticography allows the surgeon to determine the relative refractory period of the cortex after stimulation and to map accordingly. In most situations, careful use of cortical and subcortical mapping will decrease the morbidity of the surgical procedure.

Recent developments in functional MRI (*f* MRI) of the brain have made possible the preoperative anatomic correlation between tumor tissue and functional (i.e., motor, sensory, and speech) cerebral tissue. Atlas et al. (1) used a noninvasive oxygen-dependent MRI technique to map regional brain activity, which is then superimposed on conventional MR images of the tumor. The authors noted that functional brain activity could be demonstrated within the periphery of and adjacent to the tumor tissue. Although this preoperative information does not substitute for intraoperative cortical mapping, added preoperative information is gained.

When the natural history of a tumor is not predictable and tumor cells may undergo malignant transformation, it remains the bias of most surgeons to remove as much of the tumor as possible. In such cases the use of intraoperative three-dimensional (3-D) imaging technology helps to estimate the extent of the tumor. All systems allow the surgeon to better appreciate and navigate through the complex 3-D anatomy of the operative exposure. Although several types of systems are currently available, all contain fundamental elements, including a method for registration of image and physical space, an intraoperative localization device, a computer video display of digital medical images, and a mechanism for real-time intraoperative feedback (7). These frameless stereotaxy systems were developed because of the restrictions imposed by stereotactic frame methodology in which a fixed frame is screwed into the patient's skull to allow for precise stereotactic localization during the operation. With these newer technologies, one image volume is mapped onto the points in another image volume or onto physical space itself, and these volumes are then said to have been registered to one another and become true point-to-point maps capable of precise surgical guidance. Rather than applying an external frame of reference to a patient's head (i.e., standard stereotaxy) to register medical images and access preselected target points, the frameless techniques rely on removable fiducial markers attached to the skin to serve as external point of reference sources. The original method of registration involved skull surface-based registration that fit a set of points extracted from contours identified in one image set to physical coordinates of the patient's cranium. The registration accuracy of surface-based methods is inferior to that of point-based registration methods. Point-based registration systems work by defining corresponding points in different images and physical space, determining their spatial coordinates, and calculating a geometric transformation between the volumes. These points may be intrinsic (i.e., patient-specific anatomic landmarks) or extrinsic (artificially applied markers). There are two types of extrinsic markers: mobile markers taped to the soft tissue (no invasive procedure necessary) and rigid markers (felt to be superior because of accuracy) fixed to the skull or other bone.

After the patient has the fiducials placed and is scanned, the images are transferred to the preoperative computer workstation. Specific MRI pulse sequences are utilized for visualization of certain regions of interest, such as the T2-weighted MR images, which are most sensitive for defining margins of low-grade astrocytomas and oligodendrogliomas. The surgeon may preoperatively define an approach to the lesion that may optimize the bone flap and scalp incision as well as plan tumor volume resection. Once in the operating room, points are registered using the fiducials after the patient's head has been securely placed in the head holder. As the surgical procedure commences, intraoperative display supports real-time updating of surgical position by means of a cursor and corresponding radiographic images. Brain shifts ranging from millimeters to several centimeters may occur as a result of tumor resection or cyst drainage. These shifts will affect the accuracy of the localization device and require the attention of the surgical team. In our experience, parenchymal shift intraoperatively has proven less of a concern than originally anticipated for most procedures, especially if the head is positioned so that the approach to the tumor is perpendicular to the floor and the brain is parallel to the floor, thereby limiting shifts in the anterior-posterior plane. However, it may be helpful to utilize other instru-

mentation during the course of resection such as ultrasound and endoscopy in conjunction with the frameless navigational tool. Overall benefits of the intraoperative frameless stereotaxic devices include greater consistency in achieving adequate cranial exposure; navigational guidance in difficult areas, especially the skullbase; and improved appreciation of the boundaries of primary brain tumors (which are visually indistinguishable from surrounding normal brain) allowing for maximum tumor resection.

Despite the registration of image-to-physical space, digital scan information remains historical data based on the preoperative MR image and becomes outdated during the course of surgical manipulation of tissues. Most frameless stereotactic systems are not real-time devices, and after removal of a portion of the tumor, opening of cysts, or lobectomy, the image may no longer be an accurate representation of the anatomy. Experience with intraoperative ultrasound has aided the surgeon greatly with many tumor types, and its use can improve the estimate of tumor removal. Many tumors are hyperechoic (Fig. 4) and can be imaged before and after the dura has been opened (5). Hammoud et al. (5) demonstrated that low-grade gliomas are usually echogenic relative to the surrounding brain. The authors warn that with previous surgery and/or radiation the ultrasound information is less reliable. Our own experience confirms their conclusions in that the ultrasound images aid both in localization and complete removal of the lesions.

Intraoperative MRI has been investigated recently. It appears to be an accurate method for intraoperative assessment of total tumor removal (8). A novel MRI suite was developed that combines the essential features of an MRI suite with a fully functional operating room. All equipment must be MRI compatible. This technique provides near real-time (i.e., approximately a 5–10-minute image processing delay to obtain intraoperative MR images) with high-quality MR images during the surgical procedure. Surgery takes places on the MRI table, which allows MR images to be obtained at any

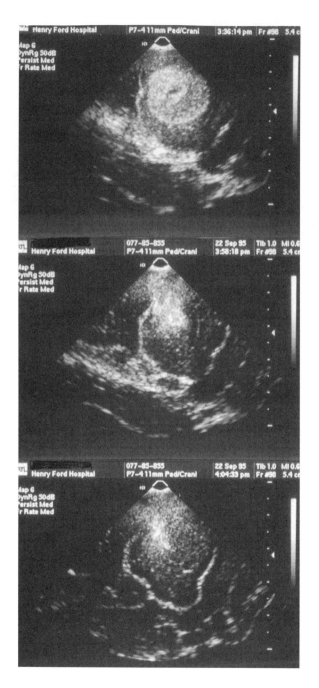

FIG. 4. Ultrasound images depicting the hyperechoic tumor (top), midway through the resection (center), and after resection (bottom). The residual hyperechoic area in the bottom picture represents blood in the tumor bed.

time during the procedure by advancing the patient's head into the MRI magnet while maintaining sterile conditions. The suite also allows for frameless stereotactic guidance with 3-D digitizer systems. The system is being piloted by several centers but is expensive and poses unique difficulties in utilization.

As technology improves and allows the surgeon to safely remove 90% or more of all primary brain tumors, prospective studies will need to determine to what extent this removal benefits the patient. The patient with a low-grade primary brain tumor differs from one with a high-grade neoplasm in two major areas. First, the major portion of a high-grade tumor can be easily differentiated from the surrounding brain tissue using the naked eye or magnification, whereas the boundary of a low-grade tumor frequently is indistinguishable from surrounding normal brain. Second, the survival of patients with high-grade tumors is variable but generally far shorter than those with low-grade tumors. Certainly optimization of surgical morbidity is always of paramount importance and is particularly critical for patients with low-grade primary brain tumors who may enjoy long, symptom-free survivals and in many instances permanent cure. Although surgical/anatomic boundaries will for now remain ill-defined and the various technologies and techniques discussed cannot alone ensure the removal of all tumor cells in most patients, progress has been made to decrease surgical morbidity and optimize the outcome for patients with low-grade primary brain tumors.

REFERENCES

1. Atlas SW, Howard RS, Maldjian J, et al. Functional magnetic resonance imaging of regional brain activity in patients with intracerebral gliomas: findings and implications for clinical management. *Neurosurgery* 1996; 38:329–337.
2. Berger MS, Cohen W, Ojemann GA. Correlation of motor cortex brain mapping data with magnetic resonance imaging. *J Neurosurg* 1990;72:383–386.
3. Bernstein M, Parent AG. Complications of CT-guided stereotactic biopsy of intraaxial brain lesions. *J Neurosurg* 1994;81:165–168.
4. Haglund MM, Berger MS, Shamseldin M, Lettich E, Ojemann GA. Cortical localization of temporal lobe language sites in patients with gliomas. *Neurosurgery* 1994;34:567–576.
5. Hammoud MA, Ligon BL, Elsouki R, Shi WM, Schomer DF, Sawaya R. Use of intraoperative ultrasound for localizing tumors and determining the extent of resection: a comparative study with magnetic resonance imaging. *J Neurosurg* 1996;84:737–757.
6. Kelly PJ. Computed tomography and histologic limits in glial neoplasms: tumor types and selection for volumetric resection. *Surg Neurol* 1993;39:458–465.
7. Maciunas RJ, Berger MS, Copeland B, Mayberg MR, Selker R, Allen GS. A technique for interactive image-guided neurosurgical intervention in primary brain tumors. *Neurosurg Clin North Am* 1996;7:245–266.
8. Moriarty TM, Kikinis R, Jolesz FA, Black PM, Alexander E. Magnetic resonance imaging therapy. *Neurosurg Clin North Am* 1996;7:323–327.
9. Ojemann GA, Ojemann JG, Lettich E, Berger MS. Cortical language localization in the left, dominant hemisphere. *J Neurosurg* 1989;71:316–326.
10. Salcman M. Intrinsic cerebral neoplasms. In: Apuzzo MLJ, ed. *Brain surgery, complication avoidance and management.* New York: Churchill Livingstone, 1993: 379–390.

The Practical Management of Low-Grade Primary Brain Tumors, edited by Jack P. Rock, Mark L. Rosenblum, Edward G. Shaw, and J. Gregory Cairncross. Lippincott Williams & Wilkins, Philadelphia, © 1999

5

Role of Radiation Therapy in the Management of Low-Grade Glioma in Adults

Edward G. Shaw

Department of Radiation Oncology, Wake Forest University School of Medicine, Winston-Salem, North Carolina 27157

One of the most controversial decisions for an adult patient with a low-grade glioma is whether to use radiation therapy. Relevant issues include the natural history of the disease with early (i.e., at the time of diagnosis) versus delayed (i.e., at the time of recurrence) radiation therapy, outcome with postoperative radiation therapy, what radiation treatment fields to use (i.e., whole versus partial brain), radiation dose, and toxicity of radiation therapy. In the following sections, each of these issues will be discussed as they relate to adults with supratentorial low-grade glioma.

NATURAL HISTORY AND OUTCOME WITH EARLY VERSUS DELAYED RADIATION THERAPY

The decision to observe an adult with a presumed supratentorial low-grade glioma, based on the clinical presentation and imaging findings or following histologic verification, is one that has been justified in the literature for several reasons, including the presumed accuracy of an imaging diagnosis, the favorable natural history of biopsy-proven disease, the lack of proven benefit for early radiation therapy, and the potential morbidities of administering radiation (6,33). Two series have addressed the accuracy of an imaging diagnosis of low-grade glioma in adult patients who present with a seizure, are neu-

rologically intact, and have a supratentorial nonoptic pathway nonenhancing lesion on a computed tomographic (CT) or magnetic resonance imaging (MRI) scan (25,72). Of 55 patients in the combined series, 36 (65%) had confirmation of a low-grade glioma, 16 (30%) had an anaplastic astrocytoma, and three (5%) had a benign process. These data imply that nearly one-third of patients with a suspected low-grade glioma based on imaging findings actually have a high-grade glioma, the standard care of which would include radiation therapy. Regarding the natural history of supratentorial low-grade glioma, Mayo Clinic studies have reported the observed versus expected survival outcome of patients, the majority of whom were adults, with histologically verified low-grade pilocytic astrocytoma, diffuse fibrillary astrocytoma, oligoastrocytoma, and oligodendroglioma (54, 55). For each of the histologic types of low-grade glioma, the observed survival (Table 1) was significantly worse than that of an age- and sex-matched control population, which had an expected survival of more than 95%. Based on these sorts of data, it has been argued, though unconvincingly to some, that all such patients should undergo biopsy or surgical resection followed by radiation therapy (52), although the survival benefit for early radiation has yet to be demonstrated in a prospective, randomized clinical trial. The European

TABLE 1. *Survival of supratentorial low-grade gliomas*

Survival	Histologic type			
	Pilo-A	Diff-A	OA	O
Median (years)	—	4.7	7.1	9.8
2 years (%)	88	80	89	93
5 years (%)	85	46	63	73
10 years (%)	79	17	33	49
15 years (%)	79	7	17	49

Key: A, astrocytoma; O, oligodendroglioma; OA, oligoastrocytoma; Pilo, pilocytic; Diff, diffuse. Modified from Ref. 45.

Organization for the Research and Treatment of Cancer (EORTC) is conducting such a study in which adults with hemispheric low-grade glioma of all histologic types are randomized to either observation (i.e., delayed radiation therapy) or initial radiation therapy using 54 Gy to localized treatment fields (20). Until the results of this trial become available, the decision regarding observation and delaying radiation therapy until the time of tumor progression versus early radiation must be based on the available retrospective literature. There are several series evaluating these strategies. In one study, Recht et al. compared the survival of 20 adult patients with histologically proven supratentorial low-grade astrocytoma who underwent surgery, with or without radiation therapy (the no-wait group), with that of 26 adults who had a presumed diagnosis of low-grade astrocytoma based on their presentation with a seizure disorder, a normal neurologic examination, and imaging evidence suggestive of a supratentorial noncontrast-enhancing low-grade glioma, who were then observed (the wait group). Ultimately, 15 of 26 patients (58%) in the wait group developed progressive disease based on a worsening of their clinical status, increasing tumor size, or the development of contrast enhancement on a CT or MRI scan. Although details of therapy at the time of progression were not given, the survival of the wait group was comparable with that of the no-wait group (median survival time, 7 years) (43). In another study, Leighton et al. compared the survival of 80

adult patients with supratentorial low-grade astrocytoma, oligoastrocytoma, or oligodendroglioma treated with postoperative radiation therapy with 87 patients who had treatment deferred until the time of progression. Ultimately, only 34% of patients in the latter group received radiation. The median survival time was 8 years in the postoperative radiation group compared with 13 years in the deferred treatment group, a difference that was statistically significant on a univariate but not a multivariate analysis. However, the two groups of patients were not comparable in that patients who received postoperative radiation had more unfavorable prognostic factors, including a shorter duration of symptoms, nonseizure symptoms at presentation, bulky residual tumor after surgery, and astrocytoma pathology (28). Realizing the inherent biases in the report, the data suggest that the timing of radiation treatment was not a significant factor. The data presented in this section, when considered together, suggest that when physician and patient plan to treat, histologic verification of a presumed low-grade glioma in an adult based on imaging data is a Practice Guideline (i.e., moderate clinical certainty exists to recommend this management strategy based on the evidence in the literature), whereas both observation (deferred radiation) and early radiation are Practice Options (i.e., the most appropriate management strategy based on the evidence is uncertain) (10).

POSTOPERATIVE RADIATION THERAPY

Numerous retrospective series contrast the survival of patients who do or do not receive radiation therapy following surgical treatment of a supratentorial low-grade glioma. Table 2 summarizes the outcome of surgery alone versus surgery plus radiation therapy in supratentorial low-grade glioma series that include primarily adult patients with astrocytomas and oligoastrocytomas (and in some cases, oligodendrogliomas) treated between 1956 and 1995 (1,19,28,36,38–40,51,58,70). Two

TABLE 2. Results of surgery ± radiation therapy for supratentorial low-grade glioma (mainly astrocytoma and oligoastrocytoma)

Authors	Years of Study	Histologies Included	S + RT × 12 Treatment	n	Survival			
					Median (Years)	5 Year (%)	10 Year (%)	Univariate p-value
Bahary et al. (1)	1974–1992	A, OA	Surgery	20	NR	66	—	NS
			S + RT	43	9.2	67	—	
Janny et al. (14)	1970–1989	A, OA	Surgery	18	4.9	50	26	0.8
			S + RT	15	3.9	45	27	
Leighton et al. (20)	1979–1995	A, OA, O	Surgery	87	13.0	84	70	0.003
			S + RT	80	8.0	62	35	
Nicolato et al. (26)	1977–1989	A	Surgery	46	—	66	—	0.12
			S + RT↓	9	—	44	—	
			S + RT↑	18	—	29	—	
Philippon et al. (28)	1978–1987	A	Surgery	61	—	65	—	0.43
			S + RT	118	—	55	—	
Piepmeier (29)	1975–1985	A, OA	Surgery	23	8.5	—	—	0.174
			S + RT	26	6.5	—	—	
Piepmeier et al. (30)	1982–1990	A	Surgery	45	NR	—	—	NS
			S + RT	10	9	—	—	
Shaw et al. (41)	1960–1982	A, OA	Surgery	19	—	32	11	0.034
			S + RT↓[b]	72	5.0	49	21	
			S + RT↑[b]	35	6.5	68	39	
Shibamoto et al. (48)	1965–1989	A	Surgery	18	—	37	11	0.048
			S + RT	101	—	60	41	
Westergard et al. (57)	1956–1991	A	Surgery	81		—	—	0.35
			S + RT	82[a]	6.7	—	—	

Key: A, astrocytoma; OA, oligoastrocytoma; O, oligodendroglioma; S, surgery; RT, radiation therapy; NR, not reached; NS, not significant.; n, number of patients.

[a] Only includes patients who received RT after 1969 when the minimum dose was 45 Gy.

[b] RT↓, low-dose RT (<53 Gy); RT↑, high-dose RT (≥53 Gy).

of them suggest a survival benefit from postoperative radiation therapy (51,58). In the Mayo Clinic series the 5- and 10-year survival rates were 32% and 11% for patients who had surgery alone (most of whom had gross total resection), 47% and 21% in those receiving low-dose radiation (<53 Gy), and 68% and 39% for those receiving high-dose radiation (≥53 Gy) (51). Shibamoto et al. reported similar results. The surgery-only patients had 5- to 10-year survival rates of 37% and 11% versus 60% and 41% with the addition of postoperative radiation therapy (58). However, seven other series have not identified a survival difference with postoperative radiation for adults with astrocytoma or oligoastrocytoma (1,19,36,38,39,40,70), and one suggested a significant decrease in survival with radiation therapy (28). In these collected series, for both irradiated and unirradiated patients, median survival times were in the range of 4.3–13.0 years, with 5- and 10-year survival rates ranging from 32% to 84% and from 11% to 70%, respectively.

Table 3 summarizes the outcome of surgery alone versus surgery plus radiation therapy in supratentorial oligodendroglioma series that include primarily adult patients with low-grade tumors treated between 1940 and 1990 (4,7,8,15,26,29,44,53,59,69). All 10 series report better survival with the addition of postoperative radiation, but in only four did the difference reach statistical significance (7,15,29,59). In two series, the apparent survival benefit was limited to patients whose tumors were subtotally resected (53,59), whereas one series found no difference in survival among patients who had gross total resection with or without radiation therapy (29). However, in the Mayo Clinic series, death due to local recurrence following gross total resection alone was 26% and 41% at 5 and 10 years, respectively (53). In summary, although the management strategies of early and delayed postoperative radiation therapy are both reasonable Practice Options (10) for patients with supratentorial low-grade oligodendroglioma, based on the evidence in the literature, the survival benefit remains controversial.

When the various retrospective series (see Tables 2 and 3) are analyzed for the effect of radiation therapy as a function of age, there does appear to be a strong suggestion that radiation therapy improves survival in older patients. The series by Philippon et al. showed no survival benefit for postoperative radiation therapy when all patients, regardless of age and extent of resection, were taken into account. However, in the subset of those more than 50 years old who underwent subtotal resection or biopsy, the 5-year survival rate was 70% with radiation versus 25% without radiation in patients with grade I tumors, and the 3-year survival rate was 50% with radiation versus 25% without in those with grade II tumors (38). Nicolato et al. also showed a difference in outcome based on an age cutoff of 50 years. Median survival time and the 5-year survival rate were 3.3 years and 36% in patients 50 years old or less, compared with 1.8 years and 0% in those more than 50, respectively, a difference that was statistically significant (36). Franzini et al. found a 100% 3-year survival rate in patients less than 40 years old who had a ^{3}H-labeling index under 5% (14). In the analysis of the Mayo Clinic study, patients ≥35 years old had significantly poorer survival if postoperative radiation therapy was not given or if the dose of radiation was less than 53 Gy. Five- and 10-year survival rates were 37% and 5% in these patients, compared with 67% and 45%, respectively, when the postoperative radiation was given in doses exceeding 53 Gy (51). Tumor size may partially explain the age effect. Bahary et al. measured an average tumor volume of 43 cm^3 in patients under 35 years old and of 72 cm^3 in those older than 35. In that series, patients with tumors of more than 50 cm^3 had a significantly poorer survival (1). Radiation may have effects other than those that affect survival. In a small series of five patients with medically intractable epilepsy due to an underlying supratentorial low-grade astrocytoma, radiation therapy in doses of 54–61.2 Gy resulted in one patient becoming seizure-free, three having more than a 90% decrease in seizure frequency, and one having a more than

TABLE 3. *Results of surgery ± radiation therapy for supratentorial oligodendroglioma (mainly low-grade)*

Authors	Years of study	Grade and histology	Treatment	n	Median (years)	5-year (%)	10-year (%)	Univariate p-value	Comments
Bullard et al. (3)	1940–1983	LG + HG	S	34	4.5	48	16	0.67	No dose-response
		O	S + RT	37	5.2	60	12	—	29.3–62 Gy
Celli et al. (5)	1953–1986	LG>HG	S	77	3.1	36	—	<0.018	No dose-response
		O<OA	S + RT	28	6.3	57	—	—	<50 vs ≥50 Gy
Chin et al. (6)	1963–1977	LG + HG	S	11	NR	82	—	—	
		O	S + RT	24	NR	100	—	—	
Gannett et al. (12)	1956–1984	LG>HG	S	14	3.9	51	36	0.032	
		O>OA	S + RT	27	7.0	83	46	—	
Kros et al. (19)	1972–1986	IG	S	10	2.0	20	0	>0.05	
		O	S + RT	23	3.8	40	0	—	
Lindegaard et al. (21)	1953–1977	LG>HG	S	62	2.2	27	12	0.039	No dose-response 40–60 Gy; no benefit with RT if GTR
		O	S + RT	108	3.2	36	8	—	
Reedy et al. (34)	1950–1980	LG + HG	S	21	—	67	—	—	
		O	S + RT	27	—	63	—	—	
Shaw et al. (41)	1960–1982	LG<HG	S	8	2.0	25	25	0.09	Dose-response @ 50 Gy; data shown are in STR/Bx pts
		O	S + RT↓	26	4.5	39	20	—	
			S + RT↑	29	7.9	62	31	—	
Shimizu et al. (49)	1957–1990	LG>HG	S	8	3.4	25	—	0.019	All pts had STR; p-value is for 5-yr survival difference
		O + OA	S + RT	23	7.0	74	—	—	
Wallner et al. (56)	1940–1983	LG + HG	S	11	5.6	57	18	0.09	RT doses were >45 Gy
		O	S + RT	14	11.2	80	56	—	

Key: LG, low-grade; HG, high-grade; O, oligodendroglioma; OA, oligoastrocytoma; n, number of patients (pts); Gy, Gray;–, data not reported; NR, not reached; RT↓, low-dose radiation therapy (RT) (<50 Gy); RT↑, high-dose RT (≥50 Gy);–, data; GTR, gross total resection; STR, subtotal resection; Bx, biopsy.

75% but less than 90% reduction in seizures (46). Radiation therapy appears not to increase the likelihood of malignant degeneration (28), and at least one series suggests it may decrease the likelihood of malignant degeneration or at least delay its onset. Reichenthal et al. observed a 9% incidence of malignant degeneration in the patients who received postoperative radiation therapy, as opposed to 18% in those who had surgery alone (45). Both Piepmeier et al. and Vertosick et al. reported an approximately 60% incidence of malignant degeneration in their series (40,68). Vertosick et al. further observed that the median time to malignant differentiation was 5.4 years for patients who received radiation therapy, contrasted with 3.7 years for those who had surgery alone (68). These data underscore the need for a well-designed prospective, randomized clinical trial in which the end points would include not only survival but also time to progression and the likelihood of malignant degeneration.

For those patients who do receive radiation therapy, a decision must be made about the appropriate treatment field as well as the dose. Several series analyzing failure patterns in irradiated patients with supratentorial low-grade glioma suggest that when tumor progression occurs, it almost always is at the site of the primary tumor within the irradiated treatment volume (37,42,50), thus implying that partial-brain treatment fields that encompass the tumor, as opposed to whole-brain radiation, are appropriate. Furthermore, with the identification of isolated tumor cells up to several centimeters beyond the margin of the tumor on a T2-weighted MRI scan (21), the appropriate radiation target volume should include the MRI extent of tumor with a 2- to 3-cm margin of surrounding brain tissue. One way to minimize the amount of radiation given to the normal brain tissue beyond the radiation target volume is through the use of three-dimensional radiation treatment planning, also referred to as conformal radiation therapy. This allows radiation beams to be directed from an infinite number of angles, permitting a more optimal beam geometry than two-dimensional treatment planning in which radiation beams are usually given from anterior, posterior, or lateral directions. Figure 1 shows an example of a low-grade glioma planned and treated with three-dimensional radiation techniques. In this example of a frontal lobe tumor, the patient's contralateral frontal lobe is spared from receiving any significant radiation dose through the use of radiation beams that are oriented in the sagittal plane on the involved side. Another conformal radiation therapy approach is called stereotactic radiotherapy. Multiple arcs of radiation are used to treat the radiation target volume with minimal margin of surrounding brain tissue, typically 0–0.5 cm (41,61).

Regarding the potential benefit of higher doses of radiation therapy compared with lower doses, the retrospective data have been mixed. Medberry et al. found tumor progression in 89% of patients receiving less than 50 Gy, compared with 53% for those who received 50 Gy or more (31). North et al. had no survivors for patients who received less than 45 Gy, compared with a 66% 5-year survival rate for those receiving 45–59 Gy and a 22% 5-year survival rate for those who had more than 59 Gy and up to 66 Gy. However, patients in the lowest-dose group died before completing radiation therapy, whereas those in the highest-dose group had only biopsy and had CT evidence of a more aggressive tumor (37). As mentioned previously, the analysis of the Mayo Clinic study also suggested an improvement in survival with doses of 53 Gy or more versus lower doses (51). There has been one published randomized clinical trial comparing a lower and a higher dose of radiation. The EORTC trial randomized 379 adult patients with supratentorial low-grade glioma of all histologic types to receive 45 or 59.4 Gy to localized treatment fields. Initial analysis has failed to demonstrate a difference in survival between the two doses. The 5-year survival rate was 58% with 45 Gy and 59% with 59.4 Gy (20). A randomized trial by the North Central Cancer Treatment Group (NCCTG), Radiation Therapy Oncology Group (RTOG), and

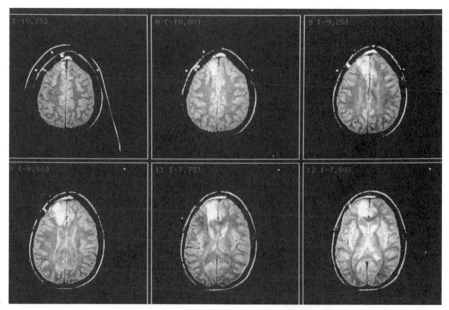

A

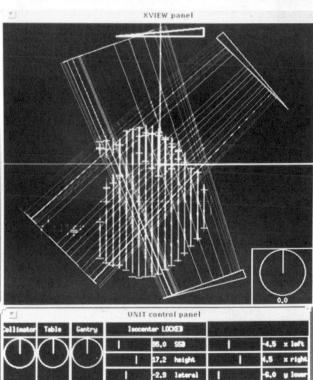

B

FIG. 1. A: Treatment planning MRI scan images of a patient with a subtotally resected low-grade astrocytoma of the right frontal lobe. **B:** Screen display from the three-dimensional treatment planning computer system used to generate a radiation treatment plan for the patient shown in Fig. 1A. Three beams are shown, including an anterior beam (AP), an anterior beam angled 45 degrees superiorly (A45S), and a posterior beam angled 30 degrees superiorly (P30S), all oriented in the sagittal plane.

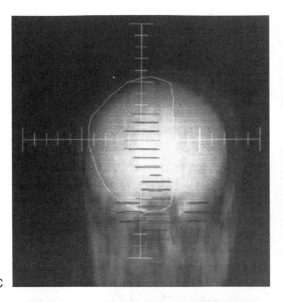

C

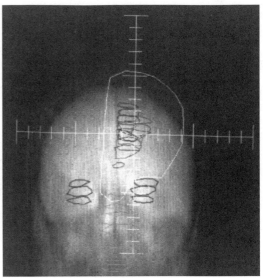

D

E

FIG. 1. *Continued.* **C–E:** Computer-generated radiographs showing the beam's eye views of the AP, A45S, and P30S beams shown in Fig. 1B. The tumor volume (and eyes) are outlined with black lines. The radiation treatment field is outlined by white lines. Note the modification of the radiation treatment fields to block the right eye on the A45S and P30S beams.

FIG. 1. *Continued.* **F–H:** Treatment setup for the AP, A45S, and P30S beams shown in Figs. 1B–E. Note the different positions of the linear accelerator and treatment couch for each of the three beams.

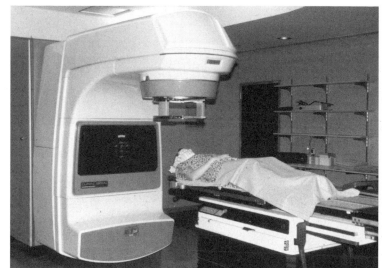

F

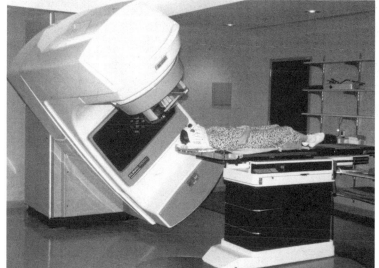

G

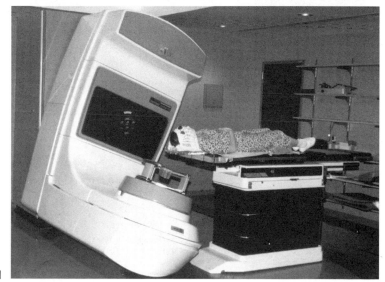

H

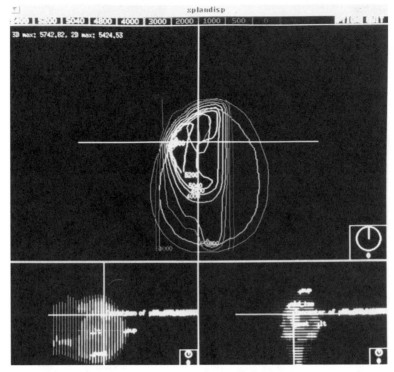

I

FIG. 1. *Continued.* **I:** Axial isodose distribution for the treatment plan shown in Figs. 1B–H. Note the rapid fall-off of dose medially, indicating that little radiation dose is being given to the patient's contralateral frontal lobe.

Eastern Cooperative Oncology Group in a similar patient population compared 50.4 Gy with 64.8 Gy, also using localized treatment fields. The trial closed in 1994 and should be reported in the near future. The schema for the next prospective randomized clinical trial in adults with supratentorial low-grade glioma, to be coordinated by the RTOG, is shown in Figure 2. The study divides patients into favorable and unfavorable risk groups, based on the known prognostic factors of age and extent of surgical resection. Favorable patients are observed, reserving radiation or other therapy until the time of tumor progression, whereas unfavorable patients are randomized to radiation therapy (a compromise dose of 54 Gy) without or with procarbazine, CCNU, and vincristine (PCV) chemotherapy.

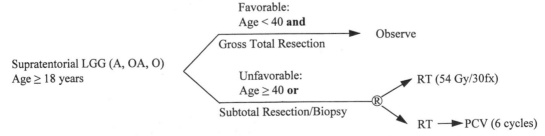

FIG. 2. Schema for the current RTOG low-grade glioma trial in adults. RTOG, radiation therapy oncology group; LGG, low-grade glioma; A, astrocytoma; OA, oligoastrocytoma; O, oligodendroglioma; RT, radiation therapy; Gy, gray; PCV, procarbazine, CCNU, and Vincristine (chemotherapy).

RADIATION THERAPY FOR FAVORABLE LOW-GRADE GLIOMA VARIANTS

There is a group of primary central nervous system (CNS) tumors that has a distinctly more favorable prognosis than the low-grade diffuse astrocytomas, oligoastrocytomas, and oligodendrogliomas. These include the pilocytic astrocytomas (World Health Organization [WHO] grade I) and the other low-grade glioma variants, including the pleomorphic astrocytomas (PXA), subependymal giant cell astrocytomas, and subependymomas.

There are also three other primary CNS tumors of neuronal or mixed neuronal/glial origin that can be grouped with the low-grade glioma variants because of their similar presentation and favorable prognosis, including the gangliogliomas, central neurocytomas, and dysembryoplastic neuroepithelial tumors (DNTs). Other than the pilocytic astrocytomas, which comprise approximately 20% of supratentorial low-grade gliomas and 80% of cerebellar gliomas (18,55), the six other variants are quite uncommon, accounting for approximately 1% or less of primary CNS tumors. From an imaging standpoint, they are typically well-circumscribed, enhancing, and sometimes cystic, calcified, or both (5,23).

Pilocytic astrocytomas typically occur in children and young adults, with common locations being the cerebellum, optic pathways, hypothalamus/third ventricle, and cerebral hemispheres. They are the most common primary brain tumor in patients with type 1 neurofibromatosis (3,23). The overall 10-year survival rate is 80% or greater, independent of location in the brain (12,16,18,23,34,67), although rarely they may behave more aggressively (67). In patients undergoing gross total resection, the 10-year disease-free and overall survival rates approach 100% (18,34,67). For those who have subtotal resection, particularly children, a reasonable strategy is observation with close follow-up (63) because there is no apparent survival benefit to routine postoperative radiation therapy (18,34), and a second surgical procedure accomplishing gross total resection appears curative (34). Radiation therapy is usually reserved for symptomatic subtotally resected or unresectable tumors, usually in the setting of tumor recurrence. When pilocytic astrocytomas require radiation, very localized treatment fields (enhancing tumor with a 1-cm margin) to moderate doses (45–54 Gy) are recommended (51).

Pleomorphic xanthoastrocytomas also occur in children and young adults, usually in the cerebral cortex (temporal lobes), sometimes with adjacent meningeal and rarely craniospinal leptomeningeal involvement. Despite their pleomorphism, they usually behave in an indolent manner (5,23). Treatment recommendations depend on the grade of the astrocytic component. When gross total resection has been achieved of a PXA that contains a low-grade diffuse astrocytoma (WHO grade II), observation is appropriate. Indications for radiation therapy (doses, treatment fields similar to the more common forms of WHO grade II low-grade gliomas) include PXAs that contain an anaplastic astrocytoma or glioblastoma (WHO grades III-IV); symptomatic, subtotally resected or unresectable tumors; or recurrent PXAs, particularly if their astrocytic component becomes more malignant-appearing (5,62,71).

Gangliogliomas consist of neoplastic ganglion (neuronal) cells as well as neoplastic glial (astrocytic) cells. They can occur in children and adults, although most present in the first two to three decades of life. Although gangliogliomas can develop anywhere in the CNS, they usually occur in the supratentorial brain, most often in a temporal location. Like the PXAs, the glial component can be low grade (WHO grade II) or higher grade (WHO grades III–IV) (5,23). Treatment principles are similar to the PXAs from both a surgical and radiotherapeutic standpoint (27).

Dysembryoplastic neuroepithelial tumors like gangliogliomas, also contain a mixture of neuronal and glial elements, although the neuronal component is mature, and the glial component is well differentiated and astrocytic or oligodendroglial in nature. As such, they are classified as WHO grade I tumors. Typically,

DNTs occur in a temporal location, are characteristically multinodular, and arise during the first two decades of life. Treatment principles are similar to the pilocytic astrocytomas from both a surgical and radiotherapeutic standpoint, although radiation is rarely necessary (5,23).

Central neurocytomas contain neuronal elements that are usually mature. They are classified as WHO grade II tumors. By definition, they arise in the ventricular system, usually as large tumors in the lateral ventricular system, and rarely have been reported to disseminate craniospinally. The typical age at presentation is the late 20s, although they can occur in children or adults (5,23). Treatment principles are similar to the pilocytic astrocytomas from both a surgical and radiotherapeutic standpoint. Subtotally resected tumors have been reported to respond to radiation therapy (22).

Subependymal giant cell astrocytomas occur in patients with tuberous sclerosis, often during their first two decades of life, but sometimes later. Characterized by large astrocyte-like cells, they are classified as WHO grade I tumors, like the pilocytic astrocytomas. Typically, they arise in an intraventricular or periventricular location (lateral ventricles, foramen of Monro) (5,23,57). Treatment recommendations parallel the pilocytic astrocytomas from a surgical and radiotherapeutic standpoint (57).

Subependymomas are also classified as WHO grade I–II tumors. They contain both low-grade astrocytic and ependymal-like cells, and usually arise in an intraventricular location (lateral or fourth ventricles, particularly in and around the foramen of Monro) in adults near the age of 50 (5,23). Treatment recommendations parallel the pilocytic astrocytomas, both surgically and radiotherapeutically (30). Subtotally resected and recurrent tumors have been reported to respond to radiation therapy (30).

OTHER RADIATION MODALITIES

Several other radiation modalities have been used selectively in patients with supra-tentorial low-grade glioma. These include stereotactic radiosurgery and brachytherapy, both interstitial and intracystic. In two series, radiosurgery employing doses of 16–50 Gy in one or two fractions for tumors with a maximum diameter of 30–40 mm resulted in radiographic responses in most patients treated without overt normal tissue damage, although follow-up was short in both reports (35,47, 48,64). Interstitial implants with temporary ^{125}I or ^{192}Ir, or permanent ^{125}I, to doses of 43–90 Gy have been used for the treatment of small, circumscribed, hemispheric, low-grade gliomas in surgically inaccessible locations. Five- and 10-year survival rates have ranged from 44% to 83% and 39% to 57%, similar to results achieved with external-beam radiation therapy (28,51,58). Chromic phosphate (^{32}P) also has been used in the management of low-grade glioma, but primarily for cystic tumors, usually of the pilocytic type, as well as for recurrent astrocytomas with cyst formation (49).

TOXICITY OF RADIATION THERAPY

A spectrum of radiation-induced toxicities can occur in patients receiving therapeutic brain irradiation. These range from neurocognitive sequelae, the pathogenesis of which is likely a white matter injury, to overt radiation necrosis, which is probably a consequence of vascular injury (9,56). Several recent studies have focused on the neurocognitive effects of radiation therapy in patients who are longer-term recurrence-free survivors, most of whom were irradiated for supratentorial low-grade astrocytomas. To assess the toxicity of radiation therapy, it is important to understand the neurologic and cognitive dysfunction that may result from having a hemispheric low-grade astrocytoma. In the series from Taphoorn et al., patients were assessed prospectively utilizing serial neurologic examinations; assessment of Karnofsky performance status (KPS); neuropsychological tests of attention, memory, language, visuospatial, and frontal lobe function; a quality-of-life questionnaire; and a profile of mood states.

Three groups of patients (about 20 patients per group) were studied. One group had histologically verified low-grade astrocytoma but did not receive postoperative radiation therapy. A second group received postoperative radiation therapy with 45–63 Gy, using multiple shaped localized treatment fields. A third (control) group consisted of patients with hematologic malignancies in the absence of brain involvement. With an average follow-up of 3.5 years, 93% of patients with low-grade astrocytoma, whether or not they received radiation therapy, had normal neurologic examinations and a KPS of 85–90, compared with 100% normal neurologic examinations and a KPS of 95 for the control group. Neuropsychological test scores were similar for the low-grade astrocytoma patients, whether or not they received radiation therapy, and were significantly worse than those of the control group, implying that the disease and not the radiation therapy was the underlying cause of cognitive dysfunction. In addition, patients with left hemispheric tumors in the group that received postoperative radiation therapy scored significantly better on several neuropsychological tests than patients with similarly located low-grade astrocytomas who did not receive radiation therapy. Other observations made in the low-grade astrocytoma patients, independent of whether postoperative radiation therapy was given, included a higher frequency of fatigue; memory, concentration, and speech difficulties; depression; tension; and impediment of the activities of daily living as compared with the control group. The authors concluded that radiotherapy had no negative impact on neurologic, functional, cognitive, and affective status (65). In a subsequent publication on the same group of patients from Taphoorn et al., endocrine dysfunction was noted in 10 of 13 (77%) long-term survivors of supratentorial low-grade glioma. Hypopituitarism occurred in the pituitary/adrenal axis in eight of the 10 affected patients, a subnormal growth hormone response was observed in four of 10, with multiple abnormal hormonal axes being present in six of the 10 patients (66). Klein-

berg et al. measured quality of life in 30 adult patients with hemispheric gliomas, 23 of whom had low- to intermediate-grade tumors. All patients were alive without evidence of recurrence 1 year or more after surgery and postoperative radiation therapy. Quality of life was measured by KPS, employment history, and memory function comparing results 1 year after treatment to the last follow-up and comparing outcome in those patients who received localized brain irradiation versus whole-brain treatment. Karnofsky performance status declined in none of 14 patients treated with localized fields versus 3 of 16 (19%) who received whole-brain radiation. Although two-thirds of patients were employed prior to their diagnosis, at 1 year or more following radiation therapy, 80% of those who received localized treatment fields were employed, compared with 38% to 46% who underwent whole-brain irradiation. Moderate to severe memory deficits occurred in 43% of patients receiving whole-brain irradiation as opposed to 6% with localized radiation therapy (24). In the NCCTG dose/response trial, a subset of 19 of 200 study patients who received either 50.4 or 64.8 Gy underwent psychometric testing prior to and up to 3 years following localized radiation therapy. No significant losses in general intellectual function, new learning function, or memory function were seen. The authors could not document significant detrimental neurocognitive effects from brain RT in the patients with low-grade glioma evaluated prospectively over time (17). In the series of North et al., 80% of short-term survivors (1–2 years) and 67% of long-term survivors (2–12 years) were intellectually and physically intact without major neurologic deficits following surgery and postoperative radiation therapy (37). The incidence of overt radiation necrosis following radiation therapy for low-grade hemispheric astrocytoma is not well-known. In those series from which reoperation data are available, the incidence of radiation necrosis is approximately 3% (19,32,37, 39,45,60). In the NCCTG dose/response trial, the 2-year actuarial incidence of radionecrosis

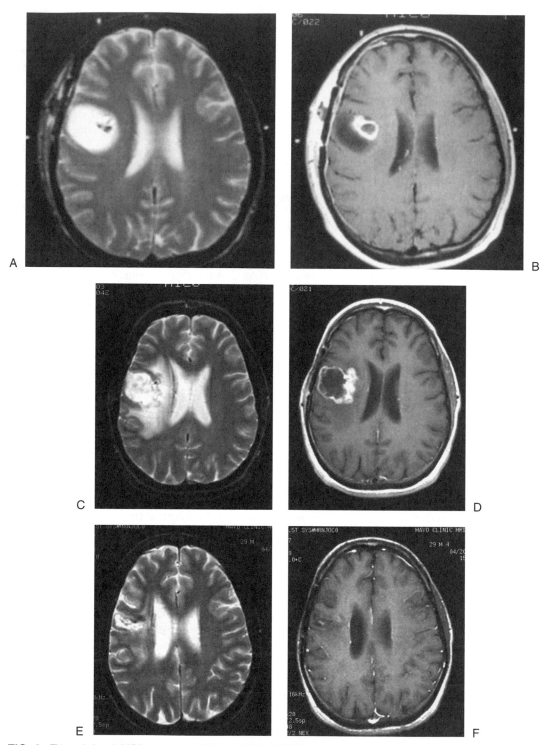

FIG. 3. T2-weighted MRI scans and T1-weighted MRI scans with contrast of a patient with a right temporal low-grade oligodendroglioma. **A,B:** Prior to radiation therapy. **C,D:** Six months following radiation localized to the tumor with a 1- to 2-cm margin. **E,F:** Sixteen and a half months later. The process represents presumed radionecrosis, which resolved without sequelae, following a brief course of oral corticosteroid medications.

was 5% with 64.8 Gy versus 1% with 50.4 Gy, given in 1.8 fractions to localized treatment fields. Fatal radionecrosis occurred in 1% of patients in each dose group (E. Shaw, unpublished data). Radionecrosis may be a transient phenomenon. Bakardjiev et al. described 28 patients aged 2–22 years who were irradiated for cerebral or optic pathway low-grade glioma. Fifteen of the patients (43%) developed worsening of their MRI scan (increased enhancement, edema, mass effect, and cyst or cavity formation) in the absence of worse neurologic symptoms or signs. The onset of these findings was 9–12 months following radiation, and resolution occurred 6–9 months after that (2). Examples of the clinical presentation, imaging changes, time course, management, and outcome in two adults with supratentorial low-grade glioma who developed radiation necrosis following postoperative treatment are shown in Figures 3 and 4.

DIAGNOSIS OF TUMOR RECURRENCE FOLLOWING RADIATION THERAPY

At some point in the illness of a typical patient with a low-grade hemispheric astrocytoma, there may be the combination of new onset or progressively worsening neurologic

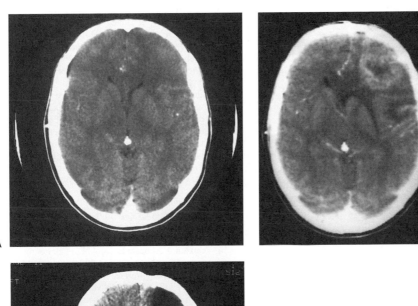

A

B

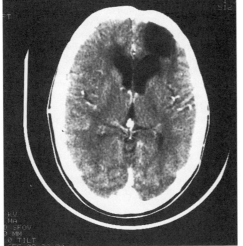

C

FIG. 4. A: Serial CT scans with contrast in a patient with a low-grade oligoastrocytoma of the left frontal lobe. **B:** One year following localized radiation therapy, the patient developed worsening neurologic symptoms, resection of which proved to be low-grade tumor and persistent radionecrosis. **C:** The patient received a one year course of BCNU chemotherapy and 5 years later remains recurrence- and toxicity-free.

symptoms and signs with imaging studies that suggest tumor recurrence. The clinical and radiographic features of tumor recurrence are indistinguishable from radiation necrosis, even by positron emission tomography (13). Rebiopsy is usually able to differentiate between these diagnostic possibilities. Seven surgical series have presented reoperation data in 100 low-grade hemispheric astrocytoma patients, in which pathology revealed low-grade tumor in 33%, high-grade tumor in 64%, and radionecrosis in 3% (19,32,37,39, 45,60). Although such patients will most likely be found to have histologically verified tumor recurrence, their prognosis is significantly affected by histology (i.e., the presence of tumor, necrosis, or both) at the time of rebiopsy. In the series of Forsyth et al., 51 previously irradiated patients (40 of whom had Kernohan grade 1–2 astrocytoma, oligoastrocytoma, or oligodendroglioma) underwent stereotactic biopsy for suspected tumor recurrence. Pathology revealed the presence of tumor alone in 30 biopsies (59%), tumor plus necrosis in 17 biopsies (33%), radionecrosis in three instances (6%), and one example of radiation-induced sarcoma. For those patients in whom tumor only was found, it was high grade in 63%. Median survival following biopsy was 10 months in patients with tumor alone versus 22 months in those with tumor plus necrosis ($p = .008$). There were no deaths among the three patients whose biopsies showed pure radionecrosis (11).

CONCLUSION

Low-grade hemispheric gliomas are a diverse group of CNS neoplasms, ones whose natural history depends primarily on the histologic type. Despite their having been considered benign historically, most of these tumors behave in an aggressive manner despite surgery and postoperative radiation therapy. Translational research—including studies of proliferation, cytogenetics, and molecular genetics—will no doubt provide much-needed insight for the next generation of biologically based therapies.

REFERENCES

1. Bahary JP, Villemure JG, Choi S, et al. Low-grade pure and mixed cerebral astrocytomas treated in the CT scan era. *J Neurooncol* 1996;27:173–177.
2. Bakardjiev AI, Barnes PD, Goumnerova LC, et al. Magnetic resonance imaging changes after stereotactic radiation therapy for childhood low-grade astrocytoma. *Cancer* 1996;78:864–873.
3. Blatt J, Jaffe R, Deutsch M, et al. Neurofibromatosis and childhood tumors. *Cancer* 1986;57:1225–1229.
4. Bullard DE, Rawlings CE, Phillips B, et al. Oligodendroglioma: an analysis of the value of radiation therapy. *Cancer* 1987;60:2179–2188.
5. Burger PC, Scheithauer BW, eds. *Atlas of tumor pathology: tumors of the central nervous system*, 3rd series, fascicle 10. Washington, DC: Armed Forces Institute of Pathology, 1994.
6. Cairncross JG, Laperriere NJ. Low-grade glioma: to treat or not to treat? *Arch Neurol* 1990;46:1238.
7. Celli P, Nofrone I, Palma L, Cantore G, Fortuna A. Cerebral oligodendroglioma: prognostic factors and life history. *Neurosurgery* 1994;35(6):1018–1035.
8. Chin HW, Hazel JJ, Kim TH, Webster JH. Oligodendrogliomas: 1. a clinical study of cerebral oligodendrogliomas. *Cancer* 1980;45:1458–1466.
9. Crossen JR, Garwood D, Glatstein E, Neuwelt EA. Neurobehavioral sequelae of cranial irradiation in adults: a review of radiation-induced encephalopathy. *J Clin Oncol* 1994;12:627–642.
10. Eddy DM. Designing a practice policy: standards, guideline, and options. *JAMA* 1990;263:3077–3084.
11. Forsyth PA, Kelly PJ, Cascino TI, et al. Radiation necrosis or glioma recurrence: is computer assisted stereotactic biopsy useful? *J Neurosurg* 1995;82:436–444.
12. Forsyth PA, Shaw EG, Scheithauer BW, et al. Supratentorial pilocytic astrocytomas: a clinicopathologic, prognostic, flow cytometric study of 51 patients. *Cancer* 1993;72:1335–1342.
13. Francavilla TL, Miletich RS, Di Chiro G, et al. Positron emission tomography in the detection of malignant degeneration of low-grade gliomas. *Neurosurgery* 1989; 24:1–5.
14. Franzini A, Leocata F, Cajola L, et al. Low-grade glial tumors in basal ganglia and thalamus: natural history and biological reappraisal. *Neurosurgery* 1994;35:817–821.
15. Gannett DE, Wisbeck WM, Silbergeld DL, Berger MS. The role of postoperative irradiation in the treatment of oligodendroglioma. *Int J Radiat Oncol Biol Phys* 1994; 30(3):567–573.
16. Garcia DM, Fulling DH. Juvenile pilocytic astrocytoma of the cerebrum in adults: a distinctive neoplasm with favorable prognosis. *J Neurosurg* 1985;63:382–386.
17. Hammack J, Shaw E, Ivnik R, et al. Neurocognitive function in patients receiving radiation therapy for supratentorial low-grade glioma: a North Central Cancer Treatment Group prospective study (Abstract). *Proc Am Soc Clin Oncol Meet* 1995;14:151.
18. Hayostek C, Shaw E, Scheithauer B et al. Astrocytomas of the cerebellum: a comparative clinicopathologic study of pilocytic and diffuse astrocytomas. *Cancer* 1993;73:856–859.
19. Janny II, Cure H, Mohr M, et al. Low-grade supratentorial astrocytomas: management and prognostic factors. *Cancer* 1994;73:1937–1945.

20. Karim A, Maat B, Hatlevoll R. A randomized trial on dose-response in radiation therapy of low-grade cerebral glioma: European Organization for Research and Treatment of Cancer (EORTC) study 22844. *Int J Radiat Oncol Biol Phys* 1996;36(3):549–556.

21. Kelly PJ, Daumas-Duport C, Scheithauer BW, et al. Stereotactic histologic correlations of computed tomography- and magnetic resonance imaging-defined abnormalities in patients with glial neoplasms. *Mayo Clin Proc* 1987;62:450–459.

22. Kim DG, Paek SH, Kim IIH, et al. Central neurocytoma: the role of radiation therapy and long-term outcome. *Cancer* 1997;79(10):1995.

23. Kleihues P and Cavanee WK. *Pathology and genetics of tumours of the nervous system.* Lyon, France: International Agency for Research on Cancer, 1998.

24. Kleinberg L, Wallner K, Malkin MG. Good performance status of long-term disease-free survivors of intracranial gliomas. *Int J Radiat Oncol Biol Phys* 1993; 26:129–133.

25. Kondziolka D, Lunsford LD, Martinez AJ. Unreliability of contemporary neurodiagnostic imaging in evaluating suspected adult supratentorial (low-grade) astrocytoma. *J Neurosurg* 1993;79:533–536.

26. Kros J, Pieterman H, van Eden CG, Avezaat CJJ. Oligodendroglioma: the Rotterdam-Dijkzigt experience. *Neurosurgery* 1994;34(6):959–966.

27. Krouwer HGJ, Davis RL, McDermott MW, et al. Gangliogliomas: a clinicopathological study of 25 cases and review of the literature. *J Neurooncol* 1993;17:139.

28. Leighton C, Fisher B, Bauman G, et al. Supratentorial low-grade glioma in adults: an analysis of prognostic factors and timing of radiation. *J Clin Oncol* 1997; 15(4):1294–1301.

29. Lindegaard KF, Mørk SJ, Eide GE, et al. Statistical analysis of clinicopathological features, radiotherapy, and survival in 170 cases of oligodendroglioma. *J Neurosurg* 1987;67:224–230.

30. Lombardi D, Scheithauer BW, Meyer FB, et al. Symptomatic subependymoma: a clinicopathologic and flow cytometric study. *J Neurosurg* 1991;75:583–588.

31. Medbery III CA, Straus KL, Steinberg SM, et al. Low-grade astrocytomas: treatment results and prognostic variables. *Int J Radiat Oncol Biol Phys* 1988;15:837–841.

32. Miralbell R, Balart J, Matias-Guiu X, et al. Radiotherapy for supratentorial low-grade gliomas: results and prognostic factors with special focus on tumor volume parameters. *Radiother Oncol* 1993;27:112–116.

33. Morantz RA. Radiation therapy in the treatment of cerebral astrocytoma. *Neurosurgery* 1987;20:975–982.

34. Morreale VM, Ebersold MJ, Quast LM, Parisi JE. Cerebellar astrocytoma: experience with 54 cases surgically treated at the Mayo Clinic, Rochester, Minnesota, from 1978 to 1990. *J Neurosurg* 1997;87.257–261.

35. Mundinger F, Ostertag CB, Birg W, et al. Stereotactic treatments of brain lesions. *Appl Neurophysiol* 1980;43: 198–204.

36. Nicolato A, Gerosa MA, Fina P, Iuzzolino P, Giorgiutti F, Bricolo A. Prognostic factors in low-grade supratentorial astrocytomas: a uni- and multivariate statistical analysis in 76 surgically treated adult patients. *Surg Neurol* 1995;44:208–23.

37. North CA, North RB, Epstein JA, et al. Low-grade cerebral astrocytomas: survival and quality of life after radiation therapy. *Cancer* 1990;66:6–14.

38. Philippon JH, Clernenceau SH, Fauchon FH, et al. Supratentorial low-grade astrocytomas in adults. *Neurosurgery* 1993;32:554–559.

39. Piepmeier JM. Observations on the current treatment of low-grade astrocytic tumors of the cerebral hemispheres. *J Neurosurg* 1987;67:177–181.

40. Piepmeier J, Christopher S, Spencer D, et al. Variations in the natural history and survival of patients with supratentorial low-grade astrocytomas. *Neurosurgery* 1996;38(5):872–879.

41. Pozza F, Colombo F, Chierego G, et al. Low-grade astrocytomas: treatment with unconventionally fractionated external beam stereotactic radiation therapy. *Radiology* 1989;171:565–569.

42. Pu A, Sandler HM, Radany EH, et al. Low-grade gliomas: preliminary analysis of failure patterns among patients treated using 3D conformal external beam irradiation. *Int J Radiat Oncol Biol Phys* 1995;31(3): 461–466.

43. Recht LD, Lew R, Smith TW. Suspected low-grade glioma: is deferring treatment safe? *Ann Neurol* 1992; 31:431–436.

44. Reedy DP, Bay JW, Hahn JF. Role of radiation therapy in the treatment of cerebral oligodendroglioma: an analysis of 57 cases and a literature review. *Neurosurgery* 1983;13(5):499–503.

45. Reichenthal E, Feldman Z, Cohen MI., et al. Hemispheric supratentorial low-grade astrocytomas. *Neurochirurgia* 1992;35:18–22.

46. Rogers LIZ, Morris HH, Lupica K. Effect of cranial irradiation on seizure frequency in adults with low-grade astrocytoma and medically intractable epilepsy. *Neurology* 1993;43:1599–1601.

47. Sceratti M, Montemaggi P, Iacoangeli M, Roselli R, Rossi GF. Interstitial brachytherapy for low-grade cerebral gliomas: analysis of results in a series of 36 cases. *Acta Neurochir (Wein)* 1994;131:97–105.

48. Schätz CR, Kreth FW, Faist M, Warnke PC, Volk B, Ostertag CB. Interstitial 125-iodine radiosurgery of low-grade gliomas in the insula of Reil. *Acta Neurochir (Wien)* 1994;130:80–99.

49. Schomberg PJ, Kelly PJ, Earle JD, Anderson JA. Phosphorus-32 therapy of cystic brain tumors (Abstract). *Int J Radiat Oncol Biol Phys* 1988;15(Suppl 1):157.

50. Shaw EG, Scheithauer BW, Gilbertson MS, et al. Postoperative radiotherapy of supratentorial low-grade gliomas. *Int J Radiat Oncol Biol Phys* 1989;16: 663–668.

51. Shaw EG, Daurnas-Duport C, Scheithauer BW, et al. Radiation therapy in the management of low-grade supratentorial astrocytomas. *J Neurosurg* 1989;70: 853–861.

52. Shaw EG. Low-grade gliomas: to treat or not to treat? A radiation oncologist's viewpoint (editorial). *Arch Neurol* 1990;47:1138–1139.

53. Shaw EG, Scheithauer BW, O'Fallon JR, Tazelaar HD, Davis DH. Oligodendrogliomas: the Mayo experience. *J Neurosurg* 1992;76:428–434.

54. Shaw E. The low-grade glioma debate: evidence defending the position of early radiation therapy. *Clin Neurosurg* 1995;42:488–494.

55. Shaw EG, Scheithauer B, O'Fallon J. Supratentorial gliomas: a comparative study by grade and histologic type. *J Neurooncol* 1997;32:273–278.

56. Sheline G, Wara WM, Smith V. Therapeutic irradiation

in brain injury. *Int J Radiat Oncol Biol Phys* 1980;6: 1215–1228.

57. Shepherd CW, Scheithauer BW, Gomez MR, et al. Subependymal giant-cell astrocytomas: a clinical pathologic and flow cytometric study. *Neurosurgery* 1991;28–864–868.

58. Shibamoto Y, Kitakabu Y, Takahashi M, et al. Supratentorial low-grade astrocytoma: correlation of computed tomography findings with effect of radiation therapy and prognostic variables. *Cancer* 1993;72:190–195.

59. Shimizu KT, Tran LM, Mark RJ, Selch MT. Management of oligodendrogliomas. *Radiology* 1993;186: 569–572.

60. Sofietti R, Chio A, Giordana MT, et al. Prognostic factors in well-differentiated cerebral astrocytomas in the adult. *Neurosurgery* 1989;24:686–692.

61. Souhami L, Olivier A, Podgorsak EB, et al. Fractionated stereotactic radiation therapy for intracranial tumors. *Cancer* 1991;68:2101–2108.

62. Strom EH, Skullerud K. Pleomorphic xanthoastrocytoma: report of 5 cases. *Clin Neuropathol* 1982;2: 188–191.

63. Sutton LN, Cnaan A, Klatt L, et al. Postoperative surveillance imaging in children with cerebellar astrocytomas. *J Neurosurg* 1996;84(5):721–725.

64. Szikla G, Schhenger M, Blond S, et al. Interstitial and combined interstitial and external irradiation of supratentorial gliomas: results of 61 cases treated 1973–1981. *Acta Neurochir* 1984;33:355–362.

65. Taphoorn MJB, Schiphorst AK, Snoek FJ, et al. Cognitive functions and quality of life in patients with low-grade gliomas: the impact of radiotherapy. *Ann Neurol* 1994;36:48–54.

66. Taphoorn MJB, Heimans JJ, van der Veen EA, Karim ABMF. Endocrine functions in long-term survivors of low-grade supratentorial glioma treated with radiation therapy. *J Neurooncol* 1995;25:97–102.

67. Tomlinson F, Scheithauer B, Hayostek C, et al. The significance of atypia and histologic malignancy in pilocytic astrocytoma of the cerebellum. *J Child Neurol* 1993;9:301–310.

68. Vertosick FT, Selker RG, Arena VC. Survival of patients with well-differentiated astrocytomas diagnosed in the era of computed tomography. *Neurosurgery* 1991; 28:496–501.

69. Wallner KE, Gonzales M, Sheline GE. Treatment of oligodendrogliomas with or without postoperative irradiation. *J Neurosurg* 1988;68:684–688.

70. Westergaard L, Gjerris F, Klinken L. Prognostic parameters in benign astrocytomas. *Acta Neurochir* 1993; 123:1–7.

71. Whittle IR, Gordon A, Misra BK, et al. Pleomorphic xanthoastrocytoma: report of four cases. *J Neurosurg* 1989;70:463–468.

72. Wilden JN, Kelly PJ. CT computerized stereotactic biopsy for low density CT lesions presenting with epilepsy. *J Neurol Neurosurg Psychiatry* 1987;50: 1302–1305.

The Practical Management of Low-Grade Primary Brain Tumors, edited by Jack P. Rock, Mark L. Rosenblum, Edward G. Shaw, and J. Gregory Cairncross. Lippincott Williams & Wilkins, Philadelphia, © 1999

6

Chemotherapy and Alternatives for Adult Low-Grade Glial Tumors

Tom Mikkelsen

Departments of Neurology and Neurosurgery, Henry Ford Hospital, Detroit, Michigan 48202

Patients with low-grade infiltrative astrocytomas and oligodendrogliomas are likely to have a relatively long survival time. When subtotally resected or when clinical progression occurs, however, limitations of conventional therapies come to light. Radiation therapy, although a mainstay of tumor management, is unfortunately associated with a significant incidence of central nervous system toxicity, especially over the long term when the treatment fields are large. As a result, controversy exists concerning appropriate management of patients with these tumors (8). Clearly, as in malignant gliomas, prognosis depends significantly on factors such as patient age, performance status, and presence of symptoms of intracranial pressure (9). In a retrospective study of 379 patients, Lote et al. (9) also noted the lack of benefit of either high-dose (greater than 55 Gy) external-beam radiation therapy or intra-arterial chemotherapy. Of course, the other feature of low-grade tumors indicative of their clinical aggressiveness is the tendency toward malignant progression, which was found at reoperation in 45% in Lote's series (9).

Issues relating to operation for low-grade gliomas have been widely published, and many retrospective studies suggest an additional benefit from postoperative radiation, whether at diagnosis or at recurrence (14,15). The efficacy of this treatment paradigm remains controversial. Few prospective clinical trials of either adjuvant or primary chemotherapy have been performed in this population, because of their relatively low incidence and prolonged survival. A pediatric trial, where prolonging time to radiation is strongly desired, showed multiagent chemotherapy capable of prolonging disease stability (17). Shibamoto et al. (19) described a series of patients radiated for supratentorial low-grade astrocytoma where 19% of the patients received chemotherapy, mostly CCNU, with no demonstrable impact on survival. Eyre et al. (4) published the only randomized trial of radiotherapy alone versus radiotherapy plus CCNU for incompletely resected low-grade gliomas in the Southwest Oncology Group. Again, no survival benefit was gained with the use of this agent. A North Central Cancer Treatment Group phase II study (2) to assess primary chemotherapy with procarbazine, vincristine, and lomustine (PCV) shows cases where both regression and progression are seen, with no relation to cellular proliferation rate. Follow-up for survival is continuing.

Another significant issue is that of the cell type of the tumor. It appears that oligodendroglioma, long known to have a more favorable prognosis, also confers chemoresponsiveness (1). In this study by Allison et al., the combination of radiation and chemotherapy increased local control of oligodendroglioma whether the tumors contained pure, mixed, or anaplastic histology. Radiation alone can offer good local control as long as 60 Gy is delivered. Chemotherapy alone, although not widely studied, appears to delay time to tumor progression and may be useful, especially for pediatric patients, but in this series, all nine patients treated with chemotherapy alone following surgery developed tumor recurrence within 40 months. Other pilot trials have also demonstrated responsiveness in the adjuvant setting. Mason et al. (10) treated nine patients (eight from the time of diagnosis) with histologically verified and subtotally resected low-grade oligodendroglioma with PCV for up to six cycles. Radiation therapy was not employed at the time of initial treatment. All patients were symptomatic, and five improved with therapy, whereas four remained stable. All patients responded with decreasing volume of T2 signal. Only one received radiation therapy at the completion of six cycles of PCV, which was not for failure but for further attempt to reduce the volume of the T2 signal. Maximum response was noted in the nine patients at a median of 9 months (range 5–22 months) after initiation of treatment. PCV therapy was associated with a mean reduction of 51% in signal intensity (range 5% to 83%). All surviving patients ($n = 7$) treated at the time of diagnosis had sustained response ranging from 22 to 45 months (median = 35 months). Two patients died from complications of disease, but neither had received more than two cycles of PCV. Although the results reported in this series are extremely encouraging, responses may be variable.

Recently, the concept of cytostatic agents being used to restrain tumor progression (rather than induce cytotoxic cytoreduction) has emerged (7). This concept questions the current therapeutic model in cancer management, derived from microbiology, in which cancer cells are considered to be different from the host, and these differences are exploited therapeutically. Continuing the analogy to infection, conventional wisdom has held that unless cells are killed and totally eliminated, they will overwhelm the host. A regulatory model has recently been proposed in which cancer can be viewed as a dynamic maladaptive process that originates within the host, is constantly in evolution, and is potentially reversible (18). This model is consistent with the molecular genetic understanding of cancer processes such as clonal evolution, as we have demonstrated in gliomas (20). One of the implications of such a model is that by reimposing biologic control on a cell population or a malignant phenotype, functional control of a tumor may be gained, and this may not require complete tumor elimination.

Invasion and angiogenesis are the newest therapeutic targets to yield agents for phase I clinical trials. Several agents identified as inhibitors of angiogenesis are now under development or in clinical trial (5). Synthetic inhibitors of the matrix metalloproteinases (21,22), thalidomide, endostatin (11), and angiostatin (13) are under active investigation. The interest in their development as clinical agents stems from their regulation of animal tumors without resistance or tachyphylaxis of angioinhibitory effects (12). Several other agents that inhibit signaling events have been shown to have anti-invasive or antiangiogenic activity. Tamoxifen, an inhibitor of protein kinase C at high concentration, is under investigation in recurrent malignant gliomas (3). Pollack and Kawecki (16) have examined the efficacy of tamoxifen as an antiproliferative agent *in vitro* for benign and malignant pediatric glial tumors. Carboxyamido-triazole (CAI), an inhibitor of non-voltage-gated calcium channels, has antitumor activity *in vitro* against human glioblastoma cell lines (6), and phase II trials in malignant gliomas are under way. Whether such dormancy therapy, where a therapeutic agent is administered on an ongoing basis to suppress malignant transformation or angiogenesis, is practical in the preventative management of low-grade gliomas will likely depend on the success of these agents in the relatively compressed natural history of malignant gliomas. Given the difficulties in long-term clinical trials for low-grade glioma, the challenges in bringing these therapies to the clinic are formidable. However, if a relatively nontoxic agent chronically administered could restrain tumor recurrence and malignant progression seen in most of these patients, the benefits accrued would be significant indeed.

REFERENCES

1. Allison RR, Schulsinger A, Vongtama V, Barry T, Shin KH. Radiation and chemotherapy improve outcome in oligodendroglioma. *Int J Radiat Oncol Biol Phys* 1997; 37:399–403.
2. Buckner J, Nelson D, Hammack J, Sebo T, Zenk D, O Fallon J. Primary chemotherapy (CT) (procarbazine, CCNU, vincristine: PCV) in low grade glioma: phase II trial (Abstract). *J Neurooncol* 1997;35:S12.
3. Couldwell WT, Hinton DR, Surnock AA, et al. Treatment of recurrent malignant gliomas with chronic high dose tamoxifen. *Clin Cancer Res* 1996;2:619–622.
4. Eyre HJ, Eltringham JR, Crowley J, Morantz RA. A randomized trial of radiotherapy versus radiotherapy plus CCNU for incompletely resected low-grade gliomas: Southwest Oncology Group study. *J Neurosurg* 1993; 78:909–914.
5. Folkman J. Clinical applications of research on angiogenesis. *N Engl J Med* 1996;333:1757–1763.
6. Jacobs W, Mikkelsen T, Smith R, Nelson K, Rosenblum ML, Kohn EC. Inhibitory effects of CAI in glioblastoma growth and invasion. *J Neurooncol* 1996;32: 93–101.
7. Kohn EC, Liotta LA. Molecular insights into cancer invasion: strategies for prevention and intervention. *Cancer Res* 1995;55:1856–1862.
8. Levin VA. Controversies in the treatment of low-grade astrocytomas and oligodendrogliomas. *Curr Opin Oncol* 1996;8:175–177.
9. Lote K, Egeland T, Hager B, et al. Survival, prognostic factors, and therapeutic efficacy in low-grade glioma: a retrospective study in 379 patients. *J Clin Oncol* 1997; 15:3129–3140.
10. Mason WP, Krol GS, DeAngelis LM. Low-grade oligodendroglioma responds to chemotherapy. *Neurology* 1996;46:203–207.
11. O'Reilly MS, Boehm T, Shing Y, et al. Endostatin: an endogenous inhibitor of angiogenesis and tumor growth. *Cell* 1997;88:277–285.
12. O'Reilly MS, Holmgren L, Chen C, Folkman J. Angiostatin induces and sustains dormancy of human primary tumors in mice. *Nature Med* 1996;2:689–692.
13. O'Reilly MS, Holmgren L, Shing Y, et al. Angiostatin: a novel angiogenesis inhibitor that mediates the suppression of metastases by Lewis lung carcinoma. *Cell* 1994;79:315–328.
14. Philippon JH, Clemenceau SH, Fauchon FH, Foncin JF. Supratentorial low-grade astrocytomas in adults. *Neurosurgery* 1993;32:554–559.
15. Piepmeier JM, Gunel M. Management of low-grade gliomas: radiation therapy at time of recurrence. *Clin Neurosurg* 1995;42:495–507.
16. Pollack IF, Kawecki S. The efficacy of tamoxifen as an antiproliferative agent *in vitro* for benign and malignant pediatric glial tumors. *Pediatr Neurosurg* 1995;22: 281–288.
17. Prados MD, Edwards MS, Rabbitt J, Lamborn K, Davis RL, Levin VA. Treatment of pediatric low-grade gliomas with a nitrosourea-based multiagent chemotherapy regimen. *J Neurooncol* 1997;32:235–241.
18. Schipper H, Goh CR, Wang TL. Shifting the cancer paradigm: Must we kill to cure? *J Clin Oncol* 1995;13: 801–807.
19. Shibamoto Y, Kitakabu Y, Takahashi M, et al. Supratentorial low grade astrocytoma: correlation of computed tomography findings with effect of radiation therapy and prognostic variables. *Cancer* 1993;72:190–195.
20. Sidransky D, Mikkelsen T, Schwechheimer K, Rosenblum ML, Cavenee W, Vogelstein B. Clonal expansion of p53 mutant cells is associated with brain tumor progression. *Nature* 1992;355:846–847.
21. Taraboletti G, Garofalo A, Belotti D, et al. Inhibition of angiogenesis and murine hemangioma growth by Batimastat, a synthetic inhibitor of matrix metalloproteinases. *J Natl Cancer Inst* 1995;87:293–298.
22. Wang X, Fu X, Brown PD, Crimmin MJ, Hoffman RM. Matrix metalloproteinase inhibitor BB-94 (Batimastat) inhibits human colon tumor growth and spread in a patient-like orthotopic model in nude mice. *Cancer Res* 1994;54:4726–4728.

The Practical Management of Low-Grade Primary Brain Tumors, edited by Jack P. Rock, Mark L. Rosenblum, Edward G. Shaw, and J. Gregory Cairncross. Lippincott Williams & Wilkins, Philadelphia, © 1999

7

Management of Cerebellar Astrocytomas in Children

Paul M. Kanev

Division of Neurosurgery, Penn State University College of Medicine; and Department of Neurosurgery, Hershey Medical Center, Hershey, Pennsylvania 17033

Second only to leukemia among pediatric neoplasms, central nervous system (CNS) tumors are the most common solid tumors in children; their incidence is 2.5–3.5 per 100,000 patients (8). Widely regarded as the most benign cerebral glioma, cerebellar astrocytomas account for nearly 40% of all posterior fossa masses in children. Astrocytomas with near identical histology are common within the optic nerves or chiasm, thalamus, and hypothalamus; and cystic or solid low-grade ependymomas may occur in or adjacent to the fourth or lateral ventricles. The clinical behavior and prognosis of these tumors, however, is more aggressive than cerebellar astrocytoma, and cure with surgery alone is unusual.

Beginning with the first patient series reported by Cushing in 1931 (6), children have enjoyed favorable and prolonged outcomes following resection of cerebellar astrocytoma. In contrast to malignant childhood tumors (including medulloblastomas, ependymomas, and malignant brain stem astrocytomas, where neuro-oncology management includes adjuvant therapy, and other less aggressive uncommon lesions, including ganglioglioma, gangliocytoma, dysembryoplastic neuroepithelial tumor, and subependymal giant cell astrocytoma, where greater controversy surrounds the potential for cure and adjuvant therapy remains undefined), the vast majority of cerebellar astrocytomas are surgically curable. This chapter reviews the clinical presentation, imaging characteristics, and surgical management of cerebellar astrocytoma.

PRESENTATION

In common with other posterior fossa tumors in children, the symptoms of cerebellar astrocytomas are linked to cerebellar dysfunction and the effects of hydrocephalus. The tumor may present at any time during the first 25 years of life, yet is most common among children 5–14 years of age. Cerebellar astrocytomas are equally common among boys and girls. In contrast with the rapid presentation of medulloblastoma, symptoms of cerebellar astrocytoma are initially vague and nonspecific, reflecting their slow growth (7). The duration of symptoms before diagnosis is typically 1–2 years, and more than 90% of cerebellar astrocytomas are discovered within 4 years from the onset of symptoms. Because of their indolent, nonspecific complaints, many children have completed evaluation by pediatricians, gastroenterologists, otolaryngologists, and ophthalmologists.

Headache, frequently frontal or suboccipital in location, is the most common presenting symptom (13). Many children will complain of neck pain and discover relief with head flexion. Linked with ventricular dilatation, which to some degree accompanies many of these lesions, there is disinterest in eating, nausea, vomiting, and lethargy. Emesis is common when awakening but may occur suddenly at other times throughout the day. Head tilt and neck stiffness reflect cerebellar tonsil herniation and pressure exerted upon the cervicomedullary junction and lower cranial nerves. Many children will complain of blurred or double vision, and report difficulty with vertical and horizontal gaze.

In younger children, hydrocephalus may lead to suture diastasis, bulging of the anterior fontanelle, and enlargement of the circumference of the head. Tapping of the skull may produce a dull percussion sound, or Macewen's sign. There may be paralysis of the abducens nerve from pressure exerted upon its long subarachnoid path toward Durello's canal and entrance into the posterior cavernous sinus.

Focal neurologic signs of cerebellar dysfunction are present in more than half of children with cerebellar astrocytoma. Similar to medulloblastoma or ependymomas, which fill the fourth ventricle, truncal ataxia and gait changes are common with midline vermis tumors, whereas clumsiness, lack of coordination, and dysmetria of the arm or leg are encountered when tumors compress the cerebellar hemisphere or deep nuclei. Symptoms occur ipsilateral to the lesion and may evolve quite slowly. Subtle decrements in

sports performance or deteriorating handwriting may be noticed by coaches or schoolteachers. Other signs of compression upon cerebellar pathways or cranial nerve nuclei may include diplopia, gaze paralysis, horizontal or vertical nystagmus, mild hemiparesis, tongue paralysis, swallowing difficulties, or other deficits of lower cranial nerve function. Seizures are extremely rare and suggest a supratentorial process rather than a cerebellar mass.

RADIOLOGICAL AND PREOPERATIVE STUDIES

Although conventional skull X-rays may be entirely normal, tumor calcifications may be demonstrated within the posterior fossa. The indirect radiologic changes of hydrocephalus may include splitting of the cranial sutures, erosion of the dorsum sellae, and thinning of the calvarium. Computed tomography (CT) and, more recently, magnetic resonance imaging (MRI) have become the studies of choice for diagnosis and localization of cerebellar astrocytomas and other posterior fossa tumors. Three characteristic tumor forms are identified with MRI. These include the largely cystic tumors with a mural enhancing nodule, and solid tumor masses, with or without central microcysts (Fig. 1). The signal voids of

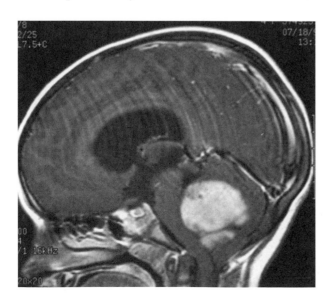

FIG. 1. Gadolinium-enhanced sagittal T1-weighted MRI sequence of a solid enhancing astrocytoma that filled the fourth ventricle. There was associated hydrocephalus and tonsillar displacement.

calcification or prominent blood vessels are common with solid tumors. Falsely cystic tumors with a thick wall surrounding a hypodense central core may also be demonstrated (Fig. 2). The cyst and mural nodule pattern is virtually pathognomonic of cerebellar astrocytoma, whereas solid tumors filling the fourth ventricle may be difficult to distinguish from medulloblastoma or astrocytoma. Sagittal T1-weighted MRI sequences may best demonstrate brain stem invasion or tonsillar herniation, whereas extension into the cerebellar peduncles is best suggested on T2-weighted sequences. The extent of hydrocephalus is readily seen on CT or MRI.

Contrast enhancement of the cyst wall on MRI or CT represents tumor infiltration in every case (1,15). Encountered in fewer than 50% of cases of cerebellar astrocytoma, the nonenhancing cyst wall adjacent to the enhancing mural nodule is nonneoplastic and represents compressed and gliotic white matter. Cystic tumors are most common lateral within the cerebellar hemispheres; no clear sided preference has been established. Solid and mixed solid and cystic tumors occur within the midline vermis and may extend toward the deep cerebellar nuclei, extend toward the middle cerebellar peduncle, or fill the fourth ventricle.

HISTOPATHOLOGY

Russel and Rubenstein introduced the most widely used histopathologic classification of cerebellar astrocytomas (14). The pilocytic tumor is composed of elongated, tapering tumor cells, a spongy glial background with glial fibrillary acidic protein-negative Rosenthal fibers, and abundant microcysts. Some tumors have a more fibrillary character with a compact arrangement of cells and modest nuclear atypia. Morphologic features of endothelial proliferation, mitotic figures, and even necrosis are not associated with an aggressive clinical behavior as when encountered within other tumors. Foci of oligodendroglioma or gangliocytoma, or leptomeningeal tumor deposits may be observed. Flow cytometry in pilocytic tumors is frequently diploid and more likely tetraploid or aneuploid in the fibrillary variant.

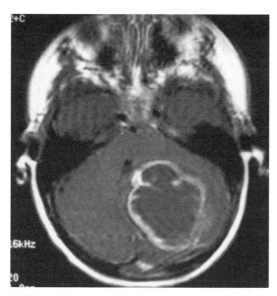

FIG. 2. Axial gadolinium-enhanced T1-weighted MRI sequence of a hypodense solid cerebellar hemisphere astrocytoma. The contrast enhancement of the thickened wall represents the falsely cystic tumor. The fourth ventricle is displaced toward the right.

SURGICAL MANAGEMENT

The initial decision confronting the pediatric neurosurgeon treating a child with a posterior fossa tumor is the management of hydrocephalus. In most cases, control of mild to moderate symptoms of increased intracranial pressure (ICP) can be achieved with dexamethasone, 1 mg/k/day, divided every 6 hours, up to a daily maximum of 24 mg. The response may be quite rapid and endures for nearly 1 week after administration. If there has been extensive vomiting and dehydration, children are better candidates for surgery after fluids and nourishment are replenished over several days. Infrequently, a child with profound elevation of ICP will present with somnolence, lethargy, or coma. An emergency ventriculostomy should be placed with a slow, judicious drainage of cerebrospinal fluid

(CSF) in the first 24 hours. The collection chamber can then be sequentially reduced from 25 cm H_2O to normal outflow pressures, typically 10 cm. In contrast to the control of spinal fluid volumes with an external collection system, there is a risk of rapid and uncontrolled drainage of CSF following placement of a ventricular peritoneal (VP) shunt. This may lead to subdural hematoma or upward herniation of the superior vermis through the tentorial incisura with respiratory compromise and potentially fatal midbrain compression. Following tumor resection, especially when located within the cerebellar hemisphere, most children will not be drainage dependent; a shunt is required postoperatively in only 30% to 40% of cases. If the ventricles are not dilated preoperatively, a ventriculostomy is not required.

After induction of general anesthesia, arterial, central venous, and bladder catheters are positioned. Perioperative intravenous antibiotics include nafcillin, 50 mg/kg, and gentamycin, 1 mg/kg. In the penicillin-allergic patient vancomycin is substituted, 10 mg/kg slowly infused over 1 hour. The use of perioperative anticonvulsants is not warranted. If hydrocephalus is present on the CT or MRI scans, an external ventriculostomy catheter is inserted through a right frontal burr hole. The catheter is brought out through a separate skin incision after passage through a long subcutaneous tunnel. If the ventricles are not dilated preoperatively, a ventriculostomy is not required.

In patients older than 2 years of age, the skull is immobilized in pin fixation, whereas in younger children the head is supported upon a padded horseshoe frame. The patient is then positioned prone upon padded chest rolls, with supplemental foam padding of all skin contact points. If the tumor extends into the cerebral aqueduct or the culmen or central lobules within the superior vermis, the head is flexed and rotated 270 degrees toward the right shoulder. This Concorde position affords the surgeon vision along the central axis of the cerebellar midline. The sitting position is an alternative that offers a superior exposure of the superior vermis and aqueduct region. Greater risks are associated with the sitting position, including air embolism and, in patients with hydrocephalus, subdural hematoma collection. The position requires the surgeon to support outstretched arms and is more fatiguing than the prone position.

For tumors located within the fourth ventricle, the vermis, or medial cerebellar hemisphere, a midline skin incision is made from just above the external occipital protuberance to the midcervical spine. There is sufficient exposure at the cephalad end of the incision to harvest autologous pericranium for later dural patch grafting. A lateral muscle-splitting incision is recommended for lateral cerebellar hemisphere tumors.

The cervical muscles are divided in the plane of the incision and elevated in a subperiosteal plane to the full lateral limits of the exposure. The foramen magnum and ring of C1 are exposed with blunt dissection and electrocautery, dividing the atlanto-occipital membrane. Burr holes are fashioned overlying the lateral cerebellar hemispheres, and a craniotomy is performed with a high-speed craniotome or rongeurs after broad clearance of the epidural space; the bone opening extends through the foramen magnum.

Beginning cephalad, the dural is opened in an I or Y fashion. Underlying the foramen magnum, a patent circular sinus must be anticipated and either coagulated with bipolar cautery or occluded with titanium vascular clips. Dural opening is made easier by drainage of spinal fluid from within the cisterna magna, or if a ventriculostomy has been positioned, with drainage of small aliquots of spinal fluid. The posterior ring of C1 is not removed unless there is extreme tonsillar impaction.

The arachnoid with the cisterna magna and overlying the cerebellar vermis is dissected, exposing the tonsils and the choroidal segments of the posterior inferior cerebellar arteries. Cystic or solid vermis astrocytomas widen the folia of the inferior vermis, displacing the cerebellar hemispheres lateral. Tumors in the hemisphere widen and obscure the cerebellar folia and frequently shift and displace the deep nuclei toward the midline (Fig. 3). If the tumor is located within the vermis or the fourth ventricle, an attempt is made to pass a small cotton patty through the foramen of Magendie for protection of the floor of the fourth ventricle. Intraoperative ultrasound readily demonstrates the solid and cystic tumor elements and the fourth ventricle, and guides the shortest path from the surface of the cerebellum toward the lesion; solid tumor is usually hyperechoic. Neurophysiologic monitoring of brain stem function is utilized when the tumor extends within the fourth ventricle.

Every attempt should be made to resect completely all contrast-enhancing tumor tissue. Enhancing cyst walls contain tumor cells and must be mobilized from the adjacent compressed cerebellum. If the cyst wall is nonenhancing, only resection of the enhanc-

ing nodule is required. To minimize retraction, a wide cortical incision overlying the meridian of the tumor can be made. Resection of the inferior vermis should be limited to minimize the incidence of postoperative cerebellar mutism, recently linked to vermis and/or tonsillar injury. The redundant vascular territories supplying the cerebellar hemisphere allow any prominent veins or arteries overlying the planned cortical incision to be coagulated safely.

Solid tumors are frequently encountered several millimeters under the surface of the cerebellum; the tumor has a granular, fleshy appearance, mimicking the cut surface of a pear. Cerebellar astrocytomas are removed with laser vaporization, suction, or ultrasonic aspiration. There may be vigorous bleeding within the tumor from enlarged veins and numerous vessels along the capsule. As the solid tumor is internally decompressed, the capsule is mobilized from the adjacent compressed cerebellum. With the illumination and magnification of the operating microscope, the interface of solid tumor and adjacent tissue is readily apparent. Intraoperative frameless stereotaxic localization is a valuable guide as the edge of the tumor is approached. Multiple frozen-section biopsies sampled along the perimeter of solid lesions may be helpful in identifying the tumor margin. Resection of tumor infiltration into the brain stem risks injury to cranial nerve nuclei, and complete tumor removal is rarely possible in these cases. Radical resection of tumor extension into the middle cerebellar peduncle is possible; the postoperative ipsilateral motor dysmetria and ataxia improve considerably over time.

At the conclusion of tumor resection, hemostasis is confirmed with valsalva maneuver after the use of peroxide and a monolayer of oxidized cellulose lining the resection cavity. Water-tight dural closure incorporates an autologous fascia graft. The cervical muscles and fascia are closed in layers, and staples are placed in the skin. If a ventriculostomy has been placed, its collection chamber is positioned at 10 cm for 3 days postoperatively. Chamber height is then sequentially elevated

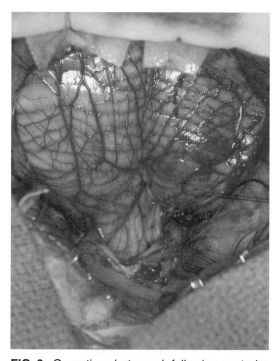

FIG. 3. Operative photograph following posterior fossa craniotomy and wide dural opening. The folia of the left cerebellar hemisphere are widened and discolored from the underlying solid astrocytoma (see Fig. 2).

while monitoring ICP. The catheter is usually removed on the fifth day postoperatively when daily output is less than 50 ml. Postoperative nafcillin, 40 mg/kg every 6 hours, is continued until the catheter is withdrawn. If the ventricles enlarge on serial postoperative CT scans, lumbar puncture further removes any residual bloody spinal fluid and promotes the circulation of CSF from the fourth ventricle. A VP shunt is placed if there is progressive pseudomeningocele formation, if there are symptoms of increased ICP, or if the ventricles continue to enlarge. Shunt placement can be avoided in nearly 60% to 70% of cases. We do not advocate catheter insertion within the cerebral aqueduct or pseudomeningocele management with cyst-peritoneal or lumbar-peritoneal shunt placement; low-pressure suboccipital headaches or acquired Chiari malformation may evolve with these shunts.

Postoperative neurologic deficits are unusual after resection of solid, cystic, or mixed tumors of the cerebellar hemispheres. Cranial nerve injury, gaze or abducens paralysis, pseudobulbar palsies, or disabling ataxia from midline nuclei injury can occur following resection of midline tumors. With contemporary pediatric anesthesia and critical-care monitoring, perioperative mortality is less than 1%.

An enhanced MRI is obtained postoperatively within the first 36 hours. At this time, any contrast enhancement represents residual tumor. The surgeon then decides whether to reoperate upon accessible tumor or to follow residual tumor if resection carries excessive neurologic risks.

LONG-TERM OUTCOME

Cerebellar astrocytoma of childhood is regarded as the most benign of all gliomas. In distinct contrast to the prognosis of other tumors of the posterior fossa in children, the 10-year prognosis exceeds 90% survival following complete resection of cerebellar astrocytoma (3,10,12). The outcome following resection of cystic tumors is more favorable than that with solid tumors, linked to the greater challenge in achieving complete resection of solid tumors. Only brain stem invasion carries a poor prognosis (3). Similar to astrocytomas within the spinal cord, pilocytic histology may afford a better prognosis than diffuse fibrillary tumors (5). In one recent study, the 10-year survival rate following resection of pilocytic tumors was 81%, compared with 7% for patients with fibrillary masses (11). Other morphologic features that appear linked to favorable prognosis include the presence of Rosenthal fibers, microcysts, subpial tumor extension, and foci of oligodendroglioma. Survival appears to be adversely influenced by the presence of necrosis, atypical nuclear features, mitoses, or increased cellular density. Unlike glioblastoma, even widespread endothelial proliferation is not associated with a poor prognosis.

Following complete tumor resection, serial MRI scans are obtained every 6 months for 3 years and then yearly until 5 years following surgery. Scans every 4 months are recommended in patients with residual disease. Like optic glioma, residual tumor may regress, involute, or remain dormant for many years (2). The recurrence rate of cerebellar astrocytoma may approach 35% (4). Reoperation is the management of choice when progression of residual disease or recurrence is demonstrated. Radiation therapy is restricted to delaying progression of brain stem extension and to adjuvant therapy of tumor recurrence inaccessible to reoperation (1,3,9). Following analysis of late recurrence, Austin and Alvord have suggested that the possibility of malignant transformation of recurrent astrocytoma is so rare that radiation therapy should not be substituted for repeat surgical excision (3).

CONCLUSION

Cerebellar astrocytomas are slow-growing tumors, and the signs and symptoms may evolve over many years. A high index of suspicion must be maintained by pediatricians or family practice physicians despite a normal neurologic examination, and a CT or MRI may be warranted before gastroenterologic or otolaryngologic evaluation. Craniotomy is performed at the time of diagnosis, and the surgical cure rate may exceed 90% following complete tumor resection. For the pediatric neurosurgeon there is little that could be more satisfying.

REFERENCES

1. Albright L. Posterior fossa tumors. *Neurosurg Clin North Am* 1992;3:881–891.
2. Alvord E, Lofton S. Gliomas of the optic nerve or chiasm: outcome by patients age, tumor site and treatment. *J Neurosurg* 1988;68:85–98.
3. Austin E, Alvord E. Recurrences of cerebellar astrocytoma: a violation of Collin's law. *J Neurosurg* 1988;68: 41–47.
4. Bruno L, Schut L, Bruce D. Cerebellar astrocytoma. In: Section of Pediatric Neurosurgery of the American Association of Neurological Surgeons, eds. *Pediatric neurosurgery: surgery of the developing nervous system.* New York: Grune and Stratton, 1982:367.
5. Crawford J, Rubenstein L, Russel D. Follow-up of cerebellar astrocytomas in relation to their pathology (Abstract). *J Neurol Neurosurg Psychiatry* 1958;21:64.
6. Cushing H. Experiences with the cerebellar astrocytomas. *Surg Gynecol Obstet* 1931;52:129–204.
7. Davis C, Joglekar V. Cerebellar astrocytomas in children and young adults. *J Neurol Neurosurg Psychiatry* 1981;44:820–828.
8. Dohrman G, Farwell J, Flannery J. Astrocytomas in childhood: a population based study. *Surg Neurol* 1985; 23:64–68.
9. Garcia D, Latifi H, Simpson J, et al. Astrocytomas of the cerebellum in children. *J Neurosurg* 1989;71:664–669.
10. Gjerris F, Klinken L. Long term prognosis in children with benign cerebellar astrocytoma. *J Neurosurg* 1978; 49:179–184.
11. Hayostek C, Shaw E, Scheithauer B, et al. Astrocytomas of the cerebellum: a comparative clinicopathologic study of pilocytic and diffuse astrocytomas. *Cancer* 1993;72:859–870.
12. Hendrick E, Hofman H, Humphreys R. Treatment of infratentorial gliomas in childhood: recent results. *Cancer Res* 1975;51:102–106.
13. Ilgren E, Stiller C. Cerebellar astrocytomas: clinical characteristics and prognostic indices. *J Neurooncol* 1987;4:293–298.
14. Russel D, Rubenstein L. *Pathology of tumors of the nervous system,* 4th ed. London: Edward Arnold, 1977:183.
15. Zimmerman R, Bilaniuk L, Bruno L, et al. Computed tomography of cerebellar astrocytoma. *J Roentgenol* 1978;130:929–940.

The Practical Management of Low-Grade Primary Brain Tumors, edited by Jack P. Rock, Mark L. Rosenblum, Edward G. Shaw, and J. Gregory Cairncross.
Lippincott Williams & Wilkins, Philadelphia, © 1999

8

Uncommon Low-Grade Primary Brain Tumors

S. Ather Enam and Jack P. Rock

Department of Neurosurgery, Henry Ford Hospital, Detroit, Michigan 48202

This chapter deals with the management issues of rare low-grade primary brain tumors. Because all the tumor varieties presented here are extremely uncommon, studies comparing the benefit of various management strategies (including surgical resection, radiation therapy, and chemotherapy) with regard to survival and recurrence are lacking. Recommendations are therefore based on personal experience and reports in the literature.

Many of these low-grade lesions are similar in respect to clinical presentation, with seizure being the most common. Radiographic imaging is sensitive but not specific for this group of tumors. In general, a pathologic diagnosis and surgical removal when feasible are recommended, but observation with or without biopsy may also be a reasonable initial strategy. Radiation can be considered especially for subtotally resected lesions, but it must be remembered that growth tends to be slow. Chemotherapy may play a role in a few of these lesions, especially in childhood.

ASTROBLASTOMA

The incidence of astroblastoma (AB) is 0.45% to 2.8% of all the primary brain tumors (25,74). Histologically, these tumors are characterized by neoplastic glial cells forming pseudorosettes with or without anaplastic features (18,142). Initially described by Bailey and Bucy (10), Bonnin and Rubinstein divided AB into two subtypes, low grade and

high grade, and suggested a correlation between histologic features and prognosis.

Astroblastoma usually presents as a cortical or subcortical mass in cerebral hemispheres, especially the parietal and frontal lobes. The pineal region, suprasellar region, corpus callosum, brain stem, and cerebellum are uncommon sites for AB (10,18,142). AB is more common in children and young adults, with a peak in the second and third decades, but it can present in middle age and beyond (18,25).

Computed tomography (CT) images of AB may vary from a cystic to solid mass, may have hypodense nodules or evidence of hemorrhage, and may show irregular enhancement (70,74). Magnetic resonance (MR) images are similarly variable. Interestingly, in two reports AB was perceived as an extra-axial mass on MR images before surgery confirmed its intra-axial location (11,199).

Clinically, AB presents with signs and symptoms of increased intracranial pressure (ICP), focal neurologic deficits, personality changes, and/or seizures (10,18). In most cases, duration of symptoms is less than a year. AB has not been found to be associated with any other disease process, except for a single case that occurred with AIDS (123).

Management

AB is almost always well-circumscribed; therefore, despite the histologic features, surgical removal may be the best form of treatment. The tumor seems to be quite radiosensitive. One of the reported cases received radiotherapy after biopsy of a suprasellar AB (18). The patient remained tumor-free during a follow-up of 12 years.

Based on the literature, either observation or radiation therapy may be considered, with radiation therapy being reserved for treatment after subtotal resection of low-grade tumors or for treatment of tumors with anaplastic histologic features. In Bonnin and Rubinstein's series (18), five patients received chemotherapy, but whether chemotherapy improved or altered the prognosis in AB of either histologic grade was not evident. At least one case of tumor regression proven by CT after chemotherapy has been reported (142). Because recurrence can occur after total resection, all patients with astroblastoma should be followed routinely with imaging for at least 5–10 years.

Prognosis correlates somewhat with histologic grade (18). Histologic evidence of necrosis did not seem to bear on the grade of AB, as it was seen in about 70% of both low-grade and high-grade AB. Anaplastic features and increased mitotic rate predicted decreased life expectancy and increased recurrence. In their series, Bonnin and Rubinstein found five of eight patients with low-grade AB survived for 3–20 years, whereas three of four with high-grade AB died within 2.5 years. Overall, of eight low-grade cases, three had recurrence, one of which was a glioblastoma multiforme (within 4.5 years), a feature shared with other types of low-grade primary brain tumors, especially the fribrillary astrocytoma. The fourth high-grade patient survived 11.5 years with a recurrence after 8.5 years that continued to be a low-grade AB.

CHOROID PLEXUS PAPILLOMA

Choroid plexus papillomas (CPs) are rare, well-differentiated, slow-growing tumors originating from the tissue that forms the choroid plexus. In most series their incidence varies from 0.4% to 1% (60,109,176). The relative frequency of CP among primary intracranial tumors in childhood is about 3%, compared with 0.5% in adults. Although the peak incidence reported in the literature occurs between the first 2 years of life to the early teen years, 50% to 70% of CP occurs in adults (41,79).

Overall, the most common site for CP is the lateral ventricles (43%), followed by the fourth ventricle (39%), third ventricle (9%), and cerebello-pontine angle (9%) (153). Considering the age of the patient, the lateral ventricle is the most frequent site in children, and the fourth ventricle is the most frequent site in adults (57,60). CP presents mostly with nonspecific signs and symptoms due to hydrocephalus. Usually the symptoms associated with CP evolve slowly. Combining both the pediatric and adult cases, headache is the most common symptom (approximately two-thirds of cases), followed by visual impairment (one-third of cases) (176). Other symptoms—such as mental changes, hemiparesis, tinnitus, or seizures—can occasionally be the main presenting symptoms (60,176). The most common sign in adult CP is papilledema, followed by gait impairment, cranial nerve palsies, and psychiatric disturbance, whereas in children gait impairment is the most common, followed by papilledema, other cerebellar signs, seizures, psychomotor retardation, and macrocephaly (176).

CP can also present with acute onset either as a result of intraventricular or intratumoral hemorrhage or as a result of sudden decompensation and herniation of insidiously developing hydrocephalus (60). CP has rarely been associated with multiple tumor diseases such as von Hippel-Lindau disease and Li-Fraumeni syndrome (109).

CT typically shows an intraventricular cauliflower-shaped mass that may vary from hypodense to hyperdense and that enhances similarly to choroid plexus. Calcification can be seen in 4% to 10% of the cases, and cystic structure can be seen within the tumor mass occasionally (176). On T1-weighted MR images, CP appears hypo- to isointense relative to brain but hyperintense relative to cerebrospinal fluid (CSF). On T2-weighted MRI it appears hyperintense relative to brain (60). Hydrocephalus with asymmetric dilatation of the ventricular system is usually evident on CT and MRI (109).

Management

CP should be excised surgically, but because of the highly vascular nature of these tumors and because of growth deep in the ventricular system, preoperative evaluation using MR angiography and/or angiogram can be informative. The risk of blood loss is high, particularly in young children, and therefore a surgical approach targeting the blood supply, such as anterior and posterior choroidal arteries, is advised (109). Although preoperative shunting for hydrocephalus is not required, intraoperative cannulation of the ventricle can be helpful. This external ventricular drainage system can then be converted to an internalized ventriculoperitoneal shunt if hydrocephalus does not resolve after surgery. In the series by Tacconi et al. (176), 14% of adult patients and 33% of pediatric patients needed shunt placement postoperatively. Harsh and Wilson recommend wide suboccipital craniotomy for fourth-ventricle CP, with control of feeding vessels prior to resection of the tumor. Tumors in the atrium of the lateral ventricle are best approached by a transcortical approach posterior to angular gyrus. A transcortical or transcallosal approach is appropriate for third-ventricular CP, and an approach through the middle temporal gyrus can be used for CP in the temporal horn.

Gross total resection is obtained in 60% to 90% of cases (57,60). Although perioperative mortality higher than 20% has been reported, with careful microsurgical technique perioperative mortality has been decreased to under 5% and transient postoperative complications to under 10% (57,60,176). Gross total resection may provide prolonged recurrence-free survival (60). In the series by Tacconi et al. (176), all recurrences were in pediatric cases, thus bringing the rate of recurrence in pediatric cases to 71% and the rate of recurrence in pediatric and adult cases combined to 4.3%.

Harsh and Wilson (60) recommend postoperative radiation therapy in almost all cases.

Because most cases of CP are histologically benign, we believe that radiotherapy should be reserved for recurrent tumors or those with anaplastic features (109,176).

DYSEMBRYOPLASTIC NEUROEPITHELIAL TUMOR

Daumas-Duport et al. initially described dysembryoplastic neuroepithelial tumor (DNT) in 1988 (32) with a report of 39 cases of unique neuroepithelial tumors associated with medically intractable seizures. The seizures usually began before the age of 20 years without any neurologic deficits and stigmata of phakomatosis. In a study of 216 patients with chronic epilepsy, DNT was the cause in 3% of the patients (193). Considering only the patients with chronic epilepsy due to neoplasia and/or dysplasia, approximately 5% to 23% harbored DNT (122,143).

The most common presenting symptoms of patients with DNT are seizure followed by headache (25). Occasionally, DNT may present with other, more rare forms of epilepsy, including infantile spasm (147). Of 16 patients studied by Raymond et al. (147), only one did not present with seizures, and electroencephalographic studies were abnormal in all patients. Frontal lobe DNT lesions can be associated with psychosis as well as seizures (162). Although not frequently associated with phakomatosis, two cases of DNT in children with neurofibromatosis type 1 have been described (99). DNT is commonly associated with cortical dysplasia. The cortical dysplasia is apparently not severe enough to cause significant mental retardation, but some delay of early developmental milestones in a small minority of patients has been reported (147).

Most cases of DNT have been supratentorial within the cortex. These lesions are usually multinodular and associated with focal cranial deformity (32). The temporal lobe nevertheless remains the most common site for DNT (131,14,147). In their study, Daumas-Duport et al. (32) found 62% of cases occurring within the temporal lobe, followed by 31% in the frontal lobe and approximately 8% in the parieto-occipital lobe. DNT has been reported in the cerebellum as well (94).

The MRI and CT scan appearance of DNT is characteristically multicystic and with a gyrus-like configuration (95,131). On CT scan DNT is mildly to profoundly hypodense and may have calcifications. On MRI, lesions are hypointense on T1-weighted images and hyperintense on T2-weighted images (95,131,147). DNT usually does not enhance with gadolinium, but a minority may show partial enhancement (147,148). Hemorrhage, edema, and mass effect are uncommon features. Bone remodeling of adjacent calvaria may also be observed.

Management

DNT is a benign lesion with no malignant recurrence reported. Before its description as a separate entity, DNT was usually diagnosed as low-grade astrocytoma, oligodendroglioma, mixed oligoastrocytoma, or ganglioglioma. As a result, patients were treated with radiotherapy and chemotherapy (147). The lesion is presumably curable by surgical excision alone, which suggests this is the treatment of choice. Adjuvant therapy is not needed (1, 32,147). Daumas-Duport et al. (32) reported that of the 17 subtotally or incompletely resected DNT followed over a mean period of 9 years (1–18 years), none showed any clinical or radiologic evidence of recurrence. Prayson et al. (144), however, reported that only four of 11 patients undergoing surgery for DNT required at least one additional surgical procedure for tumor recurrence. These recurrences followed incomplete initial excision by 2.1–4.4 years. Although none of the recurrences were malignant, it behooves the physician to follow patients clinically and radiologically after subtotal resection of DNT.

Symptomatic relief is excellent with surgery. Even partial removal has been associated with improvement in seizure activity, and there is some evidence that improvement of developmental delay may also occur after surgery. Raymond et al. (147) recommend partial or complete temporal lobectomy, or substantial corticectomy of the epileptic zone.

In their report of 16 patients, 12 were seizure-free and two had more than 80% reduction in seizure frequency. No recurrence was noted in 14 patients followed for a mean of 16 months. Kirkpatrick et al. (90) also recommend an en bloc temporal lobectomy without radiotherapy and chemotherapy.

GANGLIOCYTOMA

Gangliocytoma (GC) consists of neoplastic but well-differentiated large cells with neuronal characteristics (gangliocyte) and usually constitutes 0.1% to 0.5% of all brain tumors (40). A variant of GC occurs characteristically in the cerebellum, where it is known as Lhermitte-Duclos disease. Besides the cerebellum, GC has been found in other locations in the central nervous system, the most common of which is the temporal lobe (40,157). Other areas in which these lesions may occur with a high propensity are the floor of the third ventricle and the sellar region (40,145). Cases of GC in other regions such as the pineal region and spinal cord have also been reported (158).

On CT scan, GC is hyperdense without any significant contrast enhancement. On T1-weighted MR images, lesions appear of mixed intensity, and on T2-weighted images with hypointensity. Mass effect is not prominent in either CT or MRI (4).

Aside from commonly presenting with chronic seizure, because of its predilection for a cortical location, GC uniquely presents in association with pituitary adenomas. Nearly 50 cases of GC associated with pituitary adenoma have been reported (145). Sixty-five percent of cases of hypothalamic GC are associated with pituitary adenoma, and 74% of these patients have associated hypersecretion of pituitary hormones. Acromegaly has been reported in patients with GC (164), and other symptoms of hypothalamic dysfunction, including hyperphagia and somnolence, have been reported (14).

Management

GC is histologically benign and may actually be a dysplastic lesion-like dysplastic gangliocytoma of the cerebellum instead of a neoplastic one. Total excision of the tumor should be curative. Malignant transformation in GC has not been reported; however, after incomplete resection, clinical and radiographic follow-up is recommended. In patients who present with a long-standing history of epilepsy, particularly those with lesions in the temporal region, a comprehensive preoperative epilepsy work-up is warranted. Such an approach should improve the chances of a symptom-free postoperative course (141).

LHERMITTE-DUCLOS DISEASE

Lhermitte-Duclos disease (LD), initially described in 1920 (100), is considered to be a nonneoplastic (dysplastic) lesion in the cerebellum composed of cerebellar folia expanded by hypertrophic neurons of the internal granular layer and characterized as a mass lesion.

LD is primarily a disease of children and young adults, but an average age as high as 34 years at the time of diagnosis has been reported (5). LD commonly presents with increased ICP due to hydrocephalus (119) and/or cerebellar dysfunction (25). Rarely, other complications, such as subarachnoid hemorrhage in a recurrent mass (171) and orthostatic hypotension, possibly due to a mass effect onto the cardiorespiratory centers (155), have also been described.

Management

MRI is the imaging modality of choice because it provides better images of the posterior fossa than CT. On CT, LD is evident as a nonenhancing unilateral posterior fossa mass with or without calcifications (7). Hydrocephalus may be evident on CT or MRI. On MRI, LD typically appears as thickened folia of cerebellum, hypointense on T1-weighted images and hyperintense on T2-weighted images (62,73,118). Described classically as a nonenhancing mass, contrast enhancement on MRI has occasionally been observed and

should not be construed as evidence against the diagnosis of LD (42,62,73,118,136).

The primary objective in the treatment of LD is symptomatic relief. Symptoms are usually caused by hydrocephalus, which should be relieved by surgical excision of the mass lesion. Although resection at the margin may not be complete because of indistinct margins intraoperatively, ultrasound and particularly frameless stereotactic methods may be helpful, albeit the use of the latter may be limited in the posterior fossa. If gross total resection cannot be done, subtotal resection may be satisfactory for the short-term, with repeat debulking undertaken as deemed necessary (113).

Recurrence even after gross total resection has been described, after a period of as long as 20 years (7,73,113,171). A malignant transformation of the recurrent lesion has not been described; however, the development of malignant astrocytoma in the cerebrum 17 years after initial diagnosis of LD has been reported (38). The role of radiotherapy and chemotherapy has not been described, but these may not be necessary because malignant transformation has not been reported.

LD may occur as a sporadic disease or as a part of a newly described phakomatosis, Cowden's disease (2,181,189,192). In a review of the literature by Vinchon et al. (181), 26 of 72 cases of LD had conditions suggestive of Cowden's disease, and seven were definite cases. Cowden's disease is characterized by multiple hamartomatous lesions in the body (172). Skin, mucous membranes, thyroid, breast, gastrointestinal system, and genitourinary system may be more commonly involved. Patients with Cowden's disease have a high propensity to develop malignancy, particularly breast cancer in females (172,189). All patients with LD therefore should be carefully examined and screened for Cowden's disease. A diagnosis of Cowden's disease will necessitate life-long follow-up.

GANGLIOGLIOMA

Ganglioglioma (GG) is a variant of glial tumor that is composed of both glial cells and cells with neuronal characteristics. The term was introduced by Perkins in 1926 (138). According to Courville and Anderson (31), GGs comprise 0.4% of all intracranial tumors and 0.8% of all gliomas. The incidence in selected series, however, has been noted as high as 38% (97), probably reflecting referral bias such as predominance of pediatric cases or centers that specialize in medically intractable epilepsy. If patients with temporal lobe epilepsy secondary to a tumor are considered, then the incidence of GG has been noted to vary from 1.3% to 38% (92,122). Patients with hemispheric tumors are generally older at diagnosis than those with more midline located tumors (58). Up to 80% of GGs occur during the first three decades of life, but GGs can present as early as the first 2 years of life or as late as 70 years of age (97,156).

The most common presenting symptom is seizure. In several series of 20 or more GGs, 64% to 92% have been noted to present with epilepsy (92,169,200). Other, less common presenting symptoms were focal neurologic deficits (8% to 29%), neuro-ophthalmologic deficits, increased ICP, and impairment of higher cortical functions, including aphasia, alexia, and agraphia (58,92,200). Because of its location at other sites, such as in the posterior fossa, GG can present with less common symptoms, such as hearing loss, hemifacial spasms, or hemifacial seizures (15,35,61). In the study of Zentner et al. (200), the duration of symptoms was 3 months to 45 years (mean 11 years) prior to diagnosis.

GG is most commonly found in the temporal lobe (74% to 84% of cases), followed by the frontal lobe and the parieto-occipital lobe (92,194,200). GG has been noted at all sites in the central nervous system, including the basal ganglia, optic pathway, brain stem, spinal cord, pineal gland, and cerebellum (25,96).

Neither CT nor MRI images of GG are characteristic (92,200). On CT scan, GG is usually hypodense, and approximately half of GGs may have calcifications. Contrast enhancement is observed in most cases, but some may show inhomogeneous enhance-

ment or no enhancement at all. On T1-weighted MR images, these tumors are usually hypointense, and on T2-weighted images they are iso- to hyperintense. Rarely, CT and MRI fail to demonstrate the tumor (169,200). In both CT and MRI, cystic components can be seen in some GGs. The solid variety is more commonly located in the temporal lobe and shows better contrast enhancement (21).

Management

Gross total resection is the treatment of choice for those GGs amenable to surgical resection (58,92,97,169,200). In the combined experience of Krouwer et al. (92) and Silver et al. (169), none of the 16 tumors recurred after gross total resection, whereas of 17 patients undergoing either subtotal resection or biopsy, seven (41%) developed recurrence (92). In the experience of Silver et al. (169), of 12 patients undergoing subtotal resection or biopsy, four died of the tumor progression over a period of 4 months to 8 years. Zentner et al. observed similar recurrence-free follow-up in all patients undergoing gross total resection (200). Their perioperative mortality was 2% (one patient) secondary to a massive pulmonary embolism, and transient morbidity, such as third cranial nerve palsy or wound infection, developed in 12% of cases. Operative morbidity is related to the location of the tumor—5% for cerebral hemisphere GG versus 33% for GG in the brain stem (96). Postoperative survival and recurrence-free interval also correlate with the location of the tumor. Five-year event-free survival was 95% in cases of GG of the cerebral hemisphere, and 3-year event-free survival was 53% in cases of brain stem GG (96). Limitation in the extent of resection of tumors located in the midline (brain stem, optic tract, basal ganglia, and third ventricle) is probably the source of this difference in outcome (27,48). The experience of Haddad et al. (58) reflects a similar pattern. They found that 92% of patients with hemispheric tumors were alive and free of tumor recurrence, compared with 25% of those with midline tumors. In the opinion of

Lang et al. (96), the only variable predictive of outcome was tumor location, whereas the histologic grade did not correlate with postoperative results. However, Krouwer et al. (92) state that histologic grade was significantly related to the outcome. They found that 1- and 3-year disease-free actuarial survival was 89% and 76%, respectively, after subtotal resection or biopsy in lower-grade GG, whereas corresponding figures for high-grade GG were 63% and 33%, respectively. Of eight tumors that were examined for proliferative activity by BUdR labeling index, seven showed a value of less than 1% and did not recur, and one showed a value of more than 1% and recurred postoperatively. Krouwer et al. (92) have thus recommended that to determine the next step in the management of the patient, histologic grade and growth kinetic analysis should be studied when patients undergo subtotal resection or biopsy. If histology does not suggest anaplasia and growth potential is low, close monitoring both clinically and by neuroimaging is recommended. With anaplastic histology and/or high labeling index, adjuvant radiotherapy or, in the case of infants, chemotherapy should be considered. Regardless of histology, adjuvant radiotherapy has not provided a clear-cut survival advantage after subtotal resection; therefore reserving radiotherapy for recurrence is a treatment option (34,36,52,82,175). Lang and Miller (97) prefer to limit use of radiotherapy even further. They recommend surgery for recurrence and reserve radiotherapy for those recurrent cases where surgical resection is impossible.

The role of chemotherapy is not defined either as an adjuvant therapy after initial surgery or at recurrence (21,52,92,169). Chemotherapy may be of some use if both surgery and radiotherapy fail or if radiotherapy is needed to be deferred in a young child with an aggressive GG (92).

Because most GGs present with a longstanding chronic epileptic disorder, complete resection may improve the symptoms but not relieve them completely (58,92,122,141,200). Khajavi et al. (88) could not find any benefit of seizure surgery over gross total resection limited to the tumor. Pilcher et al. (141) argue that in many such cases the seizure was not medically intractable and that when seizures are intractable appropriate seizure surgery may result in much better outcome, providing a greater percentage improvement than the 50% to 65% reported after tumor removal only. In their report of 12 cases of GG with epileptic disorder, the patients were evaluated preoperatively with scalp or intradural electrodes with video monitoring. Neuropsychological testing as well as amytal injection of carotid was done preoperatively. Intraoperatively, most of the patients underwent functional mapping under local anesthesia, and electrocorticography was employed in guiding the extent of resection of the epileptogenic zone. The epileptogenic zone was as far as 7 cm anterior from the tumor in one of the cases. Eleven of the 12 patients who underwent complete resection of the epileptogenic zone were seizure-free postoperatively (with a mean follow-up of 3.1 years), including one patient in whom the tumor could not be resected completely. In one patient where the tumor was resected completely but the epileptogenic zone could not be removed completely, the symptoms of seizure improved by more than 90%. Wyllie et al. (195) and Otsubo et al. (132) also recommend removal of epileptogenic tissue in addition to the tumor and report a much more favorable outcome with this mode of treatment.

The outcome of patients with GG is generally favorable after gross total resection. Malignant recurrences are rare but may occur 5–23 years after resection (82,78,156,161). Diffuse leptomeningeal involvement and/or systemic dissemination of the malignancy may rarely occur (51,175,185).

NEUROCYTOMA

Since Hassoun et al. first described neurocytoma (NC) in 1982, more than 145 cases have been identified (44,63). Prior to the characterization of NC, these tumors were usually (mis)diagnosed as oligodendroglioma. NCs are characterized by their intraventricular localization, predominant occurrence in young adults, histologic similarity to oligodendrogliomas and ependymomas, expression of neuron-specific antigens, and ultrastructural features of neuronal differentiation (12,64,197). Although NC constitutes less than 1% of all the tumors of the central nervous system, nearly half of all supratentorial intraventricular tumors in adults are NC (64,197). About 77% of NCs are in the lateral ventricles, 5% are present exclusively in the third ventricle, none are present exclusively in the fourth ventricle, and two have been described with tetraventricular extension (44,150,197). In addition to their classic presentation as an intraventricular or periventricular growth, NCs have been reported at other sites in the brain, including the pons and cerebellum, and in the spinal cord (29,43,129, 170).

The clinical presentation of a classic neurocytoma is similar to that of any other intraventricular tumor. Signs and symptoms of occlusive hydrocephalus such as headache, nausea, visual and mental disturbances, and papilledema predominate (12,64,197). A few NCs may remain silent and be noticed only incidentally, whereas others located in the brain parenchyma may present with irritative symptoms such as medically intractable epilepsy (43,54,129,146). More acute presentations, such as spontaneous intraventricular hemorrhage, have also been reported (130).

Centrally located NCs usually follow a benign course, although a few cases with malignant histopathology and malignant clinical course have been described (44,63,129,184, 197).

On CT scan NCs appear as slightly hyperdense intraventricular masses with irregular margins and areas of hypodensity. Cysts may be observed in 85% and calcification in 69% of cases (22,129). On MRI, signal intensity is heterogeneous on both T1- and T2-weighted images. Signal voids, probably due to prominent veins, are observed in 62% of cases, and intratumoral hemorrhage may be seen in 15% of cases (22). Hydrocephalus due to obstruc-

tion of CSF flow is observed in many cases on both MRI and CT.

Management

Because NC is usually a slow-growing, benign tumor, complete removal of the tumor is usually curative (64,110,129,197). For NC situated in the lateral ventricles or the third ventricle, an anterior transcallosal microneurosurgical approach has been recommended (197). In a review of 127 cases from the literature, Hassoun et al. (64) found that NC could be removed totally in nearly half of the cases.

Radiotherapy has a limited role in treatment of NC. It is generally recommended for those NCs with malignant pathology. NCs may recur after incomplete surgical resection, but because of their low proliferative potential, radiotherapy is not recommended as an adjuvant treatment (64). Postoperative recurrence-free survival of up to 19 years has been reported, and of the more than 145 cases reported in the literature, only nine have recurred (44,64). Two of these eventually resulted in craniospinal dissemination through the CSF pathways. Although radiotherapy has been recommended for subtotally removed tumors (197), avoiding this therapy as an adjuvant treatment for subtotally removed NC seems reasonable. At recurrence, surgical excision should again be attempted, and adjuvant radiotherapy should be considered. Of the nine recurrences reported in literature, five occurred after gross total resection without radiotherapy and four occurred after subtotal resection, of which only two had received adjuvant radiotherapy (44). Two died of disease within 2–3 years after recurrence. The role of chemotherapy has not been tested, but in two recurrences with craniospinal dissemination, chemotherapy has been tried (44).

PILOCYTIC ASTROCYTOMA IN ADULTS

Pilocytic astrocytoma (PA) is frequently found in the cerebellum in the pediatric population with well-differentiated histology and a benign prognosis. Tumors with similar characteristics may also occur in the adult population. Based on age and associated microscopic features, some authors have divided PA into two groups (20,157). The adult form of PA is much less common than the pediatric (juvenile) form and tends to occur in the cerebral hemispheres, unlike the pediatric form, which usually occurs in the cerebellum or other midline structures. Although the adult form is well-circumscribed grossly, microscopically it infiltrates the surrounding parenchyma, unlike the juvenile form. The adult form is more uniform and consists of closely packed interwoven fascicles of relatively broad fibrillated bipolar cells (157).

The entity of adult PA is more controversial than any of the other uncommon low-grade glial tumors of the central nervous system. Some authors refer to PA as spongioblastoma (25). Because the adult form shares the indolent course and some histologic features with the juvenile form, some authors have suggested the two forms should be grouped together (91). Others disagree about the existence of an adult type of PA and claim that the term *PA* should stand solely for the juvenile variety (97). These authors claim that on further examination, the adult examples turned out to be ordinary fibrillar astrocytoma with tumor cells infiltrating in parallel with white matter tracts. Not surprisingly, given the rare occurrence of the adult PA and the controversy surrounding its existence, a large series concerned with the clinical features and the treatment outcomes of the adult form is lacking (49).

The adult form of PA presents more frequently in the cerebrum than the juvenile form and is extremely rare in the cerebellum (46). The median age at diagnosis of cerebral PA is 22 years, whereas that for more common diffuse low-grade astrocytoma is 34 years (49). In one Japanese series the adult form occurred more frequently in the cerebellum than in the cerebrum; of 15 cases of adult PA, nine (60%) were present in the cerebellum, two (13%) were in the brain stem, three (20%) were in the basal ganglia, and one was in the pineal region (83). The adult form of PA occurring in the cerebral hemispheres is more commonly (60% to 80%) located in the temporal or temporoparietal regions and can rarely extend into the optic chiasm and the walls of the third ventricle (151,157).

The clinical presentation of adult PA depends on its location. Cerebral PA can present with seizures, increased ICP, or focal neurologic deficits (151). The most common presenting symptom for cerebellar PA is hydrocephalus; cranial nerve deficits are expected when PA is noted in the brain stem. Presenting symptoms usually occur for less than 3 years prior to diagnosis, but symptoms of longer duration, even more than 50 years, have also been noted (87). Catastrophic presentation of adult PA is extremely rare, but sudden onset of symptoms due to hemorrhage into the tumor has been described (24,105).

Management

Gross total resection is the treatment of choice (47,49,50,83). The tumor is generally sharply demarcated from the surrounding parenchyma and therefore is amenable to complete excision in easily accessible regions of the brain (49,157). Ten-year survival after gross total resection or radical subtotal resection was 100% for supratentorial PA and decreased to 84% after subtotal resection, and to only 44% after biopsy alone (167). Similar results of 100% 10-year survival for supratentorial PA (both adult and pediatric combined) have been reported after gross total resection or radical subtotal resection (47). In the experience of Kyama et al. (83), which consisted of cerebellar, brain stem, basal ganglia, and pineal gland tumors, the 2-, 5-, and 10-year survival rates were 93.3%, 86.7%, and 86.7%, respectively, compared with 100%, 95.8%, and 95.8%, respectively, in pediatric cases. In the same series, the 10-year survival of the adult cerebellar PA (nine cases) was similar to pediatric cases (i.e., 100%) (83).

As in the case of juvenile PA, the role of radiotherapy in the treatment of adult PA is unclear. Radiation therapy does not seem to be of obvious benefit after complete resection but can be considered after subtotal resection (167). In the experience of Kayama et al., no recurrence was observed if patients either had gross total resection with or without radiotherapy or subtotal resection with radiotherapy (83). All patients with subtotal resection in their study received radiation therapy. The only cases of recurrence or tumor progression occurred after biopsy with or without adjuvant radiotherapy. These included two adults, both of whom received radiotherapy after biopsy, but their tumors recurred after 2–3 years. Based on a favorable outcome in the group of subtotal resection followed by radiation therapy, Kayama et al. suggest that, although radiotherapy is not necessary after total tumor resection, it should be instituted when residual tumor is present. Their series, however, lacks the data to support the conclusion that subtotal resection without radiotherapy is associated with higher recurrence rates. In the experience of Garcia and Fulling with seven cases of adult cerebral PA, in whom four had gross total resection and received no radiotherapy and three underwent subtotal resection plus radiotherapy, one death was related to radionecrosis. Two patients with subtotal resection and radiotherapy were followed without recurrence for 5–9 years. Although some authors have concluded that the value of radiotherapy is questionable even after partial excision (50,135), many do recommend radiotherapy after partial resection (112,115,167,186). Malignant transformation of the residual PA is possible and may be more likely in adult PA (3,30,151).

Besides rare instances of malignant transformation, PA may also develop multicentric spread (112). Mamelak et al. (112) reported a series of patients, including two adult patients (34 and 43 years old), with hypothalamic PA. Both underwent biopsy, and one had an adjuvant chemotherapy and the other had radiotherapy. The authors concluded that tumors in the hypothalamic region are more prone to develop multicentric spread and therefore recommend that all cases of hypothalamic PA

undergo gadolinium-enhanced MRI of the neuraxis and cytologic examination of the CSF to rule out multicentric disease at the time of initial diagnosis.

The role of chemotherapy has received much less consideration than radiation therapy in PA. A conclusive statement regarding its effect is therefore impossible, although its use is more often noted in children. Adjuvant chemotherapy after biopsy did not seem to prevent multicentric spread, although the therapy resulted in regression of recurrent tumor in one patient and arrest in growth of tumor in another (112).

PLEOMORPHIC XANTHOASTROCYTOMA

Pleomorphic xanthoastrocytoma (PXA) is an uncommon tumor, possibly of glial origin, regarded as benign despite the cellular pleomorphism (86,91). Initially described by Kepes et al. (85), about 73 cases of PXA have been reported so far (97). Before being described as a separate clinicopathologic entity, PXA was usually misdiagnosed as a mesenchymal neoplasm and categorized with fibroxanthoma, leptomeningeal xanthosarcoma (84,85). Histologically, it is characterized by markedly pleomorphic cells, with variable xanthomatous (intracellular lipid droplets) change (67,85).

This tumor occurs more commonly in the young, mainly in the second decade of life. According to one review of 66 cases, the mean age at presentation was 17 years (range 3–72 years), with 90% of the patients younger than 30 years (187). Males and females are equally represented (33). The common clinical presentation of patients with PXA is chronic seizures, occurring in 75% to 79% of patients (8,33). Headaches and other signs of increased ICP (49%) may also occur, with occasional focal neurologic deficits (55,76,85, 111,157).

PXA typically occurs in the temporo-parietal cortex and is located superficially in association with the leptomeninges. In fact, the leptomeningeal association is one of the distinguishing features of PXA (85,137). The leptomeningeal association, however, is not an invariable feature of PXA, as this tumor has been found deep in the thalamus distant to the leptomeninges (93). PXA has occasionally been found in other nonclassical locations such as the suprasellar region, cerebellum, or spinal cord alone or in association with other astrocytic variants (66,93,102,173,187).

On MRI or CT scan, the tumor usually appears as a cystic lesion situated on the surface of temporal or parietal lobes (16,86,93,103, 149,179,198). The cystic nature of the lesion is noted in 66% to 73% of cases (33,187). Involvement of dura and bone erosion of skull are rarely seen. On T1-weighted MR images the lesion appears isointense and hyperintense on T2-weighted images. Enhancement following administration of contrast material is seen both in CT and MRI. Vascularity of the mass is not prominent and is derived from the leptomeningeal plexus or rarely from external carotid circulation (198).

Management

PXA needs to be differentiated from malignant astrocytomas with xanthomatous change (53,108,160). As opposed to malignant astrocytomas, PXA has a favorable prognosis.

Because of well-defined margins, PXA lends itself to complete surgical excision in superficial regions and gross total resection is the treatment of choice (25,33,97,180,191). In their review of the literature, Davies et al. (33) found that 15 (68%) of 22 patients with gross total resection were alive without recurrence over a mean follow-up of 11 years (range 1–18 years), whereas five (45%) of 11 patients who underwent subtotal resection were alive and free of recurrence at a mean follow-up of 6 years. Macaulay et al. (107), in their review of the literature, however, failed to note any influence of completeness of excision on the rate of recurrence and survival over a 10-year follow-up period. Once a tumor has recurred, repeat surgery can provide favorable results if malignant transformation has not occurred (33).

Most authors do not recommend radiation therapy after initial resection (25,33,107,180). In their review of the literature, Davies et al. (33) did not find a significant difference in recurrence and survival rates with or without radiotherapy. Of 19 patients who underwent radiotherapy, 55% were alive and recurrence-free after a follow-up of more than 1 year, 33% had developed recurrence, and 28% had died, whereas of the 10 patients who did not receive radiotherapy, 60% were alive without recurrence after a follow-up of more than 1 year, 30% had developed recurrence, and 20% had died. Macaulay et al. (107) also did not find any improvement in survival if radiotherapy was provided as an adjuvant after initial resection, although the therapy did seem to decrease the incidence of recurrence mildly.

PXA is not always benign in its behavior; rarely, PXA can recur as glioblastoma multiforme, and occasionally tumors with clear anaplastic features have been found on initial resection (9,86,180,188). In fact, some have suggested that PXAs are not benign tumors but low-grade malignancies (97). These authors recommend close observation of those patients whose tumor shows anaplastic features. Increased mitotic activity is a stronger predictor of malignant transformation than focal infiltration of brain tissue (180). For patients with tumors that clearly show anaplastic changes on initial resection, adjuvant radiotherapy is therefore warranted, whereas for those whose tumor shows increased mitotic activity but not anaplasia, a choice between close follow-up and postoperative radiation therapy must be made. Chemotherapy has occasionally been used for more aggressive PXA, but the data are limited to assess the role of chemotherapy in the management of PXA (174,180).

Overall, despite a pleomorphic histologic picture, the tumor has a favorable prognosis (107,134). In their review of the outcome of 71 cases of supratentorial PXA, Macaulay et al. (107) found that 10- and 15-year actuarial survival from the onset of symptoms was 76% and 57%, respectively. Seizures associated with PXA are usually well controlled with resection of the tumor (25,55,85).

SUBEPENDYMAL GIANT CELL ASTROCYTOMA

Subependymal giant cell astrocytoma (SG) is a benign tumor that typically arises from the subependymal wall of the lateral ventricles near the foramen of Monro and is comprised of giant cells with eosinophilic cytoplasm of undetermined origin (19,97). SG occurs characteristically in patients with tuberous sclerosis. In a large series of 345 tuberous sclerosis patients, SG was found in 6.1% (168). Of 22 cases of SG, five were found to be associated with tuberous sclerosis (19). SG presents mostly during the second decade of life but can manifest as late as late middle age (20).

One of the distinguishing features of SG on CT or MRI is a uniformly contrast-enhancing mass at the foramen of Monro (116,124). Location other than the foramen of Monro, such as the ventricular trigone, has also been described (6). On MRI, SGs are isointense to gray matter in T1-weighted images and hyperintense on T2-weighted images. Calcifications may be detected in CT or MRI.

Clinically, SG may present as a mass effect either in isolation or in combination with other tuberous sclerosis features. Most present with hydrocephalus (39). The acute presentation of intratumoral hemorrhage is rare and can be massive and cause sudden death (13,59,81).

Management

SGs are circumscribed masses. Gross total resection should be the goal in the management of SG. For a lesion typically located at the foramen of Monro, both transcallosal and transcortical transventricular approaches have been recommended (190). Subtotal resection may also be adequate, given the benign nature of progression (25,124). For those patients with subtotal resection or in those in whom hydrocephalus persists even after gross total resection, shunting of CSF has been recommended (25,128).

Follow-up of surgically treated patients without adjuvant therapy has revealed a benign behavior of SG. In five cases of SG followed for 9 months to 7 years after total or subtotal resection without radiotherapy or chemotherapy, no progression or recurrence was noted despite findings of necrosis and mitosis in the tumor (28). Other authors also have not confirmed a clear-cut survival advantage with radiation therapy (17,25). In those pediatric cases of SG where adequate surgical resection was impossible, chemotherapy with nitrosourea-based cytotoxic regimens has been used with some success to defer potentially harmful radiotherapy (139). Periodic follow-up with CT or, preferably, MRI is needed to detect recurrence after progression and growth (25,28). Neuroimaging will also help detect an insidiously developing hydrocephalus. Overall, the outcome of SG is favorable, and residual tumor has remained stable for as long as 15 years after subtotal resection (25,124). Of 23 patients studied by Shepherd et al. (168), no correlation was noted between histologic features (such as atypia, mitoses, endothelial proliferation, and necrosis) and clinical course or survival. Approximately an 80% actuarial survival rate at 5- and 10-year intervals has been reported (97,168).

Because a significant number of the patients with SG have tuberous sclerosis, a thorough examination for signs of tuberous sclerosis is necessary. Similarly, when a patient presents with tuberous sclerosis, the possibility of SG should be kept in mind. Tuberous sclerosis is an autosomal dominant phakomatosis that usually presents with a classic triad of mental retardation, seizures, and adenoma sebacum (183). Once the diagnosis of tuberous sclerosis is made, examination of other organ systems is needed to reveal other stigmata of tuberous sclerosis such as cystic renal lesions.

EPENDYMOMA

First described by Virchow in 1864, ependymomas comprise approximately 1.2% to 3% of brain tumors (65,182). These tumors most frequently arise at or near the ventricular walls and are composed of ependymal and subependymal astroglial cells. Initially thought to be encapsulated and therefore amenable to cure, current information regarding intracranial low-grade tumors clearly establishes their invasive nature based on the relatively poor prognosis. The median age at the time of diagnosis is 25 years. Ependymomas occur more frequently in childhood, when the incidence is as high as 9% of pediatric brain tumors. By virtue of a predilection for the fourth ventricle, most of these tumors are found in the posterior fossa. Those lesions noted in the supratentorial compartment tend to be of a malignant phenotype.

Clinical presentation is generally silent until symptoms and signs of raised ICP are noted. The periventricular location allows for long-term delays in presentation, owing to the generous ventricular space into which the lesions will grow. Radiographically, calcification and cystic changes are common features of intracranial tumors and help to differentiate ependymoma from medulloblastoma. MRI usually shows a discrete cystic, heterogeneously enhancing lesion filling the ventricle. Although the median survival for patients with tumors in the posterior fossa can be twice that of those with tumors in the supratentorial compartment, the 5-year survival rate is still approximately 50% (140).

Based in part on the retrospective nature of most publications, the prognostic significance of many clinical and histologic parameters is impossible to assess, and conflicting results will be found regarding most variables. Histologic features correlate poorly with likelihood of recurrence even when frank anaplastic features are noted (152). Healy et al. (65) found that the amount of residual tumor on the postoperative scan was of prognostic significance, a finding noted for other subtypes of low-grade primary brain tumors. In this series of 29 children, all except four were treated with radiation (anaplastic features were noted in only two patients), and 19 patients were evaluated with postoperative scans. Of the nine patients with no postoperative residual tumor, a 75% 5-year freedom from disease progression was noted, whereas in 10 patients with residual tumor, the disease progressed in all ($p < .03$). Interestingly, the surgeon's estimate of residual disease did not correlate with survival. When tumor is noted to be invasive, prognosis is adversely affected (126).

Ependymomas are associated with dissemination throughout the subarachnoid space in 6% of patients, and although this event is noted more commonly with malignant tumors in the posterior fossa, CSF seeding has been noted with low-grade tumors (106). Despite positive CSF cytology, most instances remain clinically asymptomatic. In the report by Lyons et al. (106) the children were all under 5 years of age and the prognosis was far worse than that noted for adults in general. This difference cannot be explained based on histology or treatment features. Some authors suggest that the embryonal tumors are biologically different from the adult types, which have presumably evolved more slowly to their malignant counterparts (154).

Management

As with all low-grade brain tumors, the literature on ependymoma supports gross total resection when the risks of surgical intervention are low. As noted by Healy et al. (65), extent of resection is strongly correlated with extended disease-free survival. Although these results suggest that gross total resection should be recommended when feasible, most of these patients were treated with radiation therapy after surgical resection and the relative role of each of these modalities is unclear.

Given the tendency of ependymoma to spread through the CSF, adjuvant treatments seem warranted; however, one series reports no difference in survival after surgery followed by various forms of radiation, including craniospinal, whole brain, and involved field (65). After total resection in children, radiation does not offer any additional benefit (133). Systemic extranodal metastases have also been reported in 6.2% of 81 cases reported by Newton et al. (127). Three of these instances occurred with low-grade lesions. Chemotherapy has been administered for patients with malignant lesions but also for children with low-grade lesions. All four children with low-grade lesions treated by Lyons et al. died within 41 months of treatment (106). Based on the information available, multiple options for management are feasible. After gross total resection, follow-up with neuroimaging and no therapy can be considered. Follow-up neuroimaging should be advised for all clinical scenarios. When histologic indices of higher proliferative rates are noted, radiation can be recommended even after gross total resection. Others feel it reasonable to recommend craniospinal radiation for patients in whom anaplastic histology, positive CSF cytology, and/or spinal metastases have been noted (65,126).

SUBEPENDYMOMA

Subependymoma (SE) is a benign glioma usually found at autopsy (45). This astroglial variant was described by Scheinker in 1945 (163). Although SE was found in 0.4% of 1,000 autopsies, it constitutes only 0.7% of 1,000 symptomatic intracranial neoplasms (117), pointing to the fact that a majority of SE remains asymptomatic throughout life. Among third and lateral ventricle tumors, the incidence of SE may be as high as 5% (120). This tumor presents predominantly in middle-aged and elderly males (45). In one series, the median age of 21 patients with SE was 48.5 years (32–72 years) (89). The most common site is the lateral and fourth ventricle. However, it has been found at other sites, such as the third ventricle, cerebral aqueduct, suprasellar region, and spinal cord (56,68,69, 71,75,77,98,177,178).

Asymptomatic SE generally does not exceed 1.2 cm in size (45). Both symptomatic and asymptomatic SEs are more common in the fourth ventricle (58%) than in the lateral ventricle (38%), but those in the lateral ventricle are more likely to be clinically significant than those in the fourth ventricle (26,45). There is no consistent genetic predisposition to SE, but the lesion has been described in a father and a son, in three of 11 siblings, and in cases of neurofibromatosis (72,125,159).

SE is usually asymptomatic. Patients symptomatic with SE most commonly present with signs and symptoms of hydrocephalus. In one series, 80% of the 84 symptomatic SE patients presented with hydrocephalus (26,45). The median symptomatic period was approximately 1 year (45). The attacks of hydrocephalus can be intermittent (75). Besides hydrocephalus, hemorrhage into the subarachnoid space, into the ventricle, or within the tumor itself may also be the presenting factor, bringing attention to the hitherto asymptomatic tumor in an acute fashion (23, 37,101,114,166). Tumors in the fourth, third, or lateral ventricles may cause sudden unexpected death either from an acute hemorrhage or from an acute decompensation of an insidiously developing hydrocephalus (121,165). Symptoms due to local mass effect are extremely uncommon. Seizures are not a presenting feature of SE because of its common subcortical location.

On T1-weighted MR images, SE is heterogeneously isointense to hypointense relative to normal white matter, and on T2-weighted images it is slightly hyperintense, with little or no evidence of edema (71,89). Contrast enhancement on MRI also varies from no enhancement to marked enhancement. Heterogeneous contrast enhancement and calcification are observed more commonly in fourth ventricle SE than in lateral ventricle SE on MRI or CT scans (26). Besides dystrophic calcifications, focal hemorrhages can be seen in neuroimaging (89,196).

Management

Growth of SE within the ventricular lumen and its sharp demarcation from the surrounding brain tissue allows a complete removal in most cases, particularly those arising in the lateral ventricle (45). Because SE in the fourth ventricle usually arises from the floor of the ventricle, radical removal is less likely. During surgical excision of fourth ventricular SE tumors, special attention needs to be given to alteration of vital signs, such as heart rate and blood pressure, which suggests brain stem dysfunction (104). In the experience of Lombardi et al. (104), six of eight patients who showed such signs intraoperatively required tracheostomy postoperatively. Postoperative mortality as high as 42% has been reported in the fourth ventricular SE variety (80). Patients with subtotal resection and occasionally those with gross total resection may require a ventriculoperitoneal shunt. A ventriculostomy with external drainage clamped for sometime before removal may help identify those patients who will need shunting and may also avoid emergent ventriculostomy in the immediate postoperative period.

With adequate surgical excision, radiation therapy or chemotherapy is not indicated. Recurrences are very rare and spread via CSF has not been reported (45). Although SE seems to be radiosensitive, particularly with doses of 5,000 rad or more, Lombardi et al. (104) recommend postoperative radiotherapy only for those patients left with symptomatic residual disease or who develop recurrence after surgery. These authors followed 19 patients over a period of 1–27 years (mean 6 years). Of the 12 patients (10 with gross total resection and two with subtotal resection) who were not radiated, none developed tumor progression or died of direct tumor-related causes. Of the seven patients (two with gross total resection and five with subtotal resection) who were irradiated, three developed recurrences. The role for other adjuvant therapies such as interstitial brachytherapy has not been clearly defined but has been employed if pathology suggested a more aggressive nature of the tumor (75).

Most of the postoperative deaths are related to lower cranial nerve dysfunction following resection of fourth ventricular SE variety (104). The goal in the resection of the fourth ventricular tumors is to debulk the mass to improve the CSF flow and to avoid injury to the floor of the fourth ventricle. Use of microsurgical techniques and intraoperative cranial nerve monitoring during the resection of the SE in the fourth ventricle may reduce postoperative morbidity and mortality.

If operative morbidity and mortality are controlled, the prognosis of SE is good. Nonetheless, malignant changes can occur in SE (75) and therefore follow-up imaging is required, particularly after biopsy and/or subtotal resection.

CONCLUSION

Because of the low incidence of these neoplasms, the literature does not provide definitive recommendations regarding any of these tumor types. Surgical resection is generally considered to be a reasonable recommendation, largely because diagnosis requires surgery and, at the same time, it makes sense to remove as much of the lesion as safely possible. Unfortunately, this approach does not allow a valid comparison with nonsurgical follow-up. Ethically, it may be impossible to randomize these patients, even if there were enough cases to allow such a study. Therefore for the time being, surgical biopsy and resection remain the preferred recommendation, although observation with or without biopsy is not without its proponents. In addition, for most of these lesions, postoperative radiation therapy will remain controversial for similar reasons, and after total resection or subtotal resection without evidence of progressive growth, radiation may or may not be recommended. It is hoped that new insights into the fundamental biologic behavior of these neoplasms will allow more definitive treatment recommendations.

REFERENCES

1. Abe M, Tabuchi K, Tsuji T, Shiraishi T, Koga H, Takagi M. Dysembryoplastic neuroepithelial tumor: report of three cases. *Surg Neurol* 1995;43:240–245.
2. Albrecht S, Haber RM, Goodman JC, Duvic M. Cowden syndrome and Lhermitte-Duclos disease. *Cancer* 1992;70:869–876.

3. Alfa D, Mueller W, Slouch F, Fishig R. Supratentorial lobar pilocytic astrocytomas: report of 45 operated cases including 9 recurrences. *Acta Neurochir* 1986; 81:90–93.

4. Altman NR. MR and CT characteristics of gangliocytoma: a rare cause of epilepsy in children. *Am J Neuroradiol* 1988;9:917–921.

5. Ambler M, Pogacar S, Sidman. Lhermitte-Duclos disease (granule cell hypertrophy of the cerebellum): pathological analysis of the first family cases. *J Neuropathol Exp Neurol* 1969;28:622–647.

6. Andoh T, Kumagai M, Kondoh H, Sakai N, Yamada H, Shimokawa K. [Subependymal giant-cell astrocytoma arising from the trigone of the lateral ventricle. Report of an adult case]. [Japanese] *Neurol Med Chir* 1987;27:202–207.

7. Ashley DG, Zee CS, Chandrasoma PT, Segall HD. Lhermitte-Duclos disease: CT and MR findings. *J Comput Assist Tomogr* 1990;14:984–987.

8. Auer RN, Rice GPA, Hinton CG, et al. Cerebellar astrocytoma with benign histology and malignant clinical course: case report. *J Neurosurg* 1981;54:128–132.

9. Allegranza A, Ferraresi S, Bruzzone M, et al. Cerebromeningeal PXA. Report of four cases: clinical radiological and pathological features. (Including a case with malignant evolution.) *Neurosurg Rev* 1991;14: 43–49.

10. Bailey P, Bucy PC. Astroblastomas of the brain. *Acta Psychiatr Neurol* 1930;5:439–461.

11. Baka JJ, Patel SC, Roebuck JR, Hearshen DO. Predominantly extraaxial astroblastoma: imaging and proton MR spectroscopy features. *Am J Neuroradiol* 1993;14:946–950.

12. Barbosa MD, Balsitis M, Jaspan T, Lowe J. Intraventricular neurocytoma: a clinical and pathological study of three cases and review of the literature. *Neurosurgery* 1990;26:1045–1054.

13. Barbosa-Coutinho LM, Lima EL, Gadret RO, Ferreira NP. [Massive intratumor hemorrhage in tuberous sclerosis: autopsy study of a case] [Portuguese]. *Arquivos de Neuro-Psiquiatria* 1991;49:465–470.

14. Beal MF, Kleinman GM, Ojemann RG, Hochberg FH. Gangliocytoma of third ventricle: hyperphagia, somnolence, and dementia. *Neurology* 1981;31: 1224–1228.

15. Bills DC, Hanieh A. Hemifacial spasm in an infant due to fourth ventricular ganglioglioma: case report. *J Neurosurg* 1991;75:134–137.

16. Blom RJ. Pleomorphic xanthoastrocytoma: CT appearance. *J Comput Assist Tomogr* 1988;12:351–352.

17. Boesel CP, Paulson GW, Kosnik E, Earle KM. Brain hamartomas and tumors associated with tuberous sclerosis. *Neurosurgery* 1979;4:410–417.

18. Bonnin JM, Rubinstein LJ. Astroblastomas: a pathological study of 23 tumors, with a postoperative follow-up in 13 patients. *Neurosurgery* 1989;25:6–13.

19. Bonnin JM, Rubinstein LJ, Papasozomenos SC, Marangos PJ. Subependymal giant cell astrocytoma: significance and possible cytogenetic implications of an immunohistochemical study. *Acta Neuropathol* 1984;62:185–93.

20. Burger PC, Scheithauer BW, Vogel FS. *Surgical pathology of the nervous system and its coverings*, 3rd ed. New York: Churchill Livingstone, 1991.

21. Castillo M, Davis PC, Takei Y, Hoffman JC Jr. Intracranial ganglioglioma: MR, CT, and clinical findings in 18 patients. *Am J Neuroradiol* 1990;11:109–114.

22. Chang KH, Han MH, Kim DG, et al. MR appearance of central neurocytoma. *Acta Radiol* 1993;34: 520–526.

23. Changaris DG, Powers JM, Perot PL Jr, Hungerford GD, Neal GB. Subependymoma presenting as subarachnoid hemorrhage: case report. *J Neurosurg* 1981; 55:643–5.

24. Charles NC, Nelson L, Brookner AR, Lieberman N, Breinin GM. Pilocytic astrocytoma of the optic nerve with hemorrhage and extreme cystic degeneration. *Am J Ophthalmol* 1981;92:691–695.

25. Chen TC, Gonzalez-Gomez I, McComb JG. Uncommon glial tumors. In: Morantz RA, Walsh JW, eds. *Brain tumors: a comprehensive text.* New York: Marcel Dekker, 1994:525–557.

26. Chiechi MV, Smirniotopoulos JG, Jones RV. Intracranial subependymomas: CT and MR imaging features in 24 cases. *Am J Roentgenol* 1995;165:1245–1250.

27. Chilton J, Caughron MR, Kepes JJ. Ganglioglioma of the optic chiasm: case report and review of the literature. *Neurosurgery* 1990;26:1042–1045.

28. Chow CW, Klug GL, Lewis EA. Subependymal giant-cell astrocytoma in children: an unusual discrepancy between histological and clinical features. *J Neurosurg* 1988;68:880–883.

29. Coca S, Moreno M, Martos JA, Rodriguez J, Barcena A, Vaquero J. Neurocytoma of spinal cord. *Acta Neuropathol* 1994;87:537–540.

30. Crawford JV, Rubinstein LJ, Russell DS. Follow-up of cerebellar astrocytomas in relation to their pathology. *J Neurol Neurosurg Psychiatr* 1958;21:64–73.

31. Courville CB, Anderson FM. Neuro-gliogenic tumors of the central nervous system: report of two additional cases of ganglioglioma of the brain. *Bull Los Angeles Neurol Soc* 1941;6:154–176.

32. Daumas-Duport C, Scheithauer BW, Chodkiewicz JP, Laws ER Jr, Vedrenne C. Dysembryoplastic neuroepithelial tumor: a surgically curable tumor of young patients with intractable partial seizures: report of thirty-nine cases. *Neurosurgery* 1988;23:545–556.

33. Davies KG, Maxwell RE, Seljeskog E, Sung JH. Pleomorphic xanthoastrocytoma: report of four cases, with MRI scan appearances and literature review. *Br J Neurosurg* 1994;8:681–689.

34. DeMierre B, Stichnoth FA, Hori A, Spoerri O. Intracerebral ganglioglioma. *J Neurosurg* 1986;65:177–182.

35. Dhillon RS. Posterior fossa ganglioglioma—an unusual cause of hearing loss. *J Laryngol Otol* 1987;101: 714–717.

36. Diepholder HM, Schwechheimer K, Mohadjer M, Knoth R, Volk B. A clinicopathologic and immunomorphologic study of 13 cases of ganglioglioma. *Cancer* 1991;68:2192–2201.

37. DiLorenzo N, Rizzo A, Ciappetta P. Subependymoma of the septum pellucidum presenting as subarachnoid hemorrhage. *Neurochirurgia* 1991;34:125–126.

38. Domingo Z, Fisher-Jeffes ND, de Villiers JC. Malignant occipital astrocytoma in a patient with Lhermitte-Duclos disease (cerebellar dysplastic gangliocytoma). *Br J Neurosurg* 1996;10:99–102.

39. Duong H, Sarazin L, Bourgouin P, Vezina JL. Magnetic resonance imaging of lateral ventricular tumours. *Can Assoc Radiol J* 1995;46:434–442.

40. Ebina K, Suzuki S, Takahashi T, Iwabuchi T, Takei Y. Gangliocytoma of the pineal body: a case report and review of the literature. *Acta Neurochir* 1985;74: 134–40.

41. Ellenbogen RG, Winston KR, Kupsky WJ. Tumors of the choroid plexus in children. *Neurosurgery* 1989;25: 327–335.

42. Ellis PK. Case report: Lhermitte-Duclos disease: enhancement following gadolinium-DPTA. *Clin Radiol* 1996;51:222–224.

43. Enam SA, Ho K-L, Rosenblum ML. Neurocytoma in cerebellum: case report. *J Neurosurg* 1997;87: 100–102.

44. Eng DY, DeMonte F, Ginsberg L, Fuller GN, Jaeckle K. Craniospinal dissemination of central neurocytoma: report of two cases. *J Neurosurg* 1997;86:547–52.

45. Ernestus RI, Schroder R. [Clinical aspects and pathology of intracranial subependymoma: 18 personal cases and review of the literature] [German]. *Neurochirurgia* 1993;36:194–202.

46. Favre J, Deruaz JP, de Tribolet N. Pilocytic cerebellar astrocytoma in adults: case report. *Surg Neurol* 1993; 39:360–364.

47. Forsyth PA, Shaw EG, Scheithauer BW, O'Fallon JR, Layton DD Jr, Katzmann JA. Supratentorial pilocytic astrocytomas: a clinicopathologic, prognostic, and flow cytometric study of 51 patients. *Cancer* 1993;72: 1335–1342.

48. Garcia CA, McGarry PA, Collada M. Ganglioglioma of the brain stem: case report. *J Neurosurg* 1984;60: 431–434.

49. Garcia DM, Fulling KH. Juvenile pilocytic astrocytoma of the cerebrum in adults: a distinctive neoplasm with favorable prognosis. *J Neurosurg* 1985;63: 382–386.

50. Garcia DM, Fulling KH, Marks JE. The value of radiation therapy in addition to surgery for astrocytomas of the adult cerebrum. *Cancer* 1985;55:919–927.

51. Garcia Salazar FJ, Sanchez-Alarcos S, Gonzalez R, Coca S, Martinez R, Vaquero J. Brain ganglioglioma with large extension to subarachnoid space. *J Neurosurg Sci* 1990;34:61–63.

52. Garrido E, Becker LF, Hoffman HJ, et al. Gangliogliomas in children: a clinicopathological study. *Childs Brain* 1978;4:339–346.

53. Glasser RS, Rojiani AM, Mickle JP, Eskin TA. Delayed occurrence of cerebellar pleomorphic xanthoastrocytoma after supratentorial PXA removal. *J Neurosurg* 1995;82:116–118.

54. Goergen SK, Gonzales MF, McLean CA. Interventricular neurocytoma: radiologic features and review of the literature. *Radiology* 1992;182:787–792.

55. Goldring S, Rich KM, Picker S. Experience with gliomas in patients presenting with a chronic seizure disorder. *Clin Neurosurg* 1985;33:15–42.

56. Guha A, Resch L, Tator CH. Subependymoma of the thoracolumbar cord: case report. *J Neurosurg* 1989;71: 781–787.

57. Guidetti B, Spallone A. The surgical treatment of choroid plexus papillomas: the results of 27 years experience. *Neurosurg Rev* 1981;4:129–137.

58. Haddad SF, Moore SA, Menezes AH, VanGilder JC. Ganglioglioma: 13 years of experience. *Neurosurgery* 1992;31:171–178.

59. Hamamoto O, Honorato DC, Brito HL, Souza-Queiroz L. [Intratumor hemorrhage in tuberous sclerosis: a case report]. [Portuguese]. *Arquivos de Neuro-Psiquiatria* 1994;52(3):435–438.

60. Harsh GR, Wilson CB: Neuroepithelial tumors of the adult brain. In: Youmans JR, ed. *Neurological surgery*. Philadelphia: WB Saunders, 1990:3040–3136.

61. Harvey AS, Jayakar P, Duchowny M, et al. Hemifacial seizures and cerebellar ganglioglioma: an epilepsy syndrome of infancy with seizures of cerebellar origin. *Ann Neurol* 1996;40:91–98.

62. Hashimoto M, Fujimoto K, Shinoda S, Masuzawa T. Magnetic resonance imaging of ganglion cell tumours. *Neuroradiology* 1993;35:181–184.

63. Hassoun J, Gambarelli D, Grisoli F, et al. Central neurocytoma: an electron-microscopic study of two cases. *Acta Neuropathol* 1982;56:151–156.

64. Hassoun J, Soylemezoglu F, Gambarelli D, Figarella-Branger D, von Ammon K, Kleihues P. Central neurocytoma: a synopsis of clinical and histological features. *Brain Pathol* 1993;3:297–306.

65. Healy EA, Barnes PD, Kupsky WJ, et al. The prognostic significance of postoperative residual tumor in ependymoma. *Neurosurgery* 1991;28:666–672.

66. Herpers MJH, Freling G, Beuls EAM. Pleomorphic xanthoastrocytoma in the spinal cord: case report. *J Neurosurg* 1994;80:564–569.

67. Heyerdahl SE, Skullerud K. PXA: report of five cases. *Clin Neuropathol* 1983;2:188–191.

68. Ho KC, Meyer G, Caya J, Tieu TM, Prentiss A. Craniopharyngioma and "reactive" subependymoma of the third ventricle: a case report. *Clin Neuropathol* 1987; 6:12–15.

69. Ho KL. Tumors of the cerebral aqueduct. *Cancer* 1982;49:154–162.

70. Hoag G, Sima AAF, Rozdilsky B. Astroblastoma revisited: a report of three cases. *Acta Neuropathol* 1986;70:10–16.

71. Hoeffel C, Boukobza M, Polivka M, et al. MR manifestations of subependymomas. *Am J Neuroradiol* 1995;16:2121–2129.

72. Honan WP, Anderson M, Carey MP, Williams B. Familial subependymomas. *Br J Neurosurg* 1987;1: 317–321.

73. Hulcelle P, Dooms G, Vermonden J. Intramedullary subependymoma of the spinal cord. *Neurosurgery* 1996;38:251–257.

74. Husain AN, Leestma JE. Cerebral astroblastoma: immunohistochemical, ultrastructural, features. Case report. *J Neurosurg* 1986;64:657–661.

75. Iqbal Z, Sutcliffe JC. Subependymoma of the lateral ventricle: case report and literature review. *Br J Neurosurg* 1994;8:83–85.

76. Iwaki T, Fukui M, Kondo A, Matsushima T, Takeshita I. Epithelial properties of pleomorphic xanthoastrocytomas determined in ultrastructural and immunohistochemical studies. *Acta Neuropathol* 1987;74:142–150.

77. Jallo GI, Zagzag D, Epstein F. Intramedullary subependymoma of the spinal cord. *Neurosurgery* 1996; 38:251–257.

78. Jay V, Squire J, Becker LE, Humphreys R. Malignant transformation in a ganglioglioma with anaplastic neuronal and astrocytic components: report of a case with flow cytometric and cytogenetic analysis. *Cancer* 1994;73:2862–2868.

79. Jooma R, Hayward RD, Grant DN. Intracranial neo-

plasms during the first year of life: analysis of one hundred consecutive cases. *Neurosurgery* 1984;14: 31–41.

80. Jooma R, Torrens MJ, Bradshaw J, Brownell B. Sub-ependymomas of the fourth ventricle: surgical treatment in 12 cases. *J Neurosurg* 1985;62:508–512.

81. Kalina P, Drehobl KE, Greenberg RW, Black KS, Hyman RA. Hemorrhagic subependymal giant cell astrocytoma. *Pediatr Radiol* 1995;25:66–67.

82. Kalyan-Raman UP, Olivero WC. Ganglioglioma: a correlative clinicopathological and radiographic study of ten surgically treated cases with follow-up. *Neurosurgery* 1987;54:58–63.

83. Kayama T, Tominaga T, Yoshimoto T. Management of pilocytic astrocytoma. *Neurosurg Rev* 1996;19: 217–220.

84. Kepes JJ, Kepes M, Slowik F. Fibrous xanthomas and xanthosarcomas of the meninges and the brain. *Acta Neuropathol* 1973;23:187–199.

85. Kepes JJ, Rubinstein LJ, Eng LF. Pleomorphic astrocytoma: a distinctive meningocerebral glioma of young subjects with relatively favorable prognosis. A study of 12 cases. *Cancer* 1979;44:1839–1852.

86. Kepes JJ, Rubinstein LJ, Ansbacher L, Schreiber DJ. Histopathological features of recurrent PXA: further corroboration of the recurrent nature of this neoplasm. *Acta Neuropathol* 1989;78:585–593.

87. Kepes JJ, Whittker CK, Watson K, et al. Cerebellar astrocytomas in elderly patients with very long pre-operative histories: report of three cases. *Neurosurgery* 1989;25:258–264.

88. Khajavi K, Comair YG, Prayson RA, et al. Childhood ganglioglioma and medically intractable epilepsy: a clinicopathological study of 15 patients and a review of the literature. *Pediatr Neurosurg* 1995;22:181–188.

89. Kim DG, Han MH, Lee SH, et al. MRI of intracranial subependymoma: report of a case. *Neuroradiology* 1993;35:185–186.

90. Kirkpatrick PJ, Honavar M, Janota I, Polkey CE. Control of temporal lobe epilepsy following en bloc resection of low-grade tumors. *J Neurosurg* 1993;78:19–25.

91. Kleiheus P, Burger PC, Scheithauer BW. The new WHO classification of brain tumors. *Brain Pathol* 1993;3:255–268.

92. Krouwer HG, Davis RL, McDermott MW, Hoshino T, Prados MD. Gangliogliomas: a clinicopathological study of 25 cases and review of the literature. *J Neurooncol* 1993;17:139–154.

93. Kros JM, Vecht CJ, Stefanko CZ. The pleomorphic xanthoastrocytoma and its differential diagnosis: a study of five cases. *Hum Pathol* 1991;22:1128–1135.

94. Kuchelmeister K, Demirel T, Schlorer E, Bergmann M, Gullotta F. Dysembryoplastic neuroepithelial tumour of the cerebellum. *Acta Neuropathol* 1995;89: 385–390.

95. Kuroiwa T, Bergey GK, Rothman MI, et al. Radiologic appearance of the dysembryoplastic neuroepithelial tumor. *Radiology* 1995;197:233–238.

96. Lang FF, Epstein FJ, Ransohoff J, et al. Central nervous system gangliogliomas: 2. Clinical outcome. *J Neurosurg* 1993;79:867–873.

97. Lang FF, Miller DC. Astroglial variants. In: Black PM, Loeffler JS, eds. *Cancer of the nervous system.* Cambridge, MA: Blackwell Sciences, 1997:516–548.

98. Lee KS, Angelo JN, McWhorter JM, Davis CH Jr.

Symptomatic subependymoma of the cervical spinal cord: report of two cases. *J Neurosurg* 1987;67: 128–131.

99. Lellouch-Tubiana A, Bourgeois M, Vekemans M, Robain O. Dysembryoplastic neuroepithelial tumors in two children with neurofibromatosis type 1. *Acta Neuropathol* 1995;90:319–322.

100. Lhermitte J, Duclos P. Sur un ganglioneurone diffus du cortex du cervelet. *Bull Assoc French Cancer* 1920;9: 99–107.

101. Lindboe CF, Stolt-Nielsen A, Dale LG. Hemorrhage in a highly vascularized subependymoma of the septum pellucidum: case report. *Neurosurgery* 1992;31: 741–745.

102. Lindboe FL, Cappelen J, Kepes JJ. Pleomorphic xanthoastrocytoma as a component of a cerebellar ganglioglioma: case report. *Neurosurgery* 1992;31:353–355.

103. Lipper MH, Eberhard DA, Phillips CD, et al. PXA, a distinctive astroglial tumor: neuroradiologic and pathologic features. *AJNR* 1993;14:1397–1404.

104. Lombardi D, Scheithauer BW, Meyer FB, et al. Symptomatic subependymoma: a clinicopathological and flow cytometric study. *J Neurosurg* 1991;75:583–588.

105. Lones MA, Verity MA. Fatal hemorrhage in a cerebral pilocytic astrocytoma-adult type. *Acta Neuropathol* 1991;81:688–690.

106. Lyons MK, Kelly PJ. Posterior fossa ependymoma: report of 30 cases and review of the literature. *Neurosurgery* 1991;28:659–665.

107. Macaulay RJ, Jay V, Hoffman HJ, Becker LE. Increased mitotic activity as a negative prognostic indicator in pleomorphic xanthoastrocytoma: case report. *J Neurosurg* 1993;79:761–768.

108. MacKenzie JM. Pleomorphic xanthoastrocytoma in a 62-year-old male. *Neuropathol Appl Neurobiol* 1987; 13:461–487.

109. Madsen JR, Troup EC, Goumnerova LC. Miscellaneous benign tumors. In: Black PM, Loeffler JS, eds. *Cancer of the nervous system.* Cambridge, MA:Blackwell Sciences, 1997:431–437.

110. Maiuri F, Spaziante R, De Caro ML, Cappabianca P, Giamundo A, Iaconetta G. Central neurocytoma: clinico-pathological study of 5 cases and review of the literature. *Clin Neurol Neurosurg* 1995;97:219–228.

111. Maleki M, Robitaille Y, Bertrand G. Atypical xanthoastrocytoma presenting as a meningioma. *Surg Neurol* 1983;20:235–238.

112. Mamelak AN, Prados MD, Obana WG, Cogen PH, Edwards MS. Treatment options and prognosis for multicentric juvenile pilocytic astrocytoma. *J Neurosurg* 1994;81:24–30.

113. Marano SR, Johnson PC, Spetzler RF. Recurrent Lhermitte-Duclos disease in a child: case report. *J Neurosurg* 1988;69:599–603.

114. Marra A, Dario A, Scamoni C, Cerati M, Crivelli G, Dorizzi A. Intraventricular subependymoma presenting as subarachnoid hemorrhage: case report. *J Neurosurg Sci* 1991;35:213–215.

115. Marsa GW, Probert JC, Rubinstein LJ, et al. Radiation therapy in the treatment of childhood astrocytic gliomas. *Cancer* 1973;32:646–655.

116. Martin N, Debussche G, DeBroucker T, Mompoint D, Marsault C, Nahum H. Gadolinium-DTPA enhanced MR imaging in tuberous sclerosis. *Neuroradiology* 1990;31:492–497.

117. Matsumura A, Ahyai A, Hori A, Schaake T. Intracerebral subependymomas: clinical and neuropathological analyses with special reference to the possible existence of a less benign variant. *Acta Neurochir* 1989;96:15–25.

118. Meltzer CC, Smirniotopoulos JG, Jones RV. The striated cerebellum: an MR imaging sign in Lhermitte-Duclos disease (dysplastic gangliocytoma). *Radiology* 1995;194:699–703.

119. Milbouw G, Born JD, Martin D, et al. Clinical and radiological aspects of dysplastic gangliocytoma (Lhermitte-Duclos disease): a report of two cases with review of the literature. *Neurosurgery* 1988;22:124–128.

120. Morita A, Kelly PJ. Resection of intraventricular tumors via a computer-assisted volumetric stereotactic approach. *Neurosurgery* 1993;32:920–926.

121. Mork SJ, Morild I, Giertsen JC. Subependymoma and unexpected death. *Foren Sci Int* 1986;30:275–280.

122. Morris HH, Estes ML, Gilmore R, Van Ness PC, Barnett GH, Turnbull J. Chronic intractable epilepsy as the only symptom of primary brain tumor. *Epilepsia* 1993;34:1038–1043.

123. Moulignier A, Mikol J, Pialoux G, Eliaszewicz M, Thurel C, Thiebaut JB. Cerebral glial tumors and human immunodeficiency virus-1 infection: more than a coincidental association. *Cancer* 1994;74:686–692.

124. Nagib MG, Haines SJ, Erickson DL, Mastri AR. Tuberous sclerosis: a review for the neurosurgeon. *Neurosurgery* 1984;14:93–98.

125. Nakasu S, Nakasu Y, Saito A, Handa J. Intramedullary subependymoma with neurofibromatosis: report of two cases. *Neurol Med Chir* 1992;32:275–280.

126. Nazar GB, Hoffman HJ, Beker LE et al. Infratentorial ependymomas in childhood: prognostic factors and treatment. *J Neurosurg* 1990;72:408–417.

127. Newton HB, Henson J, Walker RW. Extraneural metastases in ependymoma. *J Neurooncol* 1992;14:135–142.

128. Nishizaki T, Orita T, Abiko S, Aoki H, Ito H. Subependymal giant cell astrocytoma associated with tuberous sclerosis: with special reference to cell kinetic studies—case report. *Neurol Med Chir* 1990;30:695–697.

129. Nishio S, Takeshita I, Kaneko Y, Fukui M. Cerebral neurocytoma: a new subset of benign neuronal tumors of the cerebrum. *Cancer* 1992;70:529–537.

130. Okamura A, Goto S, Sato K, Ushio Y. Central neurocytoma with hemorrhagic onset. *Surg Neurol* 1995;43:252–255.

131. Ostertun B, Wolf HK, Campos MG, et al. Dysembryoplastic neuroepithelial tumors: MR and CT evaluation. *Am J Neuroradiol* 1996;17:419–430.

132. Otsubo H, Hoffman HJ, Humphreys RP, et al. Evaluation, surgical approach and outcome of seizure patients with gangliogliomas. *Pediatr Neurosurg* 1990–91;16:208–212.

133. Palma L, Celli P, Cantore G. Supratentorial ependymomas of the first two decades of life: long-term follow-up of 20 cases (including two subependymomas). *Neurosurgery* 1993;32:169–175.

134. Palma L, Maleci A, Di Lorenzo N, et al. Pleomorphic xanthoastrocytoma with 18-year survival: case report. *J Neurosurg* 1985;63:808–810.

135. Palma L, Russo A, Mercuri S. Cystic cerebral astrocytomas in infancy and childhood: long-term results. *Childs Brain* 1983;10:79–91.

136. Parkkila AK, Herva R, Parkkila S, Rajaniemi H. Immunohistochemical demonstration of human carbonic anhydrase isoenzyme II in brain tumours. *Histochem J* 1995;27:974–982.

137. Paulus W, Peiffer J. Does the PXA exist? Problems in the application of immunological techniques to the classification of brain tumors. *Acta Neuropathol* 1988;76:245–252.

138. Perkins OC. Ganglioglioma. *Arch Pathol Lab Med* 1926;2:11–17.

139. Petronio J, Edwards MS, Prados M, et al. Management of chiasmal and hypothalamic gliomas of infancy and childhood with chemotherapy. *J Neurosurg* 1991;74:701–708.

140. Pierre-Kahn A, Hirsch JF, Roux FX, et al. Intracranial ependymomas ion childhood. *Childs Brain* 1983;10:145–156.

141. Pilcher WH, Silbergeld DL, Berger MS, Ojemann GA. Intraoperative electrocorticography during tumor resection: impact on seizure outcome in patients with gangliogliomas. *J Neurosurg* 1993;78:891–902.

142. Pizer BL, Moss T, Oakhill A, Webb D, Coakham HB. Congenital astroblastoma: an immunohistochemical study. Case report. *J Neurosurg* 1995;83:550–555.

143. Prayson RA, Estes ML, Morris HH. Coexistence of neoplasia and cortical dysplasia in patients presenting with seizures. *Epilepsia* 1993;34:609–615.

144. Prayson RA, Morris HH, Estes ML, Comair YG. Dysembryoplastic neuroepithelial tumor: a clinicopathologic and immunohistochemical study of 11 tumors including MIB1 immunoreactivity. *Clin Neuropathol* 1996;15:47–53.

145. Puchner MJ, Ludecke DK, Saeger W, Riedel M, Asa SL. Gangliocytomas of the sellar region: a review. *Exp Clin Endocrinol Diabetes* 1995;103:129–149.

146. Rabinowicz AL, Abrey LE, Hinton DR, Couldwell WT. Cerebral neurocytoma: an unusual cause of refractory epilepsy. Case report and review of the literature. *Epilepsia* 1995;36:1237–1240.

147. Raymond AA, Halpin SF, Alsanjari N, et al. Dysembryoplastic neuroepithelial tumor: features in 16 patients. *Brain* 1994;117:461–475.

148. Reiche W, Kolles H, Eymann R, Feiden W. [Dysembryoplastic neuroepithelial tumor (DNT). Pattern of neuroradiologic findings]. *Radiologe* 1996;36:884–889.

149. Rippe DJ, Boyko OB, Radi M, et al. MRI of temporal lobe PXA. *J Comput Assist Tomogr* 1992;16:856–859.

150. Roche PH, Malca S, Gambarelli D, Pellet W. Giant central neurocytoma with tetraventricular and extraaxial extension: case report. *Acta Neurochir* 1995;133:95–100.

151. Rodriguez MI, Chandrasoma P. The pathology of benign cerebral astrocytomas. In: Apuzzo MLJ, ed. *Benign cerebral glioma*, vol. I. Park Ridge, IL: American Association of Neurological Surgeons, 1995:55–82.

152. Ross GW, Rubenstein LJ. Lack of histopathologic correlation of malignant ependymomas with postoperative survival. *J Neurosurg* 1989;70:31–36.

153. Rovit RL, Schechter MM, Chordoff P. Choroid plexus papillomas: observations on radiographic diagnosis. *Am J Radiol* 1970;10:608–611.

154. Rubinstein LJ. Clinical correlations of malignant ependymomas. In: Fields WS, ed. *Primary brain tumors; a review of histologic classification*. New York: Springer-Verlag, 1989:191–194.

155. Ruchoux MM, Gray F, Gherardi R, Schaeffer A, Comoy J, Poirier J. Orthostatic hypotension from a cerebellar gangliocytoma (Lhermitte-Duclos disease): case report. *J Neurosurg* 1986;65:245–248.

156. Russell DS, Rubinstein LJ. Ganglioglioma: a case with long history and malignant evolution. *J Neuropathol Exp Neurol* 1962;21:185–193.

157. Russell DS, Rubinstein LJ. *Pathology of tumors of the nervous system*, 5th ed. London: Edward Arnold, 1989.

158. Russo CP, Katz DS, Corona RJ Jr, Winfield JA. Gangliocytoma of the cervicothoracic spinal cord. *Am J Neuroradiol* 1995;16:889–891.

159. Ryken TC, Robinson RA, VanGilder JC. Familial occurrence of subependymoma: report of two cases. *J Neurosurg* 1994;80:1108–1111.

160. Sarkar C, Roy S, Bhatia S. Xanthomatous change in tumours of glial origin. *Ind J Med Res* 1990;92:324–331.

161. Sasaki A, Hirato J, Nakazato Y, Tamura M, Kadowaki H. Recurrent anaplastic ganglioglioma: pathological characterization of tumor cells. Case report. *J Neurosurg* 1996;84:1055–1059.

162. Sato T, Takeichi M, Abe M, Tabuchi K, Hara T. Frontal lobe tumor associated with late-onset seizure and psychosis: a case report. *Jpn J Psychiatr Neurol* 1993;47:541–544.

163. Schienker IM. Subependymoma: a newly recognized tumor of the subependymal derivation. *J Neurosurg* 1945;2:232–245.

164. Scheithauer BW, Kovacs K, Randall RV, Horvath E, Laws ER Jr. Pathology of excessive production of growth hormone. *Clin Endocrinol Metab* 1986;15:655–681.

165. Schwarz KO, Perper JA, Rozin L. Sudden, unexpected death due to fourth ventricular subependymoma. *Am J Foren Med Pathol* 1987;8:153–157.

166. Seiki Y, Terao H, Shibata I, Tsukahara K, Tsutsumi S, Kudo M. [A case of subependymoma in the lateral ventricle with intraventricular hemorrhage] [Japanese]. *No Shinkei Geka* [*Neurol Surg*] 1984;12:761–765.

167. Shaw EG, Daumas-Duport C, Scheithauer BW, et al. Radiation therapy in the management of low grade supratentorial astrocytomas. *J Neurosurg* 1989;70:853–861.

168. Shepherd CW, Scheithauer BW, Gomez MR, Altermatt HJ, Katzmann JA. Subependymal giant cell astrocytoma: a clinical, pathological, and flow cytometric study. *Neurosurgery* 1991;28:864–888.

169. Silver JM, Rawlings CE 3d, Rossitch E Jr, Zeidman SM, Friedman AH. Ganglioglioma: a clinical study with long-term follow-up. *Surg Neurol* 1991;35:261–266.

170. Soontornniyomkij V, Schelper RI. Pontine neurocytoma. *J Clin Pathol* 1996;49:764–765.

171. Stapleton SR, Wilkins PR, Bell BA. Recurrent dysplastic cerebellar gangliocytoma (Lhermitte-Duclos disease) presenting with subarachnoid haemorrhage. *Br J Neurosurg* 1992;6:153–156.

172. Starnik TM, van der Veen JPW, Arwerk F, et al. The Cowden syndrome: a clinical and genetic study in 21 patients. *Clin Genet* 1986;29:222–233.

173. Stuart G, Appleton DB, Cooke R. Pleomorphic xanthoastrocytoma: report of two cases. *Neurosurgery* 1988;22:422–427.

174. Sugita Y, Kepes JJ, Shigemori M, et al. PXA with desmoplastic reaction: angiomatous variant. Report of two cases. *Clin Neuropathol* 1990;9:271–278.

175. Sutton LN, Packer RJ, Rorke LB, Bruce DA, Schut L. Cerebral gangliogliomas during childhood. *Neurosurgery* 1983;13:124–128.

176. Tacconi L, Delfini R, Cantore G. Choroid plexus papillomas: consideration of a surgical series of 33 cases. *Acta Neurochir* 1996;138:802–810.

177. Tacconi L, Johnston FG, Thomas DG. Subependymoma of the cervical cord. *Clin Neurol Neurosurg* 1996;98:24–26.

178. Tolnay M, Kaim A, Probst A, Ulrich J. Subependymoma of the third ventricle after partial resection of a craniopharyngioma and repeated postoperative irradiation. *Clin Neuropathol* 1996;15:63–66.

179. Tomita T, McLone DG, Naidich TP. Mural tumors with cysts in the cerebral hemispheres of children. *Neurosurgery* 1986;19:998–1005.

180. Tonn JC, Paulus W, Warmuth-Metz M, Schachenmayr W, Sorensen N, Roosen K. Pleomorphic xanthoastrocytoma: report of six cases with special consideration of diagnostic and therapeutic pitfalls. *Surg Neurol* 1997;47:162–169.

181. Vinchon M, Blond S, Lejeune JP, et al. Association of Lhermitte-Duclos and Cowden disease: report of a new case and review of the literature. *J Neurol Neurosurg Psychiatry* 1994;57:699–704.

182. Virchow R. Die Krankhaften Geschulste. Berlin: August Hirschwald, 1864–1865.

183. Vogt H. Zur pathologie und pathologishen Anatomie der verschiedinen idiotie-formen: tuberose sklerose. *Monatsschrift Psychiatry Neurology* 1908;24:106–150.

184. Von Deimling A, Janzer R, Kleihues P, Wiestler OD. Patterns of differentiation in central neurocytoma: an immunohistochemical study of eleven biopsies. *Acta Neuropathol* 1990;79:473–479.

185. Wacker MR, Cogen PH, Etzell JE, Daneshvar L, Davis RL, Prados MD. Diffuse leptomeningeal involvement by a ganglioglioma in a child: case report. *J Neurosurg* 1992;77:302–306.

186. Wallner KE, Gonzales MF, Edwards MS, Wara WM, Sheline GE. Treatment results of juvenile pilocytic astrocytoma. *J Neurosurg* 1988;69:171–176.

187. Wasdahl DA, Scheithauer BW, Andrews BT, Jeffrey RA. Cerebellar PXA: case report. *Neurosurgery* 1994;35:947–950.

188. Weldon-Linne CM, Victor TA, Groothius DR, Vick NA. Pleomorphic xanthoastrocytoma: ultrastructural and immunohistochemical study of a case with a rapidly fatal outcome following surgery. *Cancer* 1983;52:2055–2063.

189. Wells GB, Lasner TM, Yousem DM, Zager EL. Lhermitte-Duclos disease and Cowden's syndrome in an adolescent patient: case report. *J Neurosurg* 1994;81:133–136.

190. Whittle IR. Anterior lateral ventricular subependymal giant cell astrocytomas: microsurgical aspects of two cases. *Acta Neurochir* 1992;118:176–180.

191. Whittle IR, Gordon A, Misra BK, et al. Pleomorphic xanthoastrocytoma: report of four cases. *J Neurosurg* 1989;70:463–468.

192. Williams DW 3d, Elster AD, Ginsberg LE, Stanton C. Recurrent Lhermitte-Duclos disease: report of two

cases and association with Cowden's disease. *Am J Neuroradiol* 1992;13:287–290.

193. Wolf HK, Campos MG, Zentner J, et al. Surgical pathology of temporal lobe epilepsy: experience with 216 cases. *J Neuropathol Exp Neurol* 1993;52:499–506.

194. Wolf HK, Muller MB, Spanle M, Zentner J, Schramm J, Wiestler OD. Ganglioglioma: a detailed histopathological and immunohistochemical analysis of 61 cases. *Acta Neuropathol* 1994;88:166–173.

195. Wyllie E, Luders H, Morris HH III, et al. Clinical outcome after complete or partial cortical resection for intractable epilepsy. *Neurology* 1987;37:1634–1641.

196. Yamasaki T, Kikuchi H, Higashi T, Yamabe H, Moritake K. Two surgically cured cases of subependymoma with emphasis on magnetic resonance imaging. *Surg Neurol* 1990;33:329–335.

197. Yasargil MG, von Ammon K, von Deimling A, Valavanis A, Wichmann W, Wiestler OD. Central neurocytoma: histopathological variants and therapeutic approaches. *J Neurosurg* 1992;76:32–37.

198. Yoshino MR, Lucio R. Pleomorphic xanthoastrocytoma. *AJNR* 1992;13:1330–1332.

199. Yunten N, Ersahin Y, Demirtas E, Yalman O, Sener RN. Cerebral astroblastoma resembling an extra-axial neoplasm. *J Neuroradiol* 1996;23:38–40.

200. Zentner J, Wolf HK, Ostertun B, et al. Gangliogliomas: clinical, radiological, and histopathological findings in 51 patients. *J Neurol Neurosurg Psychiatry* 1994;57:1497–502.

Common Management Issues for the Practitioner

The Practical Management of Low-Grade Primary Brain
Tumors, edited by Jack P. Rock, Mark L. Rosenblum,
Edward G. Shaw, and J. Gregory Cairncross.
Lippincott Williams & Wilkins, Philadelphia, © 1999

9

Adult Low-Grade Gliomas: Natural History, Prognostic Factors, and Timing of Treatment

Joseph O. Bampoe, Glenn Bauman, J. Gregory Cairncross, and Mark Bernstein

*J. O. Bampoe and M. Bernstein: Division of Neurosurgery, The Toronto Hospital, Western Division,
University of Toronto, Toronto, Ontario M5T 2S8 Canada
G. Bauman and J. G. Cairncross: Departments of Clinical Neurological Sciences and Oncology,
University of Western Ontario, and London Regional Cancer Centre, London, Ontario N6A 4L6 Canada*

Approximately 12,000 brain tumors are diagnosed each year in the United States. Of the primary brain tumors of glial origin (which comprise about 50% of the total), low-grade astrocytomas constitute about 30% (16,77). Age at diagnosis is an important determinant of outcome, with low-grade tumors being more indolent in younger patients, but whether these neoplasms are biologically distinct or simply diagnosed at an earlier time in a protracted natural history is unknown. The incidence of low-grade glioma in the different age groups has been estimated at 21% to 45% of gliomas in children and 10% to 15% of gliomas in adults (11,16,78).

The management of low-grade gliomas has given rise to a considerable amount of controversy, generated in part by a higher prevalence in the younger section of the population, many of whom have demonstrated a prolonged and meaningful quality of survival with different management strategies. The advent of accurate and convenient neuroimaging, especially magnetic resonance imaging (MRI), has resulted in more patients with low-grade glioma and minimal neurologic symptoms or deficits being diagnosed at an earlier stage. The benefits of the various strategies for the management of a younger,

less symptomatic patient population have been much debated because the precise impact of various treatments on the natural history of the disease is not altogether obvious and the treatments can result in toxicity. Until the results of the randomized phase III trial by the European Organization for Research and Treatment of Cancer (EORTC trial 22845) become available, it may be impossible to set standards for the management of low-grade glioma (85,87), although the results of the first EORTC trial suggest that radiation dose is less important than other factors (43). The difficulties in designing such trials have included the relatively low incidence of low-grade gliomas, the long follow-up necessary for this indolent disease, and physician bias in recommending treatment. Current reports of their management in the world literature are predominantly descriptive and observational. Factors unrelated to treatment, such as tumor histology and size, or age of patients at presentation, being intrinsic to tumors, can theoretically be analyzed in a retrospective study as accurately as with a prospective study (93). An analysis of retrospective studies on the effects of different treatments on the natural history of low-grade glioma can, as in this chapter, only recommend options for patient management (85).

NATURAL HISTORY AND PROGNOSTIC FACTORS

Histology

The difficulties in determining the natural history of low-grade gliomas can be largely accounted for by the inclusion of subgroups of tumors with different behavior and prognosis under the same histologic diagnoses and designation (43,70,90). The natural history of low-grade gliomas in most instances is of progressive growth with eventual malignant transformation (55). Some patients do, however, die of progressive low-grade disease (42,59,96).

The most favorable subgroup is that of the pilocytic astrocytoma. These are well-circumscribed, contrast-enhancing neoplasms with solid and cystic components (32,78: 105–108). Vascular proliferation in pilocytic astrocytomas does not signify a malignant phenotype, and these tumors are designated grade I under the current World Health Organization (WHO) classification (11,46). Pilocytic astrocytomas predominate in the pediatric population, with a median age of onset at diagnosis of 14 years (36). These tumors are typically confined to the optic nerve and its radiations, hypothalamus and third ventricular regions, and the cerebellum. Less commonly, they arise in the cerebral hemispheres or brain stem. They are more amenable to complete resection than other low-grade gliomas and, even without complete resection, can behave indolently, with prolonged survival, estimated at 80% to 100% at 10 and 20 years (28,74,98).

Another subtype with a relatively favorable prognosis is the oligodendroglioma. These lesions characteristically exhibit slow growth with a long natural history (89) and tend to be relatively more common in patients presenting with seizures (43,55,91,103). Low-grade oligodendrogliomas (designated grade II by the current WHO classification) have been variably reported with, or separate from, ordi-

nary astrocytoma in the literature and may have biased the survival rates found in these studies. Tumors of mixed oligodendroglial and astrocytic content have a prognosis between that of low-grade astrocytoma and oligodendrogliomas (43,88), and are inconsistently grouped with astrocytoma and oligodendroglioma in the available reports.

Rare tumors with exceptionally good prognosis that are associated with intractable epilepsy in the younger age groups include pleomorphic xanthoastrocytomas, desmoplastic infantile ganglioglioma, and dysembryoplastic neuroepithelial tumors (5,8,45,46, 70).

Fibrillary astrocytomas are the most common low-grade glioma. They affect an older section of the population, with a median age at diagnosis of approximately 35 years (54,59, 60,69,80). They are infiltrative neoplasms that expand and distort the regions from which they originate. Cortical infiltration by low-grade astrocytoma is manifested as gyral expansion with distortion of the gray/white junction, and in the white matter neoplastic cells interdigitate with normal tissue and fiber tracts, making it impossible to define their boundaries.

Some investigators have associated the clinical behavior and rates of proliferation of low-grade astrocytomas with their astrocytic lineage: slow-growing, cortically based astrocytoma being associated with a type 1 (protoplasmic) astrocytic lineage, whereas white matter low-grade astrocytomas have been found to express antigens consistent with a type 2 (fibrillary) astrocytic lineage (72).

Microscopically, low-grade astrocytoma appears as hypercellular regions within white matter. The histologic definition of these tumors has, until recently, been largely subjective (21), with the distinction being made between benign and malignant astrocytomas and therefore the selection of individual patients for aggressive therapy remaining largely arbitrary (21). Of note, neither the previous WHO (101), the Burger (11), nor the Nelson (66) classifications use exclusive or measurable histologic criteria for the identification of low-grade glioma. In the current revised WHO classification, grading of astrocytomas is based on the presence of nuclear atypia, mitosis, endothelial proliferation, and necrosis (46). In fibrillary astrocytomas, only nuclear atypia can be present. The presence of both nuclear atypia and mitosis qualifies a neoplasm as an anaplastic astrocytoma, which requires more aggressive management with adjuvant radiation therapy and chemotherapy (84). The current WHO classification of astrocytoma is basically identical to the St. Anne/Mayo scheme and has been found to have accurate interobserver reproducibility (22), to be more accurately discriminative in predicting survival among the different grades (41,87,99), and to correlate more closely with proliferation indices than other grading systems (50,62). The importance of histologic grade in determining the natural history of nonpilocytic astrocytoma is evident in the reports of treatment of low-grade astrocytoma in the computed tomography (CT) era. Reports with the longer median survival exclude tumors with both nuclear atypia and mitosis (grade III, WHO) (Table 1).

Finally, the gemistocytic variant of diffuse fibrillary astrocytoma has been associated with poor prognosis. These tumors are often treated as malignant astrocytomas, although they may only be found as a component of an otherwise unremarkable low-grade fibrillary astrocytoma (9,25,33,54,78:111–114). An autoradiographic study of the proliferation rate of gemistocytes has indicated, however, that these cells may only secondarily indicate malignancy, reflecting profound proliferative activity in adjacent neoplastic cells. The gemistocytes themselves were found to multiply slowly, if at all (39).

Age

The age of patients at presentation is another crucial determinant of the natural history of low-grade gliomas. In perhaps the largest study of low-grade glioma in the medical literature, involving 461 patients with this disease treated at the Mayo Clinic, Laws et al. (51) found that patients who were younger than 20 years had a 5-year survival of more than 80%, with a progressive decrease in survival of 60% to 35% for those in the 20- to 50-year age group and of less than 30% for those in the over-50 age group. Several other investigators have found age to be independently related to survival in low-grade glioma (43, 60,67,70,91,103). An observation that indicates the importance of tumor biology in determining survival is the inverse relationship

TABLE 1. *Effect of histological grading on median survival of nonpilocytic astrocytoma (Grades I and II) treated in the CT era*

Author	Grading system (criteria included)	Number of patients in the study	Benefit of surgery	Benefit of radiation	Median Survival/ Years
Lunsford (1995)	Burger Nuclear atypia allowed. No mitosis	35	All patients had stereotactic biopsy	All patients had radiation	9.8
Philippon (1993)	?St Anne/Mayo Nuclear atypia allowed. No mitosis	179	Total resection beneficial	Radiation beneficial only for patients over 40 years old	9.0
Vertosick (1991)	Kernohan No pleomorphism, no mention of mitosis	25	Most only had biopsy	No effect	8.2
Leighton (1997)	Kernohan/modified Ringertz/WHO	89	Residual tumor Disadvantageous	Comparison of early radiation therapy vs late	7.5
McCormack (1992)	? Grading system. Some tumors had both nuclear atypia and mitosis	53	—	—	7.2

between age and expected median survival: 20-year-olds with low-grade glioma live for approximately 25 years; 30-year-olds, for 15 years; 40-year-olds, for 5 years; and 44-year-olds, for approximately 1 year after diagnosis despite the treatment modality. Arguably, this phenomenon represents the manifestations of the same disease in the different age groups. A possible explanation of the relationship between age and median or 5-year survival is the obvious predominance of indolent or slower-growing histologic subtypes in the younger age groups. Whether tumors in this age group are biologically distinct or just detected earlier in their natural history (lead time bias) is unknown. A few investigators have, however, found no independent relationship between age and outcome in low-grade gliomas when multivariate techniques are used to separate the two prognostic factors (33,79,92). A principle that has been established from the management of patients with glioma, taking into consideration both the age of patients at presentation and the histology of their tumors, is that younger patients with high-grade malignant glioma with identical histology have a better prognosis than elderly patients. The survival of younger patients with high-grade tumors is actually better than that of older patients with low-grade tumors at presentation (20,52,80,95). This principle is applicable to the timing of intervention for patients with presumed low-grade glioma. An observation made by some investigators that might explain to some extent the difference in biology and hence the prognosis of patients with low-grade glioma in the different age groups is the finding that the proportion of gemistocytes in benign astrocytic tumors increases with age (102). Gemistocytic tumors have been associated with inferior survival times after adjusting for the effects of other covariates (87).

Other Prognostic Factors

Method of Diagnosis

The median survival of patients with low-grade glioma reported in the various series in the literature has shown a marked improvement with the advent of noninvasive and accurate neuroimaging. This probably represents a lead-time bias, with the apparent natural history of this disease being extended, because imaging diagnosis is possible at an earlier stage of the disease (55,70,96). An analysis of the study populations of patients in the era before and after the availability of CT (and lately MRI) illustrates this difference. Recent reports have estimated the overall median survival of patients treated with a variety of modalities at more than 9 years (55,61,69,70) (see Table 1). The typical imaging features for adults with supratentorial astrocytoma (which constitute the bulk of low-grade glioma) are (a) a low-attenuation mass lesion on CT that does not enhance with contrast agents, (b) low signal intensity on T1-weighted MRI with absence of contrast enhancement, and (c) high signal intensity on T2-weighted imaging (48). These typical features, however, are only found in 60% to 70% of cases (100). Recent reports have documented a varying proportion of patients with contrast-enhancing tumors in histologically verified low-grade glioma. In the series by McCormack et al. (59) of 53 cases of adult supratentorial astrocytoma, 30% of patients had contrast-enhancing tumors, a finding noted in 21.7% of 60 patients with astrocytic tumors (includes seven patients with mixed astro/oligodendroglioma and three with pleomorphic xanthoastrocytoma) reported by Piepmeier et al. (70) and in 28% of 167 patients with low-grade glioma reported by Leighton et al. (55). A notable finding in the two series from Pittsburgh, with two of the three longest median survival times reported for the treatment of nonpilocytic astrocytic tumors, is the relatively small percentage of contrast-enhancing tumors: Vertosick et al. (96) (median survival of 25 patients was 8.2 years) reported only 8% of patients with contrast-enhancing tumors, and Lunsford et al. (56) (median survival of 35 patients was 9.8 years) reported 14% of patients with contrast-enhancing tumors.

Although some investigators have found no significance in the prognostic value of contrast enhancement for the prediction of survival of patients with low-grade glioma (69,90), it is well-established that contrast enhancement is a function of blood/brain barrier abnormality and capillary permeability (90). It is a diagnostic feature in nearly 100% of glioblastomas (grade IV astrocytomas) (12, 17), a key histologic diagnostic requirement of which is endothelial proliferation (46). Several investigators have found contrast enhancement of tumors on imaging to be an independent prognostic factor for either survival or progression-free survival (59,70,91).

Clinical Presentation

The beneficial effect of a good clinical condition on presentation on predicting outcome is apparent in several reports in the literature. Patients presenting with a normal interictal examination and chronic seizures have the best prognosis. In the study by Laws et al. (51) of 461 patients spanning the six decades before the availability of CT, only 38% of patients treated were known not to have a performance deficit preoperatively, and the proportion of patients known not to have any preoperative neurologic deficit was 47%. Only 40% of patients presented with seizures and 22% presented with papilledema. The approximate median survival of all patients was 4 years. In contrast, in the study by McCormack et al. (59) of 53 patients with low-grade astrocytoma presenting between 1977 and 1988, 66% of patients were neurologically intact preoperatively and 68% presented with

seizures. The median survival of patients treated in this study was 7.25 years. Similarly, in the study by Vertosick et al. (96) of 25 patients with astrocytoma treated from 1978 to 1988, 92% of whom presented with seizures and only 8% of whom presented with papilledema, the median survival of all patients was 8.2 years. The findings of two recently published studies from the London Regional Cancer Centre and the Yale University School of Medicine further support these observations (55,71) (Table 2).

Gender

Most reported studies show no influence of gender on the overall survival of patients with low-grade glioma (43,51,59,60,61,70,92,93). A few have suggested either a statistically significant advantage for females (67,80,87) or a disadvantage (49).

Preoperative Tumor Volume

An important finding of the recently reported randomized study by the EORTC on radiation dose in the treatment of low-grade glioma concerns the relationship of tumor size and location in predicting survival (43). The T parameters of the TNM (tumor, node, metastasis) staging classification proposed were found to be significantly discriminant for prognosis for overall survival as well as for progression-free survival. After accounting for the effects of histology, patients with the best prognosis were young patients with

TABLE 2. *The effect of deferred radiation treatment on outcome of patients with low-grade glioma*

Author/ Years of study	Number of Patients/% with seizures	Histologies included	% of patients with deferred RT	Overall median survival (years)	? Difference in outcome between initial and deferred RT
Bahary 1974–1992	63/no significance	Astrocytomas, mixed oligoastrocytomas	32	Not stated (approximately 9)	No significance
Piepmeier 1982–1990	55/94.5	Astrocytomas (possibly other histologies)	20	12	No significance
Leighton 1979–1995	167/78	Astrocytomas, mixed glioma, oligodendroglioma	52	10.5	No significance (on multivariate analysis)

unifocal tumors less than 3 cm in greatest diameter situated away from the midline and with minimal neurologic deficit. Several other investigators, some using quantitative volumetric methods, have demonstrated the tendency for larger tumors to behave differently with a less favorable prognosis (they recur sooner after excision or exhibit a greater tendency toward malignant evolution) (3,4, 49).

Proliferation Markers and Survival

The difficulties in estimating the prognosis of brain tumors have led to the increasing use of proliferation markers as an adjunct to routine histologic techniques. Theoretically, they offer a more objective way of estimating malignancy and, by implication, predicting the survival of patients with these tumors (21,62). Methods that have been used to estimate the proliferative activity of low-grade glioma (the percentage of the total number of cells in proliferative phases of the cell cycle) include silver staining of nucleolar organizer regions (AgNORs) (a measure of ribosomal gene activity that correlates with the degree of tumor malignancy [35,73]) and immunohistochemical techniques for evaluating the percentage of cells labeled by the monoclonal antibody Ki-67 or for estimating the percentage of cycling cells by targeting proliferating cell nuclear antigens (PCNAs) (2,62). Some investigators have correlated the S-phase fraction, as determined by flow cytometry, with the survival of patients with oligodendroglioma and oligoastroctyoma (18).

Hoshino et al. (37,38,40) have used immunohistochemical techniques to investigate extensively the bromodeoxyuridine and iododeoxyuridine labeling indices of low-grade glioma and their relation to survival of patients with these tumors. The association between labeling indices and other prognostic factors such as age and histologic grading systems has also been investigated (18,30,50).

A few important conclusions can be drawn from these studies. First, although several proliferative parameters have been correlated with the survival of patients with low-grade glioma, discordances are observed between the labeling indices and the clinical behavior of different histologic subgroups (21). Second, reproducibility of results is also a severe limitation on the predictive value of kinetic methods. Some investigators report interobserver deviation of up to 23% in some reports (82). This is compounded by the known problem of sampling error in glioma—the region of tumor biopsied for these studies may not have the highest proliferative activity.

Some practical points that might be applicable to the management of patients with low-grade glioma are the following:

1. Low-grade astrocytoma may be segregated according to BUdR labeling index, those with an index ≥1% representing a subset with poorer prognosis than those with an index ≤1% (38,40).
2. The tendency to malignant evolution is greater in older patients with low-grade glioma (>40 years), even though they might demonstrate low labeling indices (30).
3. The St. Anne/Mayo grading system (new WHO) (46) has been found to be more closely correlated with some proliferative indices than other systems and may reflect the proliferative potential of ordinary astrocytomas (50,62).

Detection of Malignant Evolution

A feature of the natural history of low-grade gliomas that affects the timing of their management is their tendency toward malignant degeneration. The incidence of this evolution has been quoted at rates varying between 13% and 86% (51,59,64,70). The utility of positron emission tomography (PET) in detecting malignant degeneration of low-grade glioma and in prognosticating on the survival of these patients has been reported by several investigators (1,20,29,68, 81).

Although some investigators using a larger patient population have reported the predictive ability of a single [^{18}F] fluorodeoxyglucose (FDG) tumor uptake determination in defining the probability of survival (1,23,68), when using a smaller number of subjects serial FDG-PET studies have been found to be more useful (29,81). An important finding in these studies is the demonstration that malignant degeneration in a previously low-grade lesion is usually identified as a focal area of increased glucose metabolism, which supports the hypothesis that anaplastic cells are derived from a clonal cell line (29).

Summary

Clearly, several independent prognostic factors determine the natural history/clinical behavior of low-grade glioma. These include histology, age at diagnosis, and presenting symptoms. Other reported prognostic variables include proliferation indices, volume of disease at presentation, and imaging appearance. Imbalances in these important prognostic variables may severely limit the interpretation of retrospective reports. Interaction of these variables (i.e., most patients with oligodendroglioma are younger and present with seizures) also complicates prediction of outcome. Multivariate analysis, decision tree analysis, and recursive partitioning analysis may be ways to deal with these imbalances.

TIMING OF TREATMENT

Deferred Treatment

Several investigators have noted the absence of standards for the management of patients with low-grade glioma (6,14,63,70), which is basically due to the paucity of randomized controlled trials for the management of this disease. When the management of a disease involves a choice among several treatment options, each with a similar outcome in terms of survival, the expected quality of survival with the different options can help to select the appropriate treatment, especially as our therapies are largely noncurative and sometimes toxic (47). The option of observa-

tion or nontreatment of a patient with a low-grade glioma may therefore be justified if the risks of treatment (surgery and/or radiation therapy) are deemed greater than the risks of the medical treatment of a presenting complaint—usually a seizure or intermittent neurologic complaint (76,91). The wisdom of delaying treatment assumes, of course, that the diagnosis can be confidently made on clinical and imaging grounds with the exclusion of another treatable condition and that the outcome of the patient's management is independent of the time of intervention (76).

Although the risk of incorrectly diagnosing a low-grade glioma using modern neurodiagnostic imaging has been estimated to be as high as 50% (6,17,44)—notably, in the few retrospective cohort-type studies designed to address the questions of delayed treatment of glioma or the adequacy of clinical and neurodiagnostic imaging alone in making management decisions—the management option chosen did not significantly affect the outcome. Rajan et al. (75) found an incidence of only one of 15 patients (6.7%) treated with a presumed diagnosis of glioma to have a nonglial pathology, and no difference was found in the outcome, in terms of survival, between patients with verified and unverified low-grade tumors after correcting for prognostic factors. Recht et al. (76) also found the outcome, in terms of survival or quality of life, of patients treated initially by observation not to be significantly different from cohorts who were treated *ab initio*. In addition, no significant difference was found in the rate of malignant transformation of tumors in patients of both groups if examined from the time of imaging diagnosis. Only one of 20 patients with a presumed diagnosis of low-grade glioma in Recht's series was found to have a nonglial pathology.

Patients selected for observation usually have good prognostic factors: young (less than 35–40 years old), with minimal neurologic or performance deficit, and usually presenting with seizures (43,76). Notably, all patients who developed malignant transformation in the series reported by Recht et al.

were more than 45 years old at the time of imaging diagnosis. This is consistent with the findings of Franzini et al. (30) of the proliferation rates of low-grade gliomas in the different age groups.

The reluctance of some clinicians to initiate aggressive therapy for young patients with normal interictal examination and small, presumedly low-grade tumors that do not show any mass effect on neuroimaging is partly due to the perceived risks of both surgery and radiation therapy. Although the risks of surgery have decreased with the advent of recent technological advances, such as stereotactic biopsy and resections augmented with cortical mapping and intraoperative imaging with frameless navigational devices (7,47,57,104) that help reduce surgical morbidity, morbidity and mortality are still correlated with tumor location (26). Patients with deep tumors or tumors in eloquent cortex remain at significant risk from surgical resection or biopsy (13,26, 44).

The risks of complications from modern radiotherapy have been disputed (14,86). The primary concern has been the incidence of neurocognitive impairment in long-term survivors of low-grade tumors (34). Modern techniques of delivering radiation utilizing modern neuroimaging and treatment (conformal nonopposing radiation beams and moderate doses of 45–59 Gy) are associated with only transient, mild neurocognitive deficits (94,97); however, the long-term effects are unknown. In addition to the other known risks of brain necrosis and pituitary/hypothalamic dysfunction (53,58), recent reports have associated the development of anaplastic changes in children with low-grade astrocytomas with previous radiation therapy (24, 74).

The validity of the deferred treatment policy of a patient with an imaging diagnosis of low-grade glioma is further suggested by Vertosick et al. (96). The patient selection (median age of 25 patients was 32 years, 92% presented with seizures and only 8% presented with papilledema) demonstrates that good prognostic factors are consistent with pro-

longed survival (median survival was 8.2 years), regardless of management strategy because both surgery (20 patients underwent biopsy alone) and radiation therapy were not found to be significantly related to survival, and the use of radiation therapy did not make a significant impact on the time to malignant degeneration of the tumors.

After the decision is made to observe a patient with a presumed diagnosis of low-grade glioma, follow-up usually consists of close monitoring of both clinical and imaging data (6) (Fig. 1). The accuracy of such a strategy in detecting malignant degeneration of the tumor, which would then require aggressive therapy, is suggested by the findings of Francavilla et al. (29). In their study designed to detect the malignant degeneration of low-grade gliomas, this change was generally heralded by new onset seizures, worsening seizures, or impairment of neurologic function and confirmed by PET scanning.

The risk of wrongly selecting a young patient with a noncontrast-enhancing, high-grade glioma for observation (48) seems to be mitigated by the fact that the survival of younger patients with high-grade tumors is actually better than that of older patients with low-grade tumors; in other words, age supersedes histology in prognosticating for survival when other factors are equal (small nonenhancing tumor without mass effect, supratentorial location, lack of papilledema, or other neurologic deficit) (52,80,95).

Timing of Surgery

Surgical intervention eventually becomes necessary when a patient previously selected for deferred therapy presents with imaging evidence of tumor growth or clinical and imaging evidence of malignant transformation of the tumor (76). Also evident from the literature on management of low-grade glioma is that the bulk of the reports were from institutions that either practiced or advocated proceeding with therapy after early histologic diagnosis (by stereotactic biopsy or cytoreductive surgery) (19,27,43,48,51,56,63,

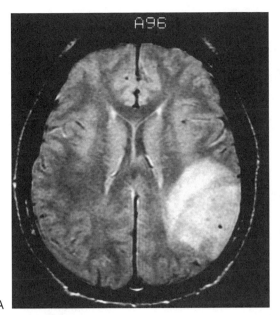
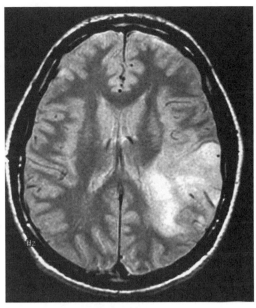

A   B

FIG. 1. A: Proton density-weighted MRI scan of left-sided temporoparietal lesion in a 38-year-old male who presented with right-sided focal sensory seizures and episodic expressive dysphasia. An imaging diagnosis of a low-grade glioma was made 3 years earlier. Patient was managed with antiepileptic medication and serial imaging only. It was decided to defer treatment of the lesion. **B:** Proton density-weighted MRI scan of the patient 6 years after scan shown in Fig. 1(A). Note that the lesion still demonstrates only minimal mass effect. Histologic diagnosis/treatment still deferred 9 years after initial recognition of the lesion, and the patient remains well.

69,83,85,87,101). Patients who have deferred therapy usually do so either because they refused surgery or because their physicians considered the risks of biopsy/resection to be greater than the risks of deferred therapy (63,76). Until the results of randomized phase III studies become available to set the standards for the management of this disease, only reasonable treatment options can be suggested from the analysis of the available literature.

The indications for neurosurgical intervention in patients with intracranial tumors are threefold: histologic, neurologic, and oncologic (19). For histologic reasons, a surgical biopsy is essential in most patients with an intracranial mass lesion. As discussed previously, however, there is no evidence that an imaging diagnosis and deferred therapy of a low-grade glioma in a young person with a single seizure impacts negatively on subsequent survival (76). Although recent reports

have suggested that the optimal treatment for low-grade glioma (least morbidity and mortality with excellent quality of life and prolonged survival) could be stereotactic biopsy *ab initio* with early radiation therapy (48,56, 104), surgical morbidity and mortality in these series are quoted as under 1%. Other investigators have found the complication rates of stereotactic biopsy to be significantly higher (6,7,65) (surgical morbidity up to 7% in some series, with the added problem of false sampling and resulting erroneous diagnosis). This should be considered when deciding on the strategy for management of low-grade glioma patients with good prognosis.

An excellent option for the management of patients with good prognosis is the practice of early histologic diagnosis with either stereotactic biopsy or cytoreductive techniques and deferred radiation therapy with or without biopsy/resection when there is evidence of tumor recurrence or progression (3,55,71). Delayed radiation may allow treatment to be postponed for extended periods or omitted for patients with indolent tumors. This strategy delays any potential side effects of treatment until treatment is clearly indicated (57). The possible risk to patients treated in this fashion is that of early tumor recurrence. Results from recently published observational or cohort type studies have shown that patients with good prognosis may benefit from this approach (see Table 2). The second randomized EORTC trial on radiation therapy of low-grade glioma was designed to address this issue, and its results will help determine the optimum timing of radiation therapy for patients with low-grade glioma (43).

There is less controversy about the value of craniotomy and tumor debulking for improving the quality of life of the patient with glioma, the neurologic indication for surgery. Surgery for tumor debulking in a lesion located in a reasonably accessible position, not crossing the midline or involving the brain stem, is recommended if a patient presents with a tumor with mass effect producing signs of increased intracranial pressure and/or focal neurologic deficit. Debulking may also result in decrease in the quantity of vasogenic edema and therefore decrease steroid requirement, avoiding the risks of chronic steroid use. Technological innovations that have been found to help reduce operative morbidity and mortality while maximizing tumor removal include stereotactic lesionectomy (15,104), awake craniotomy combined with electrophysiologic cortical mapping, and intraoperative imaging with the use of frameless navigational devices. The neurologic indication for surgery can also include surgery for intractable epilepsy caused by low-grade glial tumors. This has been found to be helpful in reducing dependence on antiepileptic medications in patients where toxic levels of medication are required to control seizures (5,8,15, 31). Good results have been reported both with and without the use of intraoperative electrocorticography.

One of the most controversial issues in the management of patients with glioma is the role of cytoreductive surgery in prolonging survival, that is, the oncologic benefit of surgery. In the absence of prospective randomized studies, opinions are varied (51,56, 63,69,70,91). The utility of cytoreductive surgery in prolonging survival in tumors with low proliferative rates has been suggested repeatedly (27,43,51,55,67,69,101). It appears to be an epiphenomenon: patients with tumors that have a low growth fraction and low proliferative rates exhibit prolonged survival with cytoreductive surgery (37,38,40). This is the rationale for the total (curative) resection of lesions in superficial cortical locations (e.g., polar lesions), where surgical morbidity can be minimized.

The importance of tumor biology in predicting outcome is demonstrated by the observation that patients with pilocytic astrocytoma have prolonged survival after gross total resection (100% 10-year survival) and subtotal resection (84% 10-year survival) (28,74, 98). A review of the literature, including results from the recently published randomized phase III trial by the EORTC (43), suggests that patients with a more aggressive tumor biology who should probably receive up-front treatment (biopsy or gross total resection with or without radiation therapy) include those demonstrating any enhancement on neuroimaging, the presence of mass effect on neuroimaging, a lesion that crosses the midline on imaging, presence of papilledema and/or focal neurologic deficit, age more than 40 years, and large lesions (greater than 3–5 cm in greatest diameter). The importance of lesion size and extent of resection in determining outcome was demonstrated by Berger et al. (4) in one of the few quantitative volumetric studies in the literature relating preoperative and postoperative tumor volume to tumor recurrence and incidence of malignant degeneration of low-grade glioma. Patients most at risk of tumor recurrence and malignant degeneration were those with larger preoperative tumors (greater than 30 cm^3) and residual tumor postoperatively.

CONCLUSION

To summarize, from the evidence in the literature:

1. Stereotactic biopsy may be the safest way to confirm the diagnosis for some patients with an imaging diagnosis of low-grade glioma. Some patients may benefit from more aggressive resections, especially those more than 40 years old with larger tumors (>3 cm in greatest diameter) and tumors causing mass effect.

2. There is presently no evidence to suggest that either initial or deferred treatment of patients with an imaging diagnosis of low-grade glioma who have good prognostic factors benefit more with one treatment strategy than with another, including no treatment (Fig. 2). The main determinant of outcome in these patients

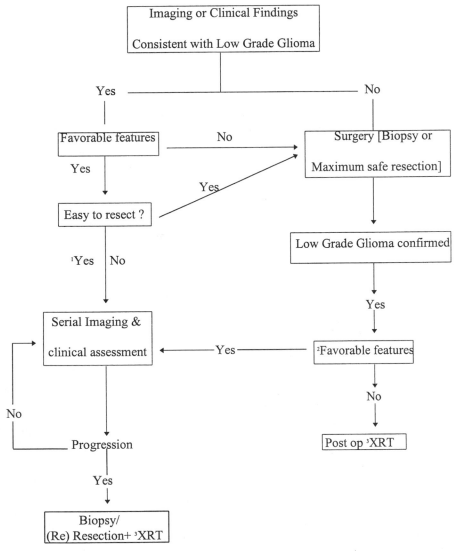

FIG. 2. Algorithm demonstrating management options for low-grade glioma. 1, indicates that serial imaging and observation may still be an option if the patient and/or lesion demonstrate favorable features; 2, favorable features: younger age (<40 yr), oligo/mixed histology, presenting with seizures; 3, XRT, radiotherapy.

(age <35 years, with a small tumor not causing mass effect, presenting with seizures, no papilledema, normal interictal examination) is the biology of the tumor.

REFERENCES

1. Alavi JB, Alavi A, Chawluk J, et al. Positron emission tomography in patients with gliomas: a predictor of prognosis. *Cancer* 1988;62:1074–1078.

2. Allegranza A, Girlando S, Arrigoni GL, et al. Proliferating cell nuclear antigen expression in central nervous system neoplasms. *Virchows Archiv [A]* 1991;419: 417–423.

3. Bahary JP, Villemure JG, Choi S. Low-grade pure and mixed cerebral astrocytomas treated in the CT scan era. *J Neurooncol* 1996;27:173–177.

4. Berger MS, Deliganis AV, Dobbins J, Keles GE. The effect of extent of resection on recurrence in patients with low grade cerebral gliomas. *Cancer* 1994;74: 1784–1791.

5. Berger MS, Ghatan S, Haglund MM, Dobbins J, Ojemann GA. Low-grade gliomas associated with intractable epilepsy: seizure outcome utilizing electrocorticography during tumor resection. *J Neurosurg* 1993;79:62–69.

6. Bernstein M, Guha A. Biopsy of low-grade astrocytomas. *J Neurosurg* 1994;80:776–777.

7. Bernstein M, Parrent AG. Complications of CT-guided stereotactic biopsy of intra-axial brain lesions. *J Neurosurg* 1994;81:165–168.

8. Boon PA, Williamson PD, Fried I, et al. Intracranial, intraaxial, space-occupying lesions in patients with intractable partial seizures: an anatomoclinical, neuropsychological, and surgical correlation. *Epilepsia* 1991;32:467–476.

9. Bouchard J, Peirce C. Radiation therapy in the management of neoplasms of the central nervous system with a special note in regard to children: twenty year's experience, 1939–1958. *Am J Roentgenol* 1960;84: 610–628.

10. Burger P, Scheithauer B. *Tumors of the central nervous system.* Washington: Armed Forces Institute of Pathology, 1994.

11. Burger PC, Vogel FS, Green SB, Strike TA. Glioblastoma multiforme and anaplastic astrocytoma. *Cancer* 1985;56:1106–1111.

12. Butler AR, Horii SC, Kricheff II, Shannon MB, Budzilovich GN. Computed tomography in astrocytomas. *Radiology* 1978;129:433–439.

13. Cabantong AM, Bernstein M. Complications of first craniotomy for intra-axial brain tumour. *Can J Neurol Sci* 1994;21:213–218.

14. Cairncross JG, Laperriere NJ. Low-grade glioma: to treat or not to treat? *Arch Neurol* 1989;46:1238–1239.

15. Cascino GD, Kelly PJ, Sharbrough FW, Hulihan JF, Hirschorn KA, Trenerry MR. Long-term follow-up of stereotactic lesionectomy in partial epilepsy: predictive factors and electroencephalographic results. *Epilepsia* 1992;33:639–644.

16. CBTRUS: 1995 Annual report. Central brain tumor registry of the United States (CBTRUS), 1996.

17. Chamberlain MC, Murovic JA, Levin VA. Absence of contrast enhancement on CT brain scans of patients with supratentorial malignant gliomas. *Neurology* 1988;38:1371–1374.

18. Coons SW, Johnson PC, Pearl DK, Astrid G, Olafsen MS. Prognostic significance of flow cytometry deoxyribonucleic acid analysis of human oligodendrogliomas. *Neurosurgery* 1994;34:680–687.

19. Curran WJ. Should patients with histologically unverified brain tumors receive cranial irradiation? *Int J Rad Oncol Biol Phys* 1993;28:549–550.

20. Curran WJ, Scott CB, Horton J, et al. Recursive partitioning analysis in three Radiation Therapy Oncology Group malignant glioma trials. *J Natl Cancer Inst* 1993;85:704–710.

21. Daumas-Duport C. Histological grading of gliomas. *Curr Opin Neurol Neurosurg* 1992;5:924–931.

22. Daumas-Duport C, Scheithauer B, O Fallon J, Kelly P. Grading of astrocytomas: a simple and reproducible method. *Cancer* 1988;62:2152–2165.

23. Di Chiro G. Positron emission tomography using [F-18] fluorodeoxyglucose in brain tumors: a powerful diagnostic and prognostic tool. *Invest Radiol* 1986;22: 360–371.

24. Dirks PB, Jay V, Becker LE, et al. Development of anaplastic changes in low-grade astrocytomas of childhood. *Neurosurgery* 1994;34:68–78.

25. Elvidge A. Long-term survival in the astrocytoma series. *J Neurosurg* 1968;28:399–404.

26. Fadul C, Wood J, Thaler H, Galicich J, Patterson RH, Posner JB. Morbidity and mortality of craniotomy for excision of supratentorial gliomas. *Neurology* 1988; 38:1374–1379.

27. Fazekas JT. Treatment of grades I and II brain astrocytomas. The role of radiotherapy. *Int J Rad Oncol Biol Phys* 1977;2:661–666.

28. Forsyth PA, Shaw EG, Scheithauer BW, O'Fallon JR, Layton DD, Katzman JA. Supratentorial pilocytic astrocytomas: a clinicopathologic, prognostic, and flow cytometric study of 51 patients. *Cancer* 1993;72: 1335–1342.

29. Francavilla TL, Miletich RS, Di Chiro G, Patronas NJ, Rizzoli HV, Wright DC. Positron emission tomography in the detection of malignant degeneration of low-grade gliomas. *Neurosurgery* 1989;24:1–5.

30. Franzini A, Leocata F, Cajola L, Servello D, Allegranza A, Broggi G. Low-grade glial tumors in basal ganglia and thalamus: natural history and biological reappraisal. *Neurosurgery* 1994;35:817–821.

31. Fried I, Kim JH, Spencer DD. Limbic and neocortical gliomas associated with intractable seizures: a distinct clinicopathological group. *Neurosurgery* 1994;34: 815–824.

32. Fulham MJ, Melisi JW, Nishimiya J, Dwyer AJ, Dichiro G. Neuroimaging of juvenile pilocytic astrocytomas: an enigma. *Radiology* 1993;189:221–225.

33. Garcia D, Fulling K, Marks J. The value of radiation therapy in addition to surgery for astrocytomas of the adult cerebrum. *Cancer* 1985;55:919–927.

34. Gregor A, Cull A, Traynor E, Stewart M, Lander F, Love S. Neuropsychometric evaluation of long-term survivors of adult brain tumours: relationship with tumour and treatment parameters. *Radiother Oncol* 1996;41:55–59.

35. Hara A, Sakai N, Yamada H, Hirayama H, Tanaka T,

Mori H. Nuclear organizer regions in vascular and neoplastic cells of human gliomas. *Neurosurgery* 1991;29:211–215.

36. Hoffman H. Supratentorial brain tumors in children. In: Youmans J, ed. *Neurological surgery*. Philadelphia: WB Saunders, 1982:2710.

37. Hoshino T. A commentary on the biology and kinetics of low-grade and high-grade gliomas. *J Neurosurg* 1984;61:895–900.

38. Hoshino T, Rodriguez LA, Kyung G. Prognostic implications of the proliferative potential of low-grade astrocytomas. *J Neurosurg* 1988;69: 839–842.

39. Hoshino T, Wilson BC, Ellis WG. Gemistocytic astrocytes in gliomas: an autoradiographic study. *J Neuropathol Exp Neurol* 1975;34:263–281.

40. Ito S, Chandler KL, Prados MD, et al. Proliferative potential and prognostic evaluation of low-grade astrocytomas. *J Neurooncol* 1994;19:1–9.

41. Janny P, Cure H, Mohr M, et al. Low grade supratentorial astrocytomas: management and prognostic factors. *Cancer* 1994;73:1937–1945.

42. Jubelirer SJ, Rubin M, Shim C. An analysis of 38 cases of low-grade cerebral astrocytoma in adults. *W Va Med J* 1993;89:102–105.

43. Karim ABMF, Maat B, Hatlevoll R, et al. A randomized trial on dose-response in radiation therapy of low-grade cerebral glioma: European Organization for Research and Treatment of Cancer (EORTC) study 22844. *Int J Rad Oncol Biol Phys* 1996;36:549–556.

44. Kelly PJ. Stereotactic biopsy and resection of thalamic astrocytomas. *Neurosurgery* 1989;25:185–194.

45. Kirkpatrick PJ, Honavar M, Janota I, Polkey CE. Control of temporal lobe epilepsy following en bloc resection of low-grade tumors. *J Neurosurg* 1993;78:19–25.

46. Kleihues P, Burger PC, Scheithauer BW. The new WHO classification of brain tumours. *Brain Pathol* 1993;3:255–268.

47. Koivukangas J, Koivukangas P. Treatment of low-grade cerebral astrocytoma: new methods and evaluation of results. *Ann Clin Res* 1986;18:115–124.

48. Kondziolka D, Lunsford DL, Martinez J. Unreliability of contemporary neurodiagnostic imaging in evaluating suspected adult supratentorial (low-grade) astrocytoma. *J Neurosurg* 1993;79:533–536.

49. Kreth FW, Faist M, Rossner R, Volk B, Ostertag CB. Supratentorial World Health Organization grade 2 astrocytomas and oligoastrocytomas: a new pattern of prognostic factors. *Cancer* 1997;79:370–379.

50. Labrousse F, Daumas-Duport C, Batorski L, Hoshino T. Histological grading and bromodeoxyuridine labeling index of astrocytomas: comparative study in a series of 60 cases. *Neurosurgery* 1991;75:202–205.

51. Laws ER, Taylor WF, Clifton MB, Okazaki H. Neurosurgical management of low-grade astrocytoma of the cerebral hemispheres. *J Neurosurg* 1984;61:665–673.

52. Leibel SA, Scott CB, Loeffler JS. Contemporary approaches to the treatment of malignant gliomas with radiation therapy. *Semin Oncol* 1994;21:198–219.

53. Leibel SA, Sheline GE. Tolerance of the central and peripheral nervous system to therapeutic irradiation. In: Lett JT, Altman KI, eds. *Advances in radiation biology*. New York: Academic Press, 1987;257–288.

54. Leibel S, Sheline G, Wara W, Boldrey E, Neilsen S. The role of radiation therapy in the treatment of astrocytomas. *Cancer* 1975;35:1551–1557.

55. Leighton C, Fisher B, Bauman G, et al. Supratentorial low-grade glioma in adults: an analysis of prognostic factors and timing of radiation. *J Clin Oncol* 1997;15:1294–1301.

56. Lunsford DL, Somaza S, Kondziolka D, Flickinger JC. Survival after stereotactic biopsy and irradiation of cerebral nonanaplastic, nonpilocytic astrocytoma. *J Neurosurg* 1995;82:523–529.

57. Macdonald DR. Low-grade gliomas, mixed gliomas, and oligodendrogliomas. *Semin Oncol* 1994;21: 236–248.

58. Marks JE, Baglan RJ, Prassad SC, Blank WF. Cerebral radionecrosis: incidence and risk in relation to dose, time, fractionation and volume. *Int J Rad Oncol Biol Phys* 1981;7:243–252.

59. McCormack BM, Miller DC, Budzilovich GN, Voorhees GJ, Ransohoff J. Treatment and survival of low-grade astrocytoma in adults: 1977–1988. *Neurosurgery* 1992;31:636–642.

60. Medberry CA, Straus KL, Steinberg SM, Cotelingam JD, Fisher WS. Low-grade astrocytomas: treatment results and prognostic variables. *Int J Radiat Oncol Biol Phys* 1988;15:837–841.

61. Miralbell R, Balart J, Matias-Guiu X, Molet J, Ariza A, Craven-Bartle J. Radiotherapy for supratentorial low-grade gliomas: results and prognostic factors with special focus on tumour volume parameters. *Radiother Oncol* 1993;27:112–116.

62. Montine TJ, Vandersteenhoven JJ, Aguzzi A, et al. Prognostic significance of Ki-67 proliferation index in supratentorial fibrillary astrocytic neoplasms. *Neurosurgery* 1994;34:674–679.

63. Morantz RA. Radiation therapy in the treatment of cerebral astrocytoma. *Neurosurgery* 1987;20:975–982.

64. Muller W, Afra D, Schroder R. Supratentorial recurrences of gliomas: morphological studies in relation to time intervals with astrocytomas. *Acta Neurochir* 1977;37:75–91.

65. Mundinger F. CT stereotactic biopsy for optimizing the therapy of intracranial processes. *Acta Neurochir Suppl* 1985;35:70–74.

66. Nelson JS, Tsukada Y, Schoenfeld D, Fulling K, Lamarche J, Peress N. Necrosis as a prognostic criterion in malignant supratentorial astrocytic gliomas. *Cancer* 1983;52:550–554.

67. North CA, North RB, Epstein JA, Piantadosi S, Wharam MD. Low-grade astrocytomas. Survival and quality of life after radiation therapy. *Cancer* 1990;66: 6–14.

68. Patronas NJ, Di Chiro G, Kufta C, et al. Prediction of survival in glioma patients by means of positron emission tomography. *J Neurosurg* 1985;62:816–822.

69. Philippon JH, Clemenceau SH, Fauchon FH, Foncin JF. Supratentorial low-grade astrocytomas in adults. *Neurosurgery* 1993;32:554–559.

70. Piepmeier JM. Observations on the current treatment of low-grade astrocytic tumors of the cerebral hemispheres. *J Neurosurg* 1987;67:177–181.

71. Piepmeier J, Christopher S, Spencer D, et al. Variations in the natural history and survival of patients with supratentorial low-grade astrocytomas. *Neurosurgery* 1996;38:872–879.

72. Piepmeier JM, Fried I, Makuch R. Low-grade astrocytoma may arise from different astrocyte lineages. *Neurosurgery* 1993;33:627–632.

73. Plate KH, Ruschoff J, Mennel HD. Cell proliferation in intracranial tumours: selective silver staining of nucleolar organiser regions (AgNORs). Application to surgical and experimental neuro-oncology. *Neuropathol Appl Neurobiol* 1991;17:121–132.

74. Pollack IF, Claasen D, al-Shboul Q, Janosky JE, Deutsch M. Low-grade gliomas of the cerebral hemispheres in children: an analysis of 71 cases. *J Neurosurg* 1995;82:536–47.

75. Rajan B, Pickuth D, Ashley S, et al. The management of histologically unverified presumed cerebral gliomas with radiotherapy. *Int J Rad Oncol Biol Phys* 1994;28:405–413.

76. Recht L, Lew R, Smith TW. Suspected low-grade glioma: Is deferring treatment safe? *Ann Neurol* 1992;31:431–436.

77. Reichenthal E, Feldman Z, Cohen ML, Loven D, Zucker G. Hemispheric supratentorial low-grade astrocytoma. *Neurochirurgia* 1992;35: 18–22.

78. Russell D, Rubinstein L. *Pathology of tumors of the nervous system.* Baltimore: Williams & Wilkins, 1989.

79. Rutten EHJM, Kazem I, Slooff JL, Walder AHK. Post operative radiation therapy in the management of brain astrocytoma: retrospective study of 142 Patients. *Int J Rad Oncol Biol Phys* 1980;7:191–195.

80. Scanlon PW, Taylor WF. Radiotherapy of intracranial astrocytomas: analysis of 417 cases treated from 1960 through 1969. Neurosurgery 1979;5:301–307.

81. Schifter T, Hoffman JM, Hanson MW, et al. Serial FDG-PET studies in the prediction of survival in patients with primary brain tumors. *J Comput Assist Tomogr* 1993;17:509–516.

82. Schroder R, Bien K, Kott R, Meyers I, Vossing R. The relationship between Ki-67 labeling and mitotic index in gliomas and meningiomas: demonstration of the variability of the intermitotic cycle time. *Acta Neuropathol* 1991;82:389–394.

83. Shapiro WR. Low-grade gliomas: When to treat? *Ann Neurol* 1992;31:437–438.

84. Shapiro W. Therapy of adult malignant brain tumors: What have the clinical trials taught us? *Semin Oncol* 1986;13:38–45.

85. Shaw E. Looking through the retrospectoscope in the era of evidence-based medicine. *J Clin Oncol* 1997;15:1289–1290.

86. Shaw EG. Low-grade gliomas: To treat or not to treat? A radiation oncologist's viewpoint. *Arch Neurol* 1990;47:1138–1139.

87. Shaw EG, Daumas-Duport C, Scheithauer BW, et al. Radiation therapy in the management of low-grade supratentorial astrocytomas. *J Neurosurg* 1989;70:853–861.

88. Shaw EG, Scheithauer BW, O'Fallon JR, Davis DH. Mixed oligoastrocytomas: a survival and prognostic factor analysis. *Neurosurgery* 1994;34:577–582.

89. Sheline GE. Radiation therapy of brain tumors. *Cancer* 1977;39:873–881.

90. Silverman C, Marks JE. Prognostic significance of contrast enhancement in low-grade astrocytomas of the adult cerebrum. *Radiology* 1981;139:211–213.

91. Smith DF, Hutton JL, Sandemann D, et al. The prognosis of primary intracerebral tumours presenting with epilepsy: the outcome of medical and surgical management. *J Neurol Neurosurg Psychiatry* 1991;54:915–920.

92. Soffietti R, Chio A, Giodana MT, Vasario E, Schiffer D. Prognostic factors in well-differentiated cerebral astrocytomas in the adult. *Neurosurgery* 1989;24:686–692.

93. Steiger HJ, Markwalder RV, Seiler RW, Ebeling U, Reulen H-J. Early prognosis of supratentorial grade 2 astrocytomas in adult patients after resection or stereotactic biopsy. *Acta Neurochir* 1990;106:99–105.

94. Taphoorn JB, Schiphorst AK, Snoek FJ, et al. Cognitive functions and quality of life in patients with low-grade gliomas: the impact of radiotherapy. *Ann Neurol* 1994;36:48–54.

95. Vecht CJ. Effect of age on treatment decisions in low-grade glioma. *J Neurol Neurosurg Psychiatry* 1993;56:1259–1264.

96. Vertosick FT, Selker RG, Arena VC. Survival of patients with well-differentiated astrocytomas diagnosed in the era of computed tomography. *Neurosurgery* 1991;28:496–501.

97. Vigliani MC, Sichez N, Poisson M, Delattre JY. A prospective study of cognitive functions following conventional radiotherapy for supratentorial gliomas in young adults: 4-year results. *Int J Rad Oncol Biol Phys* 1996;35:527–533.

98. Wallner KE, Gonzales MF, Edwards MS, Wara WM, Sheline GE. Treatment results of juvenile pilocytic astrocytoma. *J Neurosurg* 1988;69:171–176.

99. Wang HC, Ho YS. Clinicopathological evaluation of 78 astrocytomas in Taiwan with emphasis on a simple grading system. *J Neurooncol* 1992;13:265–276.

100. Weingart J, Olivi A, Brem H. Supratentorial low grade astrocytomas in adults. *Neurosurg Q* 1991;1:141–159.

101. Weir B, Grace M. The relative significance of factors affecting postoperative survival in astrocytomas grades one and two. *Can J Neurol Sci* 1976;3:47–50.

102. Westergaard L, Gjerris F, Klinken L. Prognostic parameters in benign astrocytoma. *Acta Neurochir* 1993;123:1–7.

103. Whitton AC, Bloom HJG. Low grade glioma of the cerebral hemispheres in adults: a retrospective analysis of 88 cases. *Int J Rad Oncol Biol Phys* 1990;18:783–786.

104. Wilden JN, Kelly PJ. CT computerised stereotactic biopsy for low density CT lesions presenting with epilepsy. *J Neurol Neurosurg Psychiatry* 1987;50:1302–1305.

105. Zulch KJ. Histological typing of tumours of the central nervous system. In: *International Histologic Classification of Tumours.* Geneva: World Health Organization, 1979:21.

The Practical Management of Low-Grade Primary Brain Tumors, edited by Jack P. Rock, Mark L. Rosenblum, Edward G. Shaw, and J. Gregory Cairncross. Lippincott Williams & Wilkins, Philadelphia, © 1999

10

Epilepsy and Low-Grade Gliomas

Kost Elisevich

Department of Neurosurgery, Henry Ford Hospital, Detroit, Michigan 48202

In the nineteenth century, Hughlings Jackson (77) observed the occurrence of seizures and epilepsy with primary brain tumors and pointed out that the seizure disorder could be the initial and only clinical manifestation of the condition. He correctly stated that seizure severity or type would not predict the causative tumor pathology. Seizure disorders have since been found to occur more commonly with low-grade gliomas than with the more malignant varieties (4,73,111,121,153). In their review of 703 cases of intracranial tumors and symptomatic epilepsy, Penfield et al. (111) noted seizures in 37% of patients harboring a glioblastoma, compared with 70% of patients with astrocytoma. The contrast was more striking when the comparison was made with partial seizures alone.

The primary factors underlying the development of epilepsy in the context of a low-grade glioma appear to be the slow growth kinetics of the tumor and location in the brain (50,111,121). Significantly longer disease duration is evident in patients with seizures (49,111), suggesting an inverse relationship between tumor growth rate and seizure risk (50). Several studies have observed a higher incidence of seizures associated with centrally situated (perirolandic) tumors, whereas occipital lesions were least likely to manifest with seizures (50,111).

Experimental studies are beginning to shed light on some aspects of epileptogenesis under a variety of adverse circumstances, although many more questions arise from clinical phenomenology than are answered.

BASIC MECHANISMS

Which properties are altered in the peritumoral environment to create an epileptic focus or multiple foci? Tumor-induced epileptogenicity has been studied to gain insight into the basic mechanisms underlying epileptogenesis (Table 1). References to mass effect, infiltration, or irritability lack sufficient scientific rigor to be useful explanations of the process.

An imbalance between excitatory and inhibitory controls appears to underlie epileptogenesis. Some understanding of the neuronoglial environment in this circumstance is required to determine the nature of such imbalances so as to correct them. The epileptogenic area is the site most vulnerable to ictal development by virtue of its intrinsic circuitry and/or its relationship with a neighboring structural anomaly. Individual cellular elements in the peritumoral environment have received particular attention.

Glia are involved in the uptake of the inhibitory neurotransmitter gamma aminobutyric acid (GABA), excitatory amino acid, and glutamate, and in the metabolism of glutamate to glutamine (75,136). Likewise, glioma cells studied in culture have been shown to have uptake mechanisms for GABA and glutamate

TABLE 1. *Potential mechanisms of tumor-associated epileptogenesis*

1. Glioma cells have uptake mechanisms for GABA (inhibitory transmitter), glutamate (excitatory transmitter), and glutamine, and may be capable of altering the balance of excitation/inhibition in the peritumoral tissue.
2. Decreases in GABA- and somatostatin-containing neurons in the peritumoral cerebral cortex may result in a net excitatory tendency.
3. Glioma development may interfere with the spatial buffering capacity of the normal glial syncytium, resulting in greater potassium ion concentration in the extracellular space, which renders the tissue more excitatory.
4. Alterations in the dynamics of gap junctional communication by invading glioma cells may establish greater synchrony of discharge in the neuronoglial environment of the peritumoral cerebral cortex.

(89,137). Biopsy specimens of gliomas associated with epilepsy have been shown to have a higher concentration of glutamine (10), similar to that seen in cobalt-induced epilepsy in the cat, where it has been correlated with onset and severity of epilepsy (147). Glioma cells take up and release glutamine (103,150) and thus may provide a large reservoir of precursor for peritumoral neurons to convert to glutamate (10), the primary excitatory neurotransmitter implicated in the genesis of seizures. Ostensibly, such increased excitatory influence would result in lowered seizure threshold and potentiate ictal activity.

Significant decreases in GABA- and somatostatin-containing neurons have been noted in epileptic cortex in the vicinity of low-grade gliomas (67). Neurons containing somatostatin, a modulatory neuropeptide, have been shown to be lost selectively in human hippocampal epileptic foci (30,83). Loss of somatostatin-immunoreactive neurons has also been demonstrated in animal models of experimental epilepsy (139). The finding of reduced levels of GABA- and somatostatin-immunoreactivity, some of which may have co-localized within the same neurons, suggests an alteration of neuronal phenotype in the peritumoral environment, creating a hyperexcitable cellular substrate.

Seizure activity results in an increase in extracellular potassium, which in turn promotes further excitability in this same tissue, thus creating a need for efficient spatial buffering of the ionic environment by astrocytes (72). Evidence exists of enhanced uptake of potassium by astrocytes under conditions of increased extracellular potassium concentrations (62). Astrocytes are known to form syncytial arrangements via gap junctions (35,98). Such arrangements augment the spatial buffering capacity through the creation of a large reservoir into which excess ion is allocated.

Gap junctions consist of a hexameric arrangement of connexin proteins that align in adjacent cells to form an intercellular conduit for ions and small molecules (35). Naus et al. (102) have shown an elevation of messenger RNA for connexin 43, the connexin protein subtype found in astrocytes, in peritumoral neocortex of patients presenting with acute seizures. Disturbance in the glial regulation of extracellular potassium may result, ostensibly, from disruption of the normal reactive glial syncytium in the immediate peritumoral environment. Alterations in pH will, for instance, result in the opening or closing of gap junctions and therefore a change in the reservoir capacity of the syncytium. Glioma cells ex-

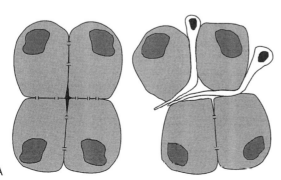

A   B

FIG. 1. A: Gap junctional (electrotonic) communication among glia allows intercellular passage of ions and small molecules. Such a syncytium may serve as a more efficient spatial buffer for potassium ion that is taken up by glia. **B:** Invasion of glioma cells, ostensibly bearing fewer gap junctions, disrupt the normal glial syncytium, therefore allowing extracellular potassium ion accumulation.

press markedly less connexin 43 mRNA (101), suggesting a lesser predilection for gap junctional communication. The invasion of a normal astrocytic syncytium by a comparatively nonsyncytial tissue may affect the balance required to maintain ionic equilibrium (Fig. 1). The reduction in potassium uptake in glia results in neuronal synchronization under circumstances of synaptic activation and can give rise to epileptiform activity (78).

There is mounting evidence that glia play an important role in the mediation of tissue excitability and that a neuronoglial model, rather than a strictly neuronal one, should be considered when postulating mechanisms underlying epileptogenesis.

RISK OF SEIZURES

Seizures will result in a variety of injuries and disabilities, including extremity fractures, vertebral compression fractures, severe burns, and cognitive impairment. The risk of death in patients experiencing a single seizure, reported as a standardized mortality ratio (SMR; ratio of observed and expected deaths), is 2.3, and when analyzed during the first 2 years after the seizure it is 4.2 (69). These figures are similar to the ratio obtained for patients with recurrent seizures due to an acquired lesion (e.g., tumor, trauma, stroke) in whom an SMR of 2.2 over 30 years was identified; in the first 2 years, the SMR was 4.3. Patients with lesion-associated epilepsy have a higher incidence of status epilepticus, an important cause of death among epileptics. The frequency of status increases from 3.8% in all patients with epilepsy to 9% in those with epilepsy secondary to an underlying lesion. The epileptic condition therefore not only limits the quality of life but, acutely and chronically, raises concern of both morbidity and mortality.

Epilepsy occurs in 6% to 21% of cases of cerebral neoplasm (16,25,29,37,41,59,95,121, 140). However, seizures of various types constitute the presenting clinical manifestation of brain tumors in 20% to 92% of patients with supratentorial intra-axial tumors (73,87,111, 121,132,164). The risk of developing seizures depends on multiple factors including tumor type, location, and proximity with the cortical gray matter (50,88,100,111,153) (Table 2). Approximately 80% to 90% of patients with oligodendrogliomas and gangliogliomas experience seizures, whereas more rapidly growing tumors impose a lower although somewhat variable incidence. Anaplastic astrocytomas carry a risk of 68% (88) and glioblastomas carry a risk of 29% to 37% (88,111,121,153). Astrocytomas have been shown to cause seizures in 66% of cases (87), suggesting that there is considerable overlap in epileptogenicity between these tumors and the anaplastic variety. This similarity is a reflection of histopathologic variability within any given tumor. The fact that anaplastic astrocytomas are likely to retain regional features of more epileptogenic lower-grade neoplasia would argue that their propensity to produce seizures may be indistinguishable from the more uniformly low-grade astrocytoma.

Metastases carry a seizure risk of about 20% (3,50,87,153), which corroborates that the rapidity of growth has an inverse relationship to the propensity for epileptogenesis. Meningiomas, however, present a 40% to 49% risk despite being extra-axial and slow growing (48,50,87,111,114,119,153,161). Of nonneoplastic lesions, arteriovenous malformations (47,66,100,109,144) and cavernous angiomas (138) have about a 35% risk of seizures. Although the slow growth of certain lesions may have a bearing upon epileptogenicity, clearly other factors unique to low-grade gliomas appear to affect seizure production more profoundly.

The primary motor cortex is most susceptible to seizure activity and the occipital lobe

TABLE 2. *Tumor-associated seizure risk factors*

1. Growth rate: low-grade tumors are more epileptogenic, perhaps as a result of length of survival.
2. Tumor type: oligodendrogliomas and gangliogliomas have a higher seizure incidence than other gliomas.
3. Location: centrally situated tumors have a higher seizure incidence, occipital tumors have the least.
4. Proximity to cortex: deeper subcortical tumors have a lesser influence upon epileptogenesis.

appears least affected (111,123). Mahaley and Dudka (88) have determined that frontal, temporal, and parietal tumors have a preoperative seizure incidence of more than 40%. Seizure frequency for astrocytomas and glioblastomas in the central region rises to 83% and 53%, respectively (36,87).

SEIZURE CHARACTER

The long-held view that the initial symptom or sign is critical in localizing the site of origin of a seizure is not always true. Some initial ictal features have more localizing value than others. Initial elementary visual hallucinations almost uniformly originate from the vicinity of the calcarine cortex (134,158), and gustatory hallucinations may be localized to the parietal operculum, uncinate region, and/or the insula (70,113). Likewise, focal clonic motor activity manifests often directly from primary motor cortex. Head and eye deviation and other forms of focal tonic activity may be lateralizing or misleading (106,118,127,162). Scalp EEG criteria alone are not sufficiently conclusive to localize focal seizure onset (16,157).

A number of cortical regions are clinically silent with regard to seizure manifestation, with initial ictal features reflecting spread of electrochemical activity into other sites at times far removed from the origin. Frontopolar, parieto-occipital, and medial parietal regions are examples of this phenomenon and may in some circumstances cloud interpretation of the extent of epileptogenicity (158). The semiology of a seizure is, in part, a reflection of its origin, although its presentation may change according to the pattern of propagation within the cerebral hemisphere(s). Seizure descriptions have been categorized by a lobar distribution (Table 3). Such descriptions serve as clinical guidelines that will aid in better defining the individual case.

TABLE 3. *Lobar seizure manifestations*

Frontal (primary generalized, absence, simple, and complex partial)
- Perirolandic: focal clonic activity; possible Jacksonian march.
- Dorsolateral: generalize rapidly; occasionally automatisms, tonic or absence like seizures; versive eye and head motion; speech arrest less common.
- Orbitofrontal: initial motor or gestural automatisms, olfactory hallucinations/illusions; autonomic signs.
- Cingulate: initial complex motor gestural automatisms; sexual automatisms, mood changes, urinary incontinence.
- Supplementary: contraversive head and eye motion with abduction and lateral rotation of contralateral arm and elbow flexion; vocalization or speech arrest.

Temporal (simple and complex partial)
- Temporobasal-limbic: aura marked by epigastric sensations, deja vu or memory flashes; impaired consciousness and arrest reaction with oroalimentary automatisms.
- Temporopolar: same; early autonomic features and oroalimentary automatisms.
- Opercular: auditory hallucinations; focal motor or sensory symptoms.
- Posterior temporal: vestibular and complex visual hallucinations.

Parietal (simple partial)
- Somatosensory auras; tonic posturing, focal clonic activity, head deviation, dysphasia, automatisms, vestibular hallucinations, metamorphosia, asomatognosia.

Occipital (simple partial)
- Elementary contralateral visual phenomena (scotoma, hemianopia, amaurosis, phosphenes); object distortion.

Frontal Lobe

A variety of seizure types manifest from the frontal lobe. These include primary generalized, absence, simple, and complex partial events (14,33,55,57,58,113,157). Seizures of frontal lobe origin tend to spread rapidly, both ipsilaterally and contralaterally, and to generalize quickly, thus confounding the ability to lateralize or localize the site of onset (8,157).

Certain clinical features help define the frontal epilepsies. Prominent motor features such as focal tonic/clonic activity, including asymmetrical tonic/adversive posturing, gen-

FIG. 2. T1-weighted MR images in coronal (**A**), axial (**B**), and sagittal (**C**) planes showing an oligodendroglioma of the inferior left frontal convexity. This 32-year-old right-handed male presented with a 6-month history of partial seizures characterized by speech arrest and more recent occasional secondary generalization. The tumor was located in the vicinity of the motor speech area anterior to the primary motor area as later determined by intraoperative electrical stimulation.

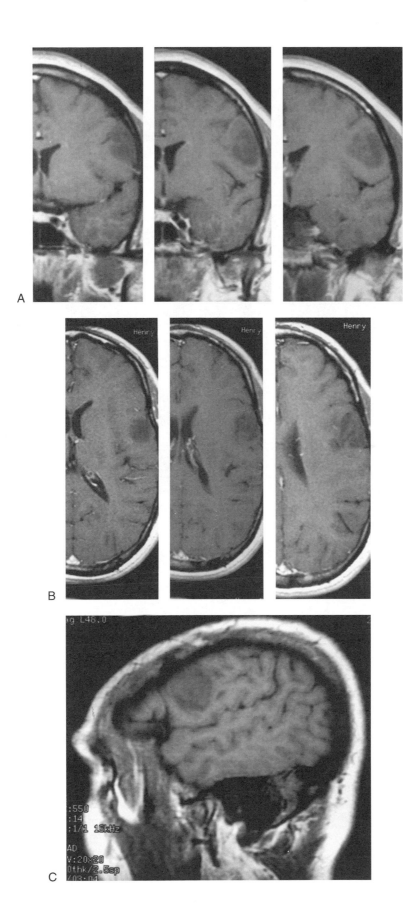

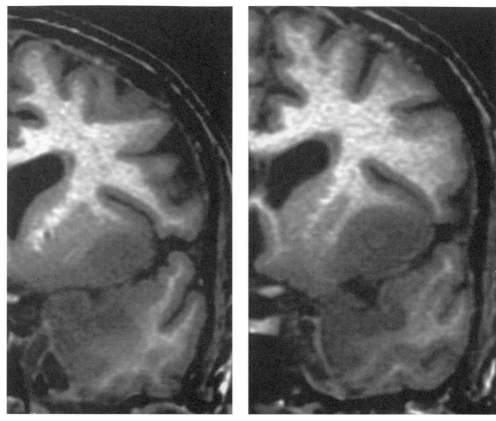

FIG. 3. A: T1-weighted MR images in the coronal plane identifying a glioma with predominantly low-grade features and isolated areas of anaplasia. The tumor occupies the left amygdalo-hippocampal and subfrontal regions. This 58-year-old male presented with an 8-month history of progressively worsening memory function and complex partial seizures consisting of brief staring episodes and lapses of consciousness without secondary generalization over at least 2 years.

eralized tonic/clonic activity, and motor automatisms (i.e., patterned bilateral arm and leg motion) are frequently evident (45,54,55, 57,58,92,113,120–122,157,159). Secondary generalization into convulsive events without evidence of focal onset is a frequent occurrence (9,105,122). Status epilepticus of the convulsive (79) or complex partial (157) variety has manifested from frontal lobe origin. Auras tend to be nonspecific (122,157) and less defined than in temporal lobe seizures.

Perirolandic seizures classically present in the form of focal clonic activity with occasional progression in a jacksonian manner. Frontal convexity (dorsolateral frontal) seizures have been reported as generalizing

rapidly without apparent focal onset (2,113), although automatisms have also manifested (113). Brief tonic and absencelike seizures have been described (32). Less commonly, versive eye and head movements and speech arrest manifest (Fig. 2). Frontopolar seizures produce no apparent clinical features (2,112, 113). Posterior spread may result in loss of consciousness, focal tonic motor activity, and generalization into tonic/clonic activity (159). Forced thinking and adversive head and eye movement with subsequent contraversive movement, axial clonic jerks, falls, and autonomic signs have been seen (26). Orbitofrontal seizures are complex partial in nature with initial motor and gestural automatisms,

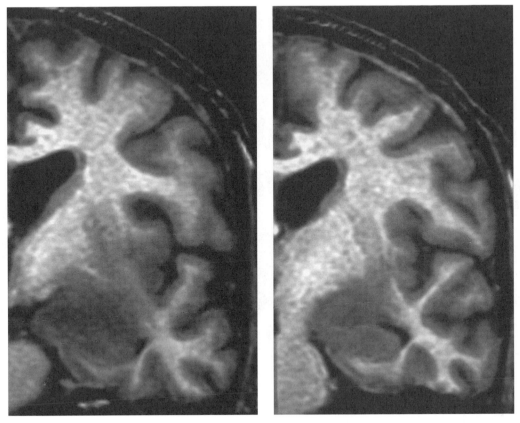

FIG. 3. A: *(Continued)*

olfactory hallucinations and illusions, and autonomic signs. Cingulate seizures are also complex partial with initial complex motor gestural automatisms (26). Sexual automatisms, mood changes, and urinary incontinence have been described as well (27,142, 159). Supplementary motor seizures typically consist of contraversive head and eye motion with abduction and external rotation of the contralateral arm and flexion at the elbow (2,8,113,154). The patient often appears to be looking at the postured hand while the legs are flexed, extended, or elevated. Vocalization or speech arrest is apparent, and consciousness is maintained. Synergistic coordinated motor action has been described (e.g., bicycling) (31,157). In addition to their asymmetric tonic character, seizures are brief (30–40 sec), are frequent (3–10/day), and begin and end abruptly (104).

Temporal Lobe

Complex partial seizures—typically characterized by an initial aura, impaired consciousness, and automatic behavior—are most often of temporal lobe origin (40,53), although extratemporal origins have also been recognized (112,113). With medial temporal onset, an arrest reaction or a motionless stare is followed by stereotyped automatisms with oroalimentary behavior predominating during which impaired consciousness is maximal (31,32) (Fig. 3). Those complex partial seizures arising from extratemporal sites often begin with semipurposeful motor activity and do not manifest arrest reactions or stereotypical automatisms. Most such seizures arise from the frontal lobe (34,149).

Wieser (154) established four types of temporal lobe complex partial seizures: temporo-

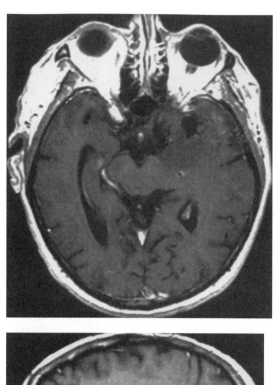

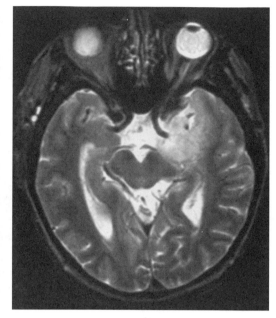

B

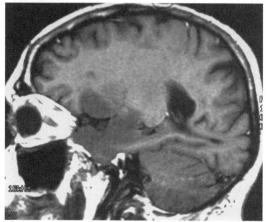

C

FIG. 3. *(Continued)* **B:** T1-weighted (left) and T2-weighted (right) MR axial images showing the expansile tumor occupying the medial temporal region and distorting the adjacent cerebral peduncle. **C:** T1-weighted MR sagittal images showing the anteroposterior extent of the tumor and its ascendance within the temporal stem.

basal/limbic, temporopolar, opercular, and posterior temporal neocortical. The temporobasal/limbic variety was the most common, with auras presenting in 80% of patients. The latter included epigastric sensations, déjà vu experiences, and memory flashes. Impaired consciousness and an arrest reaction occurred later with oroalimentary automatism (i.e., lip smacking, chewing motions). Uni- or bilateral tonic/clonic or dystonic posturing were commonly observed (155). The temporopolar seizure type was similar but included early autonomic features and oroalimentary automatisms. The opercular type included auditory hallucinations likely originating in or near Heschl's gyrus. Focal motor or sensory symptoms were also a distinguishing feature. Aphasia was rare. Posterior temporal neocortical seizures were characterized by vestibular and complex visual hallucinations. All types of temporal lobe complex partial seizures show a tendency to spread to involve first ipsilateral and subsequently the contralateral medial temporal lobe so that they tend to show similar characteristics beyond the first 10–30 seconds of onset.

In a review of 1,210 temporal excisions at the Montreal Neurological Institute, Rasmussen (122) identified gliomas, mostly astrocytomas, in 12%. An indolent glioma was often reported histopathologically (90). In cases where a definitive diagnosis was possible, tumors constituted 22%, corresponding to previous reports (44).

Parietal Lobe

Seizures of parietal lobe origin are of a simple partial and secondary generalized nature (Fig. 4). Complex partial seizures may develop after spread out of the parietal lobe (26). Somatosensory auras commonly manifest (1,156). Tingling or a feeling of electricity may remain contained in a particular location or spread in a jacksonian fashion. The sensation of motion or a need to move a body part may be noted. A loss of muscle tone, tonic postural changes, epigastric sensations, visual hallucinations, automatisms, and arrest reactions have also occurred (1,8,26,56,121). Vestibular hallucinations with violent vertigo, originating in the posterior temporal and parietal region, have been reported (8,104,154). Receptive or conductive language disturbance may manifest with dominant parietal seizures. Lateralized genital sensations imply paracentral involvement (26). Metamorphosia (distortion of shape and size) and asomatognosia (loss of awareness of a body part) may occur with nondominant parietal seizures.

In their review of 34 patients with tumoral parietal lobe epilepsy, Salanova et al. (134) found an aura in 79%, with 62% having somatosensory symptoms. Clinical manifestations were a reflection of the pattern of spread of the seizure, with 21% showing tonic posturing; 82%, focal clonic activity; 15%, head deviation; 9%, automatisms; and 6%, speech difficulty.

Occipital Lobe

Visual manifestations are frequently evident in occipital lobe seizures. Elementary visual seizures may manifest as negative (i.e., scotoma, hemianopia, amaurosis) (38,74, 108,131) or positive (i.e., phosphenes) (7,8,131) events in the contralateral visual field. Illusions of object distortion may present as a change in size, distance, inclination,

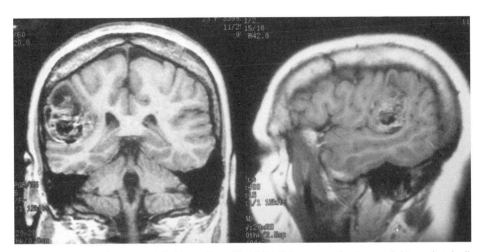

FIG. 4. T1-weighted MR coronal (left) and sagittal (right) images of a large right parietal oligodendroglioma. This 22-year-old female presented with an 11-year history of simple and complex partial seizures manifesting as brief tingling of the face and arm and as staring episodes with oroalimentary automatisms, respectively. The tumor is situated predominantly in the supramarginal gyrus, displacing the postcentral gyrus anteriorly.

or shape (26). Complex visual perceptions may occur.

Contralateral head and eye deviation is often observed at the beginning of occipital lobe seizures (99,129). Rapid forced blinking, eyelid closure or flutter, or palpebral jerks have also been reported at the onset of seizures (143). A sensation of oscillation of the eyes or the entire body may occur (26). Spread to the contralateral occipital lobe may be rapid. Alternately, lateral infra-Sylvian spread may be followed by confusion and stereotypic automatisms with invasion of medial temporal structures (108,143,159). Lateral supra-Sylvian spread may result in sensorimotor phenomena, whereas medial supra-Sylvian spread to the supplementary motor region could result in a variety of tonic motor seizures.

In a review of the characteristics of occipital lobe epilepsy, Salanova et al. (133) found that in 70% of 42 patients the clinical manifestations indicated an occipital onset. Visual auras were present in 73% of cases, of which elementary hallucinations were the most common and 29% had ictal blindness. Lateralizing clinical features were also evident in almost two-thirds of patients. More than one seizure type was exhibited in more than one-third of patients, which was suggestive of spread in a variety of directions.

MEDICAL THERAPY AND PROPHYLAXIS

The surgical approach and the extent of operative manipulation have some bearing on the risk of postoperative seizures. For instance, the subtemporal/transtentorial approach to acoustic tumors has met with a 22% incidence of seizures, with 70% occurring within 4 months, whereas no seizures occurred among patients undergoing the translabyrinthine approach (18). Surgery for middle cerebral artery aneurysms that require cerebral resection and/or retraction was shown to have an incidence of 37%, with almost all presenting within the first year (17). With other operated aneurysms, 62% of patients suffered seizures more than 1 year postoperatively.

In the case of anaplastic gliomas, Mahaley and Dudka (88) identified 36% of patients without preoperative seizures experiencing seizures postoperatively. Prophylaxis against seizures in patients with supratentorial astrocytomas undergoing surgery and irradiation (55–60 Gy) has been suggested to be beneficial in a nonrandomized study (15). The incidence of all seizure types was lower in patients receiving antiepileptic medication (Dilantin and/or phenobarbital), and no impairment of consciousness was reported with seizures in this group, whereas 18% of untreated patients had impaired consciousness. Untreated patients had a 39% incidence of seizures, compared with 21% in the treated group. Fewer seizures overall were seen in older patients, females, patients with higher-grade malignancy, and those who had more aggressive tumor resection.

Franceschetti et al. (50) studied patients with supratentorial neoplasms with and without preoperative seizures. The incidence of early postoperative seizures, mostly within the first 48 hours, was similar in the two groups. Postoperative complications (hemorrhage, edema) raised the likelihood of seizures during this period by more than twofold. Five of the 18 patients with postoperative seizures developed a status epilepticus, four of whom had received diphenylhydantoin. A decrease in serum diphenylhydantoin level postoperatively is a recognized problem and may explain the lack of response to antiepileptic coverage at an early stage. Late postoperative seizures occurred in 34% of patients with preoperative seizures who remained on antiepileptic therapy and in 15% of patients without preoperative seizures, some of whom were managed postoperatively with antiepileptic medication. Overall, the incidence of late-onset epilepsy appeared lower in the treated patients (12% versus 21%), although a significant difference was not demonstrated. In 52% of cases, the interval between surgery and the first late postoperative seizure was less than 6 months.

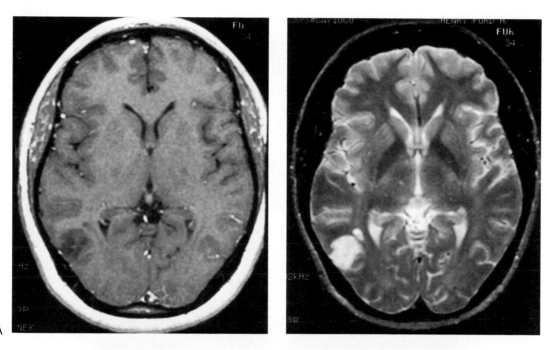

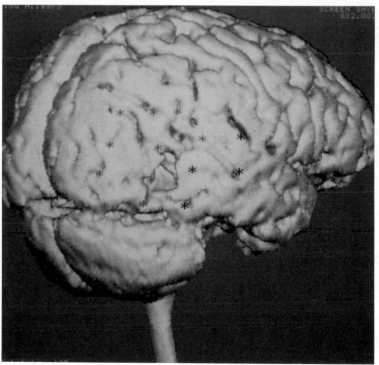

FIG. 5. A: T1-weighted (left) and T2-weighted (right) MR axial images of a right posterior temporal convexity oligodendroglioma. This 36-year-old right-handed female presented with simple partial seizures manifesting as a sensation of motion and vertigo with rare secondary generalization. **B:** Three-dimensional surface rendering of the posterior right hemisphere of the same patient reconstructed from MR axial images showing the positions of electrodes placed over the cortical surface for intraoperative electrocorticography (*asterisks*). The red asterisks mark the locations of spiking activity of various amplitudes in the vicinity of the subcortical tumor.

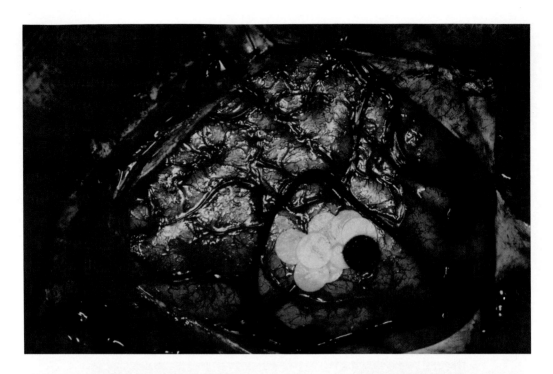

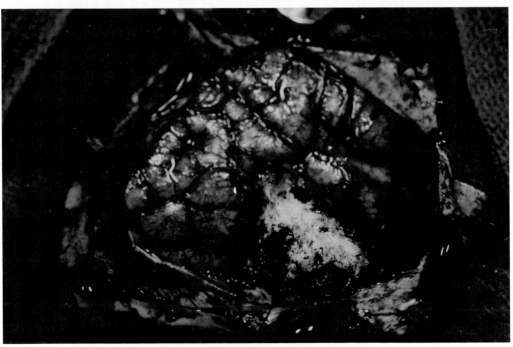

C

FIG. 5. *(Continued)* **(C)** Top: Intraoperative photograph of a cerebral exposure showing the electrode positions that demonstrated spiking activity (*black markers*) and the location of the tumor subcortically (*white markers*). The border designates the intended resection of cerebral tissue, incorporating the sites where spiking activity was of the highest amplitude. Bottom: Postresection photograph showing resection volume to the depth of the medial gliotic margin.

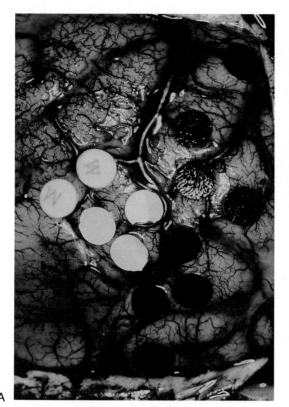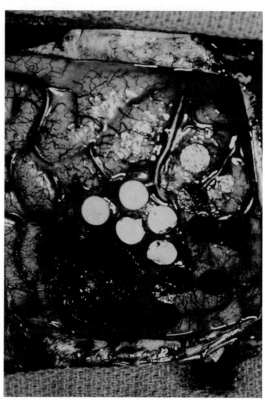

A

FIG. 6. A: Left: Intraoperative photograph of a left cerebral exposure of the patient also depicted in Fig. 2 showing the sites of electrical stimulation resulting in elementary motor activity of the face and arm (*black markers*) and therefore designating the primary motor area. The lighter-colored markers show sites of speech arrest with stimulation. The subcortical tumor is situated anteroinferiorly in the left lower corner of the photograph where the gyral surface appears widened. Right: Postresection photograph showing the extent of removal of tumor and surrounding epileptogenic cortex. Although the patient had difficulty with word-finding and disarticulate speech during the first 2 months postoperatively, his speech returned to baseline as judged by comparison of pre- and postoperative language assessment. His functional speech was sufficient for him to return to work 3 weeks postoperatively. He has remained seizure-free for 2 years at last follow-up.

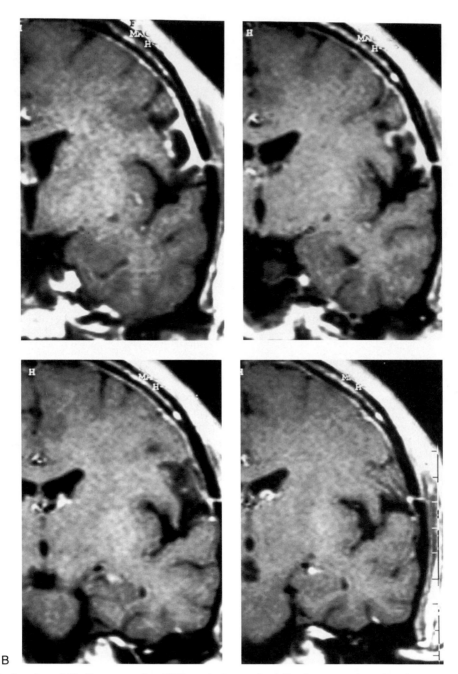

B

FIG. 6. *Continued.* **B:** Postoperative MRI study 2 months following resection showing an anteroposterior series of T1-weighted coronal images of the left frontal lobe. The resection cavity is situated in the inferior frontal gyrus and extends to the Sylvian fissure in the classically designated motor speech area.

Malignant gliomas were most common among patients with late postoperative seizures.

Seizure prophylaxis is recommended for those situations in which there is a risk of repeated seizures that exceeds the risk of prophylactic management (36). This likelihood appears most evident in situations where seizures have occurred preoperatively, the tumor and adjacent cortex is central in location, and there is associated edema or hemorrhage. The duration of antiepileptic therapy will vary according to whether a seizure disorder was apparent preoperatively and the extent to which peritumoral epileptogenicity was addressed surgically. When a single seizure heralded the presence of tumor prior to surgery, antiepileptic prophylaxis is continued for 6 months postoperatively and reduced during the last 6 weeks in the absence of any ictal activity or tumor recurrence on MRI study. Where no seizures have occurred but the patient appears at greater risk because of tumor location and associated edema, prophylaxis should be considered for at least 3 months and reconsidered if MRI study shows persistence of tumor in the surgical bed.

The maintenance of therapeutic levels of antiepileptic medications must be attempted in all cases. The efficacy of antiepileptic monotherapy can be judged only after maximizing serum levels within a tolerable limit.

Antiepileptic Medications

Discussion regarding antiepileptic drug therapy will be restricted to those medications most frequently used as monotherapy for generalized, simple, or complex partial and secondarily generalized seizures. The addition or substitution of a second antiepileptic drug should only be considered when the drug in use has been advanced to the point of side effect. The commonly used antiepileptic medications are listed in Table 4.

Dilantin (Diphenylhydantoin)

Phenytoin sodium is related to the barbiturates. The primary site of action is the motor

TABLE 4. Common Antiepileptic Medications

Generic Name	Trade Name
Carbamazepine	Tegretol (Tegretol XR)
Diphenylhydantoin	Dilantin (Fosphenytoin)
Lamotrigine	Lamictal
Phenobarbital	—
Divalproex sodium	Depakote
Gabapentin	Neurontin
Primidone	Mysoline
Clonazepam	Klonopin
Ethosuximide	Zarontin

cortex in which the spread of seizure activity is inhibited. Phenytoin stabilizes cell membrane threshold against hyperexcitability brought about by a reduction of the sodium gradient. The activation of cerebello–cerebral inhibitory pathways has also been supported as a means of anticonvulsant action (68,81). It promotes sodium efflux from neurons and appears to reduce the maximal activity of brain stem centers responsible for the tonic phase of tonic/clonic seizures.

The plasma half-life after oral administration is 22 hours (7–42 hours). Peak plasma concentrations after a single oral dose vary from 3–12 hours (60). Phenytoin is 70% to 95% bound to plasma proteins. More than 95% of phenytoin is metabolized by hepatic microsomal enzymes (160). Decreased plasma concentrations may occur with the concurrent use of carbamazepine, ethanol (chronic), barbiturates, antacids, folic acid, theophylline, enteral feeding, and oral electrolytes. Increased concentrations may occur with cimetidine, valproate, carbamazepine, fluconazole, isoniazide, disulfiram, and diazoxide. Adverse reactions include nystagmus, ataxia, dysarthria and lethargy when plasma levels exceed 20 μg/ml. A phenytoin hypersensitivity syndrome characterized by fever, rash, lymphadenopathy, and hepatitis requires prompt discontinuation of phenytoin to avoid life-threatening complications such as Stevens-Johnson syndrome. Most patients present with symptoms within 4 weeks of starting phenytoin, usually during the second and third weeks. Other adverse reactions include diabetes insipidus, thrombocytopenia, leukopenia, granulocytopenia, or pancytopenia. Steady-state serum levels are achieved after 5–7 half-lives or 7–10 days at the recommended daily regimen of 300 mg/day. Effective serum concentrations are 10–20 µg/ml (total) or 0.5–3.0 µg/ml (free) and should be determined at trough level.

An intravenous loading dose of 18 mg/kg generally achieves therapeutic serum levels in most individuals. Care is taken to ensure a delivery rate of less than 50 mg/min to avoid cardiovascular collapse. Otherwise, it may be given in 0.9% sodium chloride solution (1–10 mg/ml) by intravenous piggyback at a rate of less than 20 mg/ml. Loading by oral administration may be accomplished by administering 300-mg or 400-mg capsules in varying amounts according to body weight every 2 hours for a total of three doses. A daily maintenance dose of 300 mg is commonly prescribed. This may be delivered in 100-mg doses three times daily, two daily doses of 100 mg in the morning and 200 mg nightly, or as a single 300-mg dose nightly. The daily dose is adjusted according to serum level and the presence or absence of adverse effect.

The newly released phenytoin prodrug fosphenytoin (Cerebyx) avoids some of the difficulty associated with the parenteral use of phenytoin, such as its poor aqueous solubility and highly irritating properties (12). It is rapidly hydrolyzed to phenytoin and is promptly and completely absorbed after intramuscular administration with 100% bioavailability within 3 hours of injection. Tissue reactions do not appear after either intramuscular or intravenous administration (85). Because of the relative ease of administration and bioavailability, a combination of fosphenytoin (25 mg/kg) and lorazepam (0.1 mg/kg) appears ideal for the treatment of status epilepticus (145).

Tegretol (Carbamazepine)

Carbamazepine is effective against complex partial and generalized seizures. Its antiepileptic properties resemble those of phenytoin by reducing polysynaptic responses and blocking post-tetanic potentiation. It is 76% bound to plasma proteins. Adult therapeutic levels are between 4 and 12 µg/ml. Because the drug can induce its own metabolism, the half-life is variable and initially ranges from 25–65 hours, but with repeated doses it will drop to 12–17 hours. After oral administration, about 70% of the drug is excreted in urine. Transplacental passage is rapid (30–60 min) with accumulation of the drug in fetal tissues. The medication is available as tablet or suspension and should be delivered as a low initial daily dose to avoid gastrointestinal upset. A suggested regimen for adults is 100 mg once or twice daily, increasing at weekly intervals by 100–200 mg/day. The dosage is adjusted a minimum effective level of 800–1,200 mg daily divided into three or four doses; in children 6–12 years of age, 400–800 mg daily usually suffices.

Simultaneous administration of phenobarbital, phenytoin, or primidone can markedly lower serum levels of carbamazepine. Both valproic acid and lamotrigine will increase serum concentrations of an active metabolite, carbamazepine-10,11-epoxide. The half-life of phenytoin can be significantly shortened when concurrently administered. The serum level of valproic acid may be reduced when given with carbamazepine. Elevated plasma levels of total and/or free carbamazepine may result with coadministration with cimetidine, erythromycin, propoxyphene, or calcium channel blockers. A new extended-release preparation of carbamazepine (Tegretol XR) allows administration only twice daily to maintain therapeutic levels. Mean steady-state carbamazepine plasma levels following a standard regimen of four daily doses of Tegretol and following a twice-daily regimen of Tegretol XR in equivalent total daily amounts provided similar results in both adult and pediatric patients.

Lamictal (Lamotrigine)

Lamotrigine has an antiseizure profile similar to that of phenytoin and carbamazepine, and shares their spectrum of antiepileptic activity. It is thought to act by inhibiting release of glutamate (24,93,94,107,117,125) and has less sedative effect than phenytoin and carbamazepine. Its pharmacokinetic properties include a rapid and complete absorption orally, long elimination half-life, relatively low protein binding, lack of effect on drug-metabolizing enzymes, and lack of active or toxic metabolites (96). Its oral bioavailability is about 98% and is 55% protein-bound. Peak plasma levels are reached 1–5 hours after administration (24). Lamotrigine is primarily (94%) eliminated in the urine (110). The steady-state serum half-life is approximately 25–30 hours. After a twice-daily regimen for 6 days, this half-life remains unchanged, indicating that it does not induce its own metabolism. Therapeutic plasma concentrations have been estimated in the range of 1–3 μg/ml. These levels have been shown to inhibit photoconvulsive responses and interictal EEG changes in epileptic patients (24).

The drug may cause fatigue, ataxia, dizziness, headache, diplopia, and rash. It should be administered with caution with other antiepileptic drugs, because some have been shown to enhance or interfere with its elimination. For patients receiving liver enzyme-inducing antiepileptic drugs (carbamazepine, phenytoin, phenobarbital, primidone) without valproic acid, the recommended initial dose of lamotrigine is 50 mg daily for 2 weeks. The dose is then advanced to 50 mg twice daily for 2 weeks and thereafter by 100 mg/day every week. The usual maintenance dose is 300–500 mg daily in two divided doses, although doses of up to 700 mg daily have been used. Patients taking valproic acid should begin lamotrigine at a lower dose of 25 mg on alternate days for 2 weeks, followed by the same dose taken daily. The regimen is advanced by 25–50 mg/day every 1 or 2 weeks to a maximum of 150–200 mg daily.

SURGICAL APPROACH

The use of electrocorticography during tumor resection to define regions of epilepto-genicity in the peritumoral surround has been under debate for some time. A number of authors have indicated that resection of the tumor alone may result in good postoperative seizure control in those patients presenting with a tumor-associated seizure disorder (19,42, 43,50,64,73). It is inevitable that during tumor removal a variable amount of surrounding epileptogenic cortical tissue is removed. Incomplete removal of this peritumoral tissue may result in a slightly reduced or unaltered seizure frequency (5,19,21,50,64,73,135,140, 153). Alternatively, good seizure control with lesion removal alone may be dependent upon antiepileptic medication (19,21,50,73). The purest sampling of lesionectomy cases, performed under image-guided stereotactic means, achieved long-term seizure-free outcomes in 57% of cases (20,21,22). Of patients with temporal lobe lesions, only 22% were seizure-free. These results can be compared with those of Boon et al. (16) and Kirkpatrick et al. (84), who undertook the removal of some peritumoral cerebral tissues and achieved 83% and 81% seizure-free outcomes, respectively.

In a review of the natural history of 55 patients with supratentorial low-grade gliomas, those with chronic epilepsy had the best prognoses (115). No known recurrences or deaths were reported in 27 patients regardless of the extent of surgery. Moreover, tumors associated with chronic epilepsy were much less likely to become malignant over time. This feature emphasizes the need for adequate seizure control in this population to improve upon quality of life in the long term.

Intraoperative electrocorticography has been used by a number of authors to define epileptogenic regions (Fig. 5, see insert following page 158.) and define functional areas (Fig. 6, see insert following page 158.) of cerebral cortex in the vicinity of the tumor using electrical stimulation. Greater success with seizure control has been reported by these authors (65,116, 121,126,146). Rasmussen (121) reported that 79% of 91 patients with low-grade gliomas and intractable epilepsy had either no seizures or a marked reduction, with a median follow-up of 7 years. Favorable seizure control following resection with electrocorticography has been documented even when less than total tumor resection has been accomplished (5,163). Berger et al. (13) reviewed 45 patients with low-grade gliomas and intractable epilepsy and found 53% of patients seizure-free and no longer requiring antiepileptic medications after a mean follow-up of 54 months. An additional 38% of patients were seizure-free but required reduced doses of antiepileptic medications. Although most adults (88%) were seizure-free, 47% remained on antiepileptic medication despite 7 of 17 patients qualifying for withdrawal of medication. In contrast, 85% of children were seizure-free and off antiepileptic medications. In another study, Drake et al. (37) reviewed outcomes in 16 pediatric patients with temporal lobe mass lesions, 12 of which were tumors. In nine of 10 patients in which the hippocampus was found not to be invaded by tumor, there was concomitant medial temporal sclerosis. Of the 16 patients who were followed for more than 1 year, 56% were seizure-free and the remainder experienced a greater than 50% reduction in seizure frequency. Postresection electrocorticography resulted in extension of the original cortical resection because of persistent epileptiform activity in a certain number of cases. Minimal to moderate epileptiform disturbance sometimes remained. Postresection electrocorticography has been advocated (13) because persistent epileptiform activity after tumor resection has been associated with seizure recurrence (61).

In another study reviewing complex partial seizures associated with temporal tumors and other masses, a comparison was made of cases undergoing lesionectomy with those cases having electrocorticography with delineation of an epileptogenic zone and resection of this tissue along with the lesion (80). In those cases of lesionectomy alone, only 18.8% achieved a seizure-free status, compared with a 92.8% seizure-free outcome in the electrocorticography group. Moreover, a 62.5% seizure-free outcome was achieved in a second operation (temporal lobectomy) in the

lesionectomy group. A meta-analysis of studies that have summarized the results of simple lesion excision (lesionectomy) and those that have addressed cases wherein resection of epileptogenic cortex has been carried out has indicated a higher proportion of postoperative seizures following simple excision (56 ± 5% versus 33 ± 4%; $p < .0001$) (151). For low-grade astrocytomas alone, the outcome was more dramatic (63% versus 18%), as was the case for gangliogliomas (58% versus 14%). A feature that has become apparent in patients with low-grade gliomas is the finding of multiple seizure foci in those patients with longer seizure histories (13,126). Such findings further support the use of electrocorticography during resection.

Awad et al. (5) reviewed 47 patients with structural brain lesions and intractable partial epilepsy. The epileptogenic area, defined as the zone of maximum interictal epileptiform activity from which the patient's typical seizure arose on ictal recordings (163), was found to involve the region adjacent to the lesion in 11 patients and extended beyond the lesion in 18 patients. However, in the remaining 18 patients, remote noncontiguous zones of epileptogenicity were demonstrated. Where convergent data suggested the vicinity of the lesion to be the primary site of epileptogenicity, complete lesion excision resulted in a 90% seizure-free outcome. In a number of cases where prolonged recording and mapping have been carried out, the source of epileptic activity was remote from a structural lesion (39,63,76,91,97). These cases may demonstrate multifocal independent foci. Generally, good correlation is found between clinical seizure characteristics and lesion location with tumors in all cerebral lobes except parietal (16), although in their review of 34 cases of tumoral parietal lobe epilepsy, Salanova et al. (134) identified 75% of patients to be seizure-free or to experience seizures rarely.

Favorable outcomes have been reported with regard to seizure reduction or elimination following resections of cerebral tissue remote from the site of tumor (108,141). Overall, seizure control has proven difficult in larger series (46). The recommendation in most such cases has been to remove the ostensibly causative lesion in addition to the epileptogenic area, whether remote or not.

PATHOLOGY

The nature and location of a tumor are important in determining the occurrence of an associated seizure disorder. Most epileptogenic intra-axial tumors occur in the centro-parietal region, and the further away the tumor, the less epileptogenic it is, regardless of its histology (82). Most astrocytomas have been situated in the centro-parietal region (32%), but the incidence of seizures caused by this tumor type has been the same at all sites. Although oligodendrogliomas are more common in the frontal region (35%), the propensity to seizures has been shown to be greater in the temporal (76%) and temporoparietal regions (83%).

A special circumstance has been identified regarding certain limbic and neocortical gliomas that seem to set them apart as a distinct clinicopathologic group. In a review of 65 patients with intractable seizures and gliomas, Fried et al. (52) found most of these tumors confined to the temporal (63%) or occipital lobe (18%), occupying limbic or perilimbic neocortical locations. Most of these gliomas (83%) involved the gray matter of neocortex, transitional cortex, or allocortex. Although the majority (61%) were classified as low-grade astrocytomas, 17% were found to be anaplastic, even though patients had had a remarkably stable clinical history with chronic seizures (mean 15 years). With resection of the tumor, 82% of 60 patients with more than 1 year of postoperative follow-up were seizure-free. The authors suggest that limbic and perilimbic gliomas associated with intractable seizures and further characterized by a young host age and cortical location constitutes a distinctive glioma subgroup bearing a better prognosis. Low-grade cortical astrocytomas associated with a long history of seizures may arise from an astrocyte lineage

that is different from those limited to white matter, in which patients commonly present with a short history of symptoms (115). Daumas-Duport et al. (28) have also described a group of neuroepithelial tumors associated with intractable epilepsy and characterized by an intracortical location but with a heterogeneous cellular composition of astrocytes, oligodendrocytes, and neurons and no malignant features. These were also suggested to be surgically curable.

Many patients with temporal lobe tumors present with complex partial seizures (16,140), raising questions about the mechanism by which this occurs. An associated atrophy of the hippocampus with demonstrated cell loss, particularly in the CA4 region, has raised concerns of a dual pathology in some of the patients (6,51). Of 17 patients studied in this manner, Fried et al. (51) found 12 to bear gliomas, of which three were low-grade astrocytomas, two were cellular astrocytomas, and four were mixed astrocytoma-oligodendrogliomas. Neuronal densities in all hippocampal fields and in the granule cell layer of the dentate gyrus were significantly lower in patients with these tumors than in autopsy controls. Patients with lateral tumors and late onset of seizures were more likely to have only minimal neuronal cell loss compared with those with medially placed tumors. In the latter group, a resection sparing the hippocampus could be advised in most circumstances.

Where an atrophic hippocampus has been found by MR volumetry, resection of both the lesion and the hippocampus is more likely to achieve a seizure-free status (86). Only 20% of patients with dual pathology undergoing resection of either the lesion or hippocampus alone became seizure-free, although another 40% demonstrated significant improvement.

EFFECT OF IONIZING RADIATION

Ionizing radiation has been found to influence epileptic behavior, commonly reducing its clinical and electrographic expression (11,71,128,130,148). In the case of cerebral arteriovenous malformations with an associated seizure disorder, Heikkinen et al. (71) found seizures to cease altogether in 55% of patients treated by radiosurgery. The seizure-free interval in follow-up was 2–8 years. This antiepileptic effect was independent of angiographic evidence of obliteration of the vascular malformation. Interstitial brachytherapy (low-energy gamma irradiation) for cerebral low-grade gliomas has been found to eliminate seizure activity in 53% of patients, with a marked reduction in the frequency of seizures in an additional 40% (130). Goldring et al. (64) reported four patients with frontal lobe gliomas and seizures who underwent biopsy and external radiation therapy. Three patients became seizure-free during a follow-up of 4 years. Another 23 patients with seizures who had resection followed by radiation therapy achieved a similar favorable outcome and 83% became seizure-free. Seizures attributable to malignant tumors have also appeared to be amenable to control by ionizing radiation (23). Five of nine patients with biopsy-proven malignancy and intractable partial seizures responded with seizure-free outcomes for the duration of their survival, whereas the remainder showed a reduction in frequency of more than 75%.

The treatment of nonlesional partial epilepsy with radiosurgery has accomplished seizure-free outcomes in a number of cases (71,124,152), although the status of such treatment remains anecdotal for the present.

SUMMARY

Seizures will herald the presence of a supratentorial low-grade neoplasm in a significant number of patients and will manifest accordingly, depending upon its location in most cases. Antiepileptic therapy is necessary in particular for those who experience seizures preoperatively, in cases where the tumor is central in location and where there is associated edema or hemorrhage. Duration of therapy will vary according to whether seizures manifest preoperatively, the success with which they are controlled postopera-

tively, and the extent to which peritumoral epileptogenicity was managed surgically.

In cases where an established seizure disorder has accompanied a low-grade glioma, the use of intraoperative electrocorticography to delineate the territory of epileptogenicity in the peritumoral area is appropriate and appears to afford a more favorable outcome in seizure control. Cortical electrostimulation of the cerebral surface in cases where the tumor and/or the territory of epileptogenicity overlaps functionally eloquent cerebral areas affords maximal resection of both while maintaining a safe margin that preserves functional integrity.

Certain gliomas occupying gray matter predominantly and found in limbic or perilimbic (temporal or occipitotemporal) neocortical locations are found preferentially in younger patients. These neoplasms, generally associated with a long history of seizures, may carry a better prognosis overall, even in the case of histologic malignancy. Where an atrophic hippocampus is identified accompanying an adjacent temporal glioma, resection of both the tumor and the hippocampus bears a greater opportunity for a seizure-free outcome.

Often the sole clinical manifestation of a cerebral neoplasm is that of a seizure disorder. Proper management should address not only the neoplasm, which may be at times effectively treated by surgery alone to offer the patient a survival approximating the norm, but the associated epileptogenicity to provide the patient an optimal quality of life.

REFERENCES

1. Ajmone-Marsan C, Goldhammer L. Clinical ictal patterns and electrographic data in cases of partial seizures of fronto-central-parietal origin. In: Blazier MAB, ed. *Epilepsy: its phenomenon in man.* New York: Academic Press, 1973:235–258.
2. Ajmone-Marsan C, Ralston BL. *The epileptic seizure: its functional morphology and diagnostic significance.* Springfield, IL: Charles C Thomas, 1957.
3. Arseni C, Constantinsescu AI. Considerations on the metastatic tumours of the brain with reference to statistics of 1217 cases. *Schweiz Arch Neurol Psychiatr* 1975;117:179–195.
4. Arseni C, Petrovici IN. Epilepsy in temporal lobe tumors. *Eur Neurol* 1971;5:201–214.
5. Awad IA, Rosenfeld J, Ahl J, Hahn JF, Luders H. In-

tractable epilepsy and structural lesions of the brain: mapping, resection strategies, and seizure outcome. *Epilepsia* 1991;32:179–186.

6. Babb TL, Brown WJ, Pretorius J, et al. Temporal lobe volumetric cell densities in temporal lobe epilepsy. *Epilepsia* 1984;25:729–740.

7. Bancaud J. Les crises épileptiques d'origine occipitale (étude stéréo-electroencephalographique). *Rev Oto-neuroophthalmol* 1969;41:299–315.

8. Bancaud J, Talairach J, Bonis A, et al. La stéréo-electroencephalographie dans l'épilepsie. Paris: Masson, 1965.

9. Bancaud J, Talairach J, Morel P, et al. Generalized epileptic seizures elicited by electrical stimulation of the frontal lobe in man. *Electroencephalogr Clin Neurophysiol* 1974;37:275–282.

10. Bateman DE, Hardy JA, McDermott JR, Parker DS, Edwardson JA. Amino acid neurotransmitter levels in gliomas and their relationship to the incidence of epilepsy. *Neurol Res* 1988;10:112–114.

11. Baudoin MM, Stuhl L, Perrard AC. Un cas d'épilepsie focale traité par la radiothérapie. *Rev Neurol* 1951;84: 60–63.

12. Bebin M, Bleck TP. New anticonvulsant drugs. Focus on flunarizine, fosphenytoin, midazolam and stiripentol. *Drugs* 1994;48:153–171.

13. Berger MS, Ghatan A, Haglund MM, Dobbins J, Ojemann GA. Low-grade gliomas associated with intractable epilepsy: seizure outcome utilizing electrocorticography during tumor resection. *J Neurosurg* 1993; 79:62–69.

14. Bladin PF, Woodward J. Epilepsy and the frontal lobe. *Proc Aust Assoc Neurol* 1974;11:229–237.

15. Boarini DJ, Beck DW, Van Gilder JC. Postoperative prophylactic anticonvulsant therapy in cerebral gliomas. *Neurosurgery* 1985;16:290–292.

16. Boon PA, Williamson PD, Fried I, et al. Intracranial, intraaxial, space-occupying lesions in patients with intractable partial seizures: an anatomoclinical, neuropsychological and surgical correlation. *Epilepsia* 1991;32:467–476.

17. Cabral R, King TT, Scott DF. Epilepsy after two different neurosurgical approaches to the treatment of ruptured intracranial aneurysms. *J Neurol Neurosurg Psychiatry* 1976;39:1052–1056.

18. Cabral R, King TT, Scott DF. Incidence of post-operative epilepsy after transtentorial approach to acoustic nerve tumors. *J Neurol Neurosurg Psychiatry* 1976;39:663–665.

19. Cascino GD. Epilepsy and brain tumors: implications for treatment. *Epilepsia* 1990;31(Suppl 3):37–44.

20. Cascino GD, Boon PAJM, Fish DR. Surgically remediable lesional syndromes. In: Engel J Jr, ed. *Surgical treatment of the epilepsies.* New York: Raven Press, 1993:77–86.

21. Cascino GD, Kelly PJ, Hirschorn KA, et al. Stereotactic resection of intra-axial cerebral lesions in partial epilepsy. *Mayo Clin Proc* 1990;65:1053–1060.

22. Cascino GD, Kelly PJ, Sharbrough, Hulihan JF, Hirschorn, Trenerry MR. Long-term follow-up of stereotactic lesionectomy in partial epilepsy: predictive factors and electroencephalographic results. *Epilepsia* 1992;33:639–644.

23. Chalifoux R, Elisevich K. Effect of ionizing radiation on partial seizures attributable to malignant cerebral

tumors. *Stereotact Funct Neurosurg* 1996–97;67: 169–182.

24. Cohen AF, Land GS, Breimer DD, et al. Lamotrigine, a new anticonvulsant: pharmacokinetics in normal humans. *Clin Pharmacol Ther* 1987;42:535–541.

25. Collard M, Dupont H, Noel G. Computerized transverse axial tomography in epilepsy: summary. *Epilepsia* 1976;17:339–342.

26. Commission on Classification and Terminology of the International League against Epilepsy. Proposal for revised classification of epilepsies and epileptic syndromes. *Epilepsia* 1989;30:389–399.

27. Crandall PH. Developments in direct recordings from epileptogenic regions in the surgical treatment of partial epilepsies. In: Blazier MAB, ed. *Epilepsy: its phenomena in man.* New York: Academic Press, 1973: 287–310.

28. Daumas-Duport C, Scheithauer BW, Chodkiewicz JP, Laws ER, Vedrenne C. Dysembryoplastic neuroepithelial tumor: a surgically curable tumor of young patients with intractable partial seizures. *Neurosurgery* 1988; 23:545–556.

29. Davidson S, Falconer MA. Outcome of surgery in 40 children with temporal-lobe epilepsy. *Lancet* 1975;1: 1260–1263.

30. De Lanerolle NC, Kim JH, Robbins RJ, et al. Hippocampal interneuron loss and plasticity in human temporal lobe epilepsy. *Brain Res* 1989;495:387–395.

31. Delgado-Escueta AV, Bacsal FE, Treiman DM. Complex partial seizures on closed-circuit television and EEG: a study of 691 attacks in 79 patients. *Ann Neurol* 1981;11:292–300.

32. Delgado-Escueta AV, Nashold B, Freedman M, et al. Videotaping epileptic attacks during stereoelectroencephalography. *Neurology* 1979;29:473–489.

33. Delgado-Escueta AV, Swartz B, Maldonado H, Walsh GO, Rand RW, Halgren E. Complex partial seizures of frontal lobe origin. In: Wieser HD, Elger CE, eds. *Presurgical evaluation of epileptics: basics, techniques, implications.* Berlin: Springer-Verlag, 1987: 268–299.

34. Delgado-Escueta AV, Walsh GO. Type I complex partial seizures of hippocampal origin: excellent results of anterior temporal lobectomy. *Neurology* 1985;35: 143–154.

35. Dermietzel R, Traub O, Hwang TK, et al. Differential expression of three gap junction proteins in developing and mature brain tissue. *Proc Natl Acad Sci USA* 1986;86:10148–10152.

36. Deutschman CS, Haines SJ. Anticonvulsant prophylaxis in neurological surgery. *Neurosurgery* 1985;17: 510–517.

37. Drake J, Hoffman HJ, Kobayashi J, et al. Surgical management of children with temporal lobe epilepsy and mass lesions. *Neurosurgery* 1987;21:792–797.

38. Engel J Jr, Crandall PH. Falsely localizing ictal onsets with depth EEG telemetry during anticonvulsant withdrawal. *Epilepsia* 1983;24:344–355.

39. Engel J Jr, Driver MV, Falconer MA. Electrophysiological correlates of pathology and surgical results in temporal lobe epilepsy. *Brain* 1975;98:129–156.

40. Falconer MA. Mesial temporal (Ammon's horn) sclerosis as a common cause of epilepsy: aetiology, treatment and prevention. *Lancet* 1974;2:767–770.

41. Falconer MA, Cavanagh JB. Clinico-pathological con-

siderations of temporal lobe epilepsy due to small focal lesions: a study of cases submitted to operation. *Brain* 1959;82:483–504.

42. Falconer MA, Driver MV, Serafetinides EA. Temporal lobe epilepsy due to distant lesions: two cases relieved by operation. *Brain* 1962;85:521–534.

43. Falconer MA, Kennedy WA. Epilepsy due to small focal temporal lesions with bilateral independent spike-discharging foci. *J Neurol Neurosurg Psychiatry* 1961; 24:205–212.

44. Falconer MA, Serafetinides EA. A follow-up study of surgery in temporal lobe epilepsy. *J Neurol Neurosurg Psychiatry* 1963;26:154–165.

45. Fegerstein L, Roger A. Frontal epileptogenic foci and their clinical correlations. *Electroencephalogr Clin Neurophysiol* 1961;13:905–913.

46. Fish DR, Andermann F, Olivier A. Complex partial seizures and posterior temporal or extratemporal lesions: surgical strategies. *Neurology* 1991;41: 1781–1784.

47. Forster DM, Steiner L, Hakanson S. Arteriovenous malformations of the brain. A long-term clinical study. *J Neurosurg* 1972;37:562–570.

48. Foy PM, Copeland GP, Shaw MDM. The natural history of postoperative seizures. *Acta Neurochir (Wien)* 1981;55:253–264.

49. Franceschetti S, Battaglia G, Lodrini S, Aranzini G. Relationship between tumors and epilepsy. In: Broggi G., ed. *The rational basis of the surgical treatment of epilepsies.* London: John Libbey, 1988:47–51.

50. Franceschetti S, Binelli S, Casazza N, et al. Influence of surgery and antiepileptic drugs on seizures symptomatic of cerebral tumors. *Acta Neurochir (Wien)* 1990;103:47–51.

51. Fried I, Kim JH, Spencer DD. Hippocampal pathology in patients with intractable seizures and temporal lobe masses. *J Neurosurg* 1992;76:735–740.

52. Fried I, Kim JH, Spencer DD. Limbic and neocortical gliomas associated with intractable seizures: a distinct clinicopathological group. *Neurosurgery* 1994;34: 815–823.

53. Gastaut H. Clinical and electroencephalographic classification of epileptic seizures. *Epilepsia* 1970;11: 102–113.

54. Geier S, Bancaud J, Bonis A, Enjelvin M. Non-motor frontal epilepsy: study of electrographic and clinical features using tele-EEG and tele-stereo-EEG (Abstract). *Electroencephalogr Clin Neurophysiol* 1973; 34:699.

55. Geier S, Bancaud J, Talairach J, Bonis A, Enjelvin M, Hossard-Bouchaud H. Automatisms during frontal lobe epileptic seizures. *Brain* 1976;99:447–458.

56. Geier S, Bancaud J, Talairach J, Bonis A, Hossard-Bouchaud H, Enjelvin M. Ictal tonic postural changes and automatisms of the upper limb during epileptic parietal lobe discharges. *Epilepsia* 1977;18:517–524.

57. Geier A, Bancaud J, Talairach J, Bonis A, Szikla G, Enjelvin M. Clinical note: clinical and tele-stereo-EEG findings in a patient with psychomotor seizures. *Epilepsia* 1975;16:119–125.

58. Geier S, Bancaud J, Talairach J, Bonis A, Szikla G, Enjelvin M. The seizures of frontal lobe epilepsy: a study of clinical manifestations. *Neurology* 1977;27: 951–958.

59. Glaser GH. Treatment of intractable temporal lobe-

limbic epilepsy (complex partial seizures) by temporal lobectomy. *Ann Neurol* 1980;8:455–459.

60. Glazko AJ. Diphenylhydantoin. *Pharmacology* 1972; 8:163–177.

61. Gloor P. Contributions of electroencephalography and electrocorticography to the neurosurgical treatment of the epilepsies. *Acta Neurol* 1975;8:59–105.

62. Glotzner FL. Membrane properties of neuroglia in epileptogenic gliosis. *Brain Res* 1973;55:154–171.

63. Goldring S, Gregorie GM. Experience with gliomas and lesions which mimic them in patients presenting with chronic seizure disorder, part II. *Clin Neurosurg* 1986;33:43–70.

64. Goldring S, Rich KM, Picker S. Experience with gliomas in patients presenting with a chronic seizure disorder. *Clin Neurosurg* 1986;33:15–42.

65. Gonzalez D, Elvidge AR. On the occurrence of epilepsy caused by astrocytomas of the cerebral hemispheres. *J Neurosurg* 1962;19:470–482.

66. Guidetti B, Delitala A. Intracranial arteriovenous malformations. Conservative and surgical treatment. *J Neurosurg* 1980;53:149–152.

67. Haglund MM, Berger MS, Kunkel DD, Franck JE, Ghatan S, Ojemann GA. Changes in gamma-aminobutyric acid and somatostatin in epileptic cortex associated with low-grade gliomas. *J Neurosurg* 1992;77: 209–216.

68. Halpern LM, Julien RM. Augmentation of cerebellar Purkinje cell discharge rate after diphenylhydantoin. *Epilepsia* 1972;13:337–385.

69. Hauser WA, Annegers JF, Elveback LR. Mortality in patients with epilepsy. *Epilepsia* 1980;21:339–412.

70. Hausser-Hauw C, Bancaud J. Gustatory hallucinations in epileptic seizures: electrophysiological, clinical and anatomical correlates. *Brain* 1987;110:339–359.

71. Heikkinen ER, Yalynych N, Zubkov YN, Garmashov YA, Pak VA. et al. Relief of epilepsy by radiosurgery of cerebral arteriovenous malformations. *Stereotact Funct Neurosurg* 1989;53:157–166.

72. Hertz L. Potassium transport in astrocytes and neurons in primary culture. *Ann N Y Acad Sci* 1986;481: 318–333.

73. Hirsch JF, Sainte Rose C, Pierre-Khan A, et al. Benign astrocytic and oligodendrocytic tumors of the cerebral hemispheres in children. *J Neurosurg* 1989;70: 568–572.

74. Huott AD, Madison DS, Niedermeyer A. Occipital lobe epilepsy: a clinical and electroencephalographic study. *Eur Neurol* 1974;11:325–339.

75. Hutchinson HT, Werrback K, Vance C, Haber B. Uptake of neurotransmitters by clonal lines of astrocytoma and neuroblastoma in culture. *Brain Res* 1974; 66:265–274.

76. Ives JR, Gloor P. A long-term time-lapse video system to document the patient's spontaneous clinical seizure synchronized with the EEG. *Electroencephalogr Clin Neurophysiol* 1978;45:412–416.

77. Jackson JH. Localized convulsions from tumor of the brain. *Brain* 1882;5:364–374.

78. Janigro D, Gasparini S, D'Ambrosio R, McKhann G, DiFrancesco D. Reduction of K+ uptake in glia prevents long-term depression maintenance and causes epileptiform activity. *J Neurosci* 1997;17:2813–2824.

79. Janz D. Status epilepticus and frontal lobe lesions. *J Neurol Sci* 1964;1:446–457.

80. Jooma R, Yeh HS, Privitera MD, Gartner M. Lesionectomy versus electrophysiologically guided resection for temporal lobe tumors manifesting with complex partial seizures. *J Neurosurg* 1995;83:231–236.

81. Julien RM, Halpern LM. Effects of diphenylhydantoin and other antiepileptic drugs on epileptiform activity and Purkinje cell discharge rates. *Epilepsia* 1972;13: 387–400.

82. Ketz E. Brain tumours and epilepsy. In: Vinken PJ, Bruyn GW, eds. *Tumours of the brain and skull: handbook of clinical neurology.* Part I. Amsterdam: North-Holland, 1974:254–269.

83. Kim JH, Guimaraes PO, Shen MY, et al. Hippocampal neuronal density in temporal lobe epilepsy with and without gliomas. *Acta Neuropathol* 1990;80:41–45.

84. Kirkpatrick PJ, Honavar M, Janota I, Polkey CE. Control of temporal lobe epilepsy following en bloc resection of low-grade tumors. *J Neurosurg* 1993;78:19–25.

85. Leppik IE, Boucher R, Wilder BJ, et al. Phenytoin prodrug: preclinical and clinical studies. *Epilepsia* 1989; 30(Suppl 2):S22–S26.

86. Li LM, Cendes F, Watson C, et al. Surgical treatment of patients with single and dual pathology: relevance of lesion and of hippocampal atrophy to seizure outcome. *Neurology* 1997;48:437–444.

87. Lund M. Epilepsy in association with intracranial tumors. *Acta Psychiatr Neurol Scand Suppl* 1952;8: 1–149.

88. Mahaley MS, Dudka L. The role of anticonvulsant medication in the management of patients with anaplastic gliomas. *Surg Neurol* 1981;16:399–401.

89. Martin DL, Schain W. High affinity transport of taurine and alanine and low affinity transport of aminobutyric acid by a single transport system in cultured glioma cells. *J Biol Chem* 1979;254:7076–7084.

90. Mathieson G. Pathological aspects of epilepsy with special reference to the surgical pathology of focal cerebral seizures. In: Purpura DP, Perry JK, Walter RD, eds. *Advances in neurology,* vol. 8. New York: Raven Press, 1975:107–138.

91. Mattson RH. Value of intensive monitoring. In: Wada JA, Perry JK, eds. *Advances in epileptology,* 10th Epilepsy International Symposium. New York: Raven Press, 1980:43–51.

92. Mazars G. Cingulate gyrus epileptogenic foci as an origin for generalized seizures. In: Gastaut H, Jasper H, Bancaud J, Waltregny A, eds. *The physiopathogenesis of the epilepsies.* Springfield, IL: Charles C Thomas, 1969:186–189.

93. McGeer EG, Zhu SG. Lamotrigine protects against kainate but not ibotenate lesions in rat striatum. *Neurosci Lett* 1990;112:348–351.

94. Meldrum BS. Excitatory amino acid transmitters in epilepsy. *Epilepsia* 1991;32(Suppl 2):51–53.

95. Meyer FB, Marsh WR, Laws ER Jr, et al. Temporal lobectomy in children with epilepsy. *J Neurosurg* 1986;64:371–376.

96. Micromedex, Inc. (1974–1997). *Lamotrigine drug evaluation monograph,* vol 92, 1997.

97. Morris HH III, Luders H, Hahn JF, Lesser RP, Dinner DS, Estes ML. Neuropysiological techniques as an aid to surgical treatment of primary brain tumors. *Ann Neurol* 1986;19:559–567.

98. Mugnaini E. Cell junctions of astrocytes, ependyma and related cells in the mammalian nervous system with emphasis on the hypothesis of a generalized functional syncytium of supporting cells. In: Federoff S, Vernadakis A, eds. *Astrocytes,* vol. 1. *Development, morphogenesis and regional specialization of astrocytes.* Orlando: Academic Press, 1986:329–391.

99. Munari C, Bonis A, Kochen S, et al. Eye movements and occipital seizures in man. *Acta Neurochir* 1984; 33(Suppl):47–52.

100. Murphy MJ. Long-term follow-up of seizures associated with arteriovenous malformations: results of therapy. *Arch Neurol* 1985;42:477–479.

101. Naus CCG, Bechberger JF, Paul DL. Gap junction gene expression in human seizure disorder. *Exp Neurol* 1991;111:198–203.

102. Naus CCG, Bechberger JF, Caveney S, Wilson JX. Expression of gap junction genes in astrocytes and C6 glioma cells. *Neurosci Lett* 1991;112:33–36.

103. Nicklas WJ, Browning ET. Amino acid metabolism in glial cells: homeostatic regulation of intra- and extracellular milieu by C6 glioma cells. *J Neurochem* 1978;30:955–963.

104. Niedermeyer E. Compendium of the epilepsies. Springfield, IL: Charles C Thomas, 1974.

105. Niedermeyer E, Laws ER Jr, Walker AE. Depth EEG findings in epileptics with generalized spike-wave complexes. *Arch Neurol* 1969;21:51–58.

106. Ochs R, Gloor P, Quesney LF, Ives J, Olivier A. Does head-turning during a seizure have lateralizing or localizing significance? *Neurology* 1984;34:884–890.

107. O'Donohoe NV. Use of antiepileptic drugs in childhood epilepsy. *Arch Dis Child* 1991;66:1173–1179.

108. Olivier A, Gloor P, Andermann F. Occipitotemporal epilepsy studied with stereotactically implanted depth electrodes and successfully treated by temporal resection. *Ann Neurol* 1982;11:428–432.

109. Paterson JH, McKissock W. A clinical survey of intracranial angiomas with special reference to their mode of progression and surgical treatment: a report of 110 cases. *Brain* 1956;79:233–266.

110. Peck AW. Clinical pharmacology of lamotrigine. *Epilepsia* 1991; 32(Suppl 2):S9–S12.

111. Penfield W, Erickson TC, Tarlov I. Relation of intracranial tumors and symptomatic epilepsy. *Arch Neurol Psychiatry* 1940;44:300–315.

112. Penfield W, Kristiansen K. *Epileptic seizure patterns.* Springfield, IL: Charles C Thomas, 1951.

113. Penfield W, Jasper H. Epilepsy and the functional anatomy of the human brain. Boston: Little, Brown, 1954.

114. Peserico L, Nori A, Ravenna C. L'epilessia postoperatoria nei meniniomi endocranici. *Acta Neurochir (Wien)* 1965;13:196–211.

115. Piepmeier J, Christopher S, Spencer D, et al. Variations in the natural history and survival of patients with supratentorial low-grade astrocytomas. *Neurosurgery* 1996;38:872–878.

116. Pilcher WH, Silbergeld DL, Berger MS, Ojemann GA. Intraoperative electrocorticography during tumor resection: impact on seizure outcome in patients with gangliogliomas. *J Neurosurg* 1993;78:891–902.

117. Porter RJ. Mechanisms of action of new antiepileptic drugs. *Epilepsia* 1989; 30(Suppl 1):529–534.

118. Quesney LF. Clinical and EEG features of complex partial seizures of temporal lobe origin. *Epilepsia* 1986;27(Suppl 2):527–545.

119. Ramamurthi B, Ravi R, Ramachandran V. Convulsions with meningiomas: incidence and significance. *Surg Neurol* 1980;14:415–416.

120. Rasmussen T. Surgical therapy of frontal lobe epilepsy. *Epilepsia* 1963;4:181–198.

121. Rasmussen T. Surgery of epilepsy associated with brain tumors. In: Purpura DP, Penry JK, Walter RD, eds. *Neurosurgical management of the epilepsies advances in neurology,* vol. 8. New York: Raven Press, 1975:227–239.

122. Rasmussen T. Characteristics of a pure culture of frontal lobe epilepsy. *Epilepsia* 1983;24:482–493.

123. Rasmussen T, Blundell J. Epilepsy and brain tumor. *Clin Neurosurg* 1961;7:138–158.

124. Regis J, Peragut JC, Rey M, et al. First selective amygdalohippocampal radiosurgery for mesial temporal lobe epilepsy. *Stereotact Funct Neurosurg* 1995;64: 193–201.

125. Reynolds JEF, ed. Martindale: the extra pharmacopoeia (electronic version). Denver: Micromedex, Inc, 1993.

126. Ribaric I. Excision of two and three independent and separate ipsilateral potentially epileptogenic cortical areas. *Acta Neurochir Suppl* 1983;33:145–148.

127. Robillard A, Saint-Hilaire JM, Mercier M, Bouvier G. The lateralizing and localizing value of adversion in epileptic seizures. *Neurology* 1983;33:1241–1242.

128. Rogers L, Morris H, Lupica K. Effect of cranial irradiation on seizure frequency in adults with low grade astrocytomas and medically intractable epilepsy. *Neurology* 1993;43:1599–1601.

129. Rosenbaum DH, Siegel M, Rowan AJ. Contraversive seizures in occipital epilepsy: case report and review of the literature. *Neurology* 1986;36:281–284.

130. Rossi GF, Scerrati M, Roselli R. Epileptogenic cerebral low-grade tumors: effect of interstitial stereotactic irradiation on seizures. *Appl Neurophysiol* 1985;48: 127–132.

131. Russell WR, Whitty CWM. Studies in traumatic epilepsy. 3. Visual fits. *J Neurol* 1955;18:79–96.

132. Sachs E, Furlow FC. The significance of convulsion in the diagnosis of brain tumor. *J Missouri State Med Assoc* 1936;33:121–127.

133. Salanova V, Andermann F, Olivier A, Rasmussen T, Quesney LF. Occipital lobe epilepsy: electroclinical manifestations, electrocorticography, cortical stimulation and outcome in 42 patients treated between 1930 and 1991. *Brain* 1992;115:1655–1680.

134. Salanova V, Andermann F, Rasmussen T, Olivier A, Quesney LF. Tumoural parietal lobe epilepsy: clinical manifestations and outcome in 34 patients treated between 1934 and 1988. *Brain* 1995;118:1289–1304.

135. Schisano G, Tovi D, Nordenstam H. Spongioblastoma polare of the cerebral hemisphere. *J Neurosurg* 1963; 20:241–251.

136. Schonsboe A, Svenneby G, Hertz L. Uptake and metabolism of glutamate in astrocytes cultured from dissociated mouse brain hemispheres. *J Neurochem* 1977; 29:999–1005.

137. Schrier BK, Thompson EJ. On the role of glial cells in the mammalian nervous system. *J Biol Chem* 1974; 249:1769–1780.

138. Simard JM, Garcia-Bengochea F, Ballinger WE Jr, Micklc JP, Quisling RG. Cavernous angioma: a review

139. Sloviter RS. Decreased hippocampal inhibition and a selective loss of interneurons in experimental epilepsy. *Science* 1987;235:73–76.

140. Spencer DD, Spencer SS, Mattson RH, et al. Intracerebral masses in patients with intractable partial epilepsy. *Neurology* 1984;34:432–436.

141. Sperling MR, Cahan LD, Brown WJ. Relief of seizures from a predominantly posterior temporal tumor with anterior temporal lobectomy. *Epilepsia* 1989;30:559–563.

142. Stoffels C, Munari C, Bonis A, Bancaud J, Talairach J. Manifestations génitales et sexuelles lors des crises épileptiques partielles chez l'homme. *Rev Electroencephalogr Neurophysiol Clin* 1981;10:386–392.

143. Takeda A, Bancaud J, Talairach J, Bonis A, Bordas-Ferrer M. Concerning epileptic attacks of occipital origin. *Electroenceph Clin Neurophysiol* 1970;28:647–648.

144. Trumpy JH, Eldevik P. Intracranial arteriovenous malformations: conservative or surgical treatment? *Surg Neurol* 1977;8:171–175.

145. Uthman BM, Wilder BJ. Emergency management of seizures: an overview. *Epilepsia* 1989;30(Suppl 2): S33–S37.

146. Van Buren JM, Ajmone-Marsan C, Matsuga N. Temporal lobe seizures with additional foci treated by resection. *J Neurosurg* 1975;43:596–607.

147. Van Gelder NM, Courtois A. Close correlation between changing content of specific amino acids in epileptogenic cortex of cats and severity of epilepsy. *Brain Res* 1972;43:477–484.

148. Von Wieser W. Die Roentgentherapie der traumatischen Epilepsie. *Monatsschr Psychiatr Neurol* 1939; 101:171–179.

149. Walsh GO, Delgado-Escueta AV. Type II complex partial seizures: poor results of anterior temporal lobectomy. *Neurology* 1984;34:1–13.

150. Walum E. Counter transport of glutamine and choline in cultures of human glioma cells. *Biochem Biophys Res Comm* 1979;88:1271–1274.

151. Weber JP, Silbergeld DL, Winn HR. Surgical resection of epileptogenic cortex associated with structural lesions. *Neurosurg Clin North Am* 1993;4:327–336.

152. Whang CJ, Kim CJ. Short-term follow-up of stereotactic gamma knife radiosurgery in epilepsy. *Stereotact Funct Neurosurg* 1995;64:202–208.

153. White JC, Liu CT, Mixter WJ. Focal epilepsy: a statistical study of its causes and the results of surgical treatment. I. Epilepsy secondary to intracranial tumors. *N Engl J Med* 1948;238:891–899.

154. Wieser HG. Stereoelectroencephalographic correlates of focal motor seizures. In: Speckman EJ, Elger CE, eds. *Epilepsy and motor system.* Munich: Urban & Schwarzenberg, 1983:287–309.

155. Wieser HG. Psychomotor seizures of hippocampal-amygdalar origin. In: Pedley TA, Meldrum BS, eds. *Recent advances in epilepsy.* Edinburgh: Churchill Livingstone, 1986:57–79.

156. Williamson PD, Boon PA, Thadani VM, et al. Parietal lobe epilepsy: diagnostic considerations and results of surgery. *Ann Neurol* 1992;31:193–201.

157. Williamson PD, Spencer DD, Spencer SS, Novelly RA, Mattson RH. Complex partial seizures of frontal lobe origin. *Ann Neurol* 1985;18:497–504.

of 126 collected and 12 new clinical cases. *Neurosurgery* 1986;18:162–172.

158. Williamson PD, Thadani VM, Darcey TM, Spencer DD, Spencer SS, Mattson RH. Occipital lobe epilepsy: clinical characteristics, seizure spread patterns, and results of surgery. *Ann Neurol* 1992;31:3–13.

159. Williamson PD, Wieser H-G, Delgado-Escueta AV. Clinical characteristics of partial seizures. In: Engel J Jr, ed. *Surgical treatment of the epilepsies.* New York: Raven Press, 1987:101–120.

160. Woodbury DM, Fingl E. Drugs effective in the therapy of the epilepsies. In: Goodman LS, Gilman A, eds. *The pharmacological basis of therapeutics.* New York: Macmillan, 1975:201–226.

161. Wyler AR, Richey ET, Hermann BP. Comparison of scalp to subdural recordings for localizing epileptogenic foci. *J Epilepsy* 1989;2:91–96.

162. Wyllie E, Luders H, Morris HH. The lateralizing significance of versive head and eye movements during epileptic seizures. *Neurology* 1986;36:606–611.

163. Wyllie E, Luders H, Morris HH III, et al. Clinical outcome after complete or partial cortical resection for intractable epilepsy. *Neurology* 1987;37:1634–1641.

164. Youmans JR, Cobb CA. Glial and neuronal tumors of the brain in adults. In: Youmans JR, ed. *Neurological surgery.* Philadelphia: WB Saunders, 1982:2759–2835.

The Practical Management of Low-Grade Primary Brain Tumors, edited by Jack P. Rock, Mark L. Rosenblum, Edward G. Shaw, and J. Gregory Cairncross. Lippincott Williams & Wilkins, Philadelphia, © 1999

11

Genetics and Genetic Counseling

Paula M. Czarnecki and Daniel L. Van Dyke

Department of Medical Genetics, Henry Ford Hospital, Detroit, Michigan 48202

A heritable component to cancer has been recognized for more than a century (2,37,38). Evidence from the epidemiology of retinoblastoma, which can either arise sporadically or be inherited in an autosomal dominant pattern, led Alfred Knudson (19) to postulate that the development of this cancer is caused by two mutational events, one of which may be inherited. It is now clear that numerous other genes can act in a similar fashion (i.e., a tumor suppressor gene), including the neurofibromatosis gene, where two mutational events are required for the development of myeloid leukemia in affected subjects (34).

The explosive growth of knowledge in genetics has advanced the field to one of central importance in medical science (27). Genetics is no longer viewed as the obscure cataloging of rare disorders; indeed, genetic factors play a role in most forms of disease. Molecular genetics research is providing insights into the mechanisms of disease that apply to classic Mendelian genetic disorders and to areas not usually considered genetic such as infectious disease.

New technology is strengthening the armamentarium of the clinical geneticist. In the past the only intervention for most genetic diseases was informing the family about risks of recurrence. Today's technology allows prenatal testing for many disorders, often during the first trimester of pregnancy, and presymptomatic and predictive assessment of the risk for heritable disorders of adult onset, such as Huntington disease and breast cancer. Insight

into pathogenesis has generated specific forms of therapy, and experimental approaches based on organ transplantation and gene replacement therapy are under way.

The literature on brain tumors reveals considerably more information concerning high-grade or malignant tumors and little about low-grade tumors. Several heritable syndromes (e.g., tuberous sclerosis, neurofibromatosis types I and II) are associated with low-grade brain tumors and have yielded important information for clinicians and patients and their families (Table 1). Ikizler et al. (17) reported a 6.7% incidence of familial glioma in an unselected consecutive series of 178 newly diagnosed patients. None of the cases had associated tuberous sclerosis, neurofibromatosis types I and II, or other heritable disorders. Excluding the high-grade lesions from this series, the incidence of low-grade tumors was 1.3%.

This chapter reviews clinical genetics issues relevant to hereditary predisposition to low-grade brain tumors.

GENETIC COUNSELING

Genetic counseling is a communication process that deals with the occurrence, or the risk of occurrence or recurrence, of a genetic disorder in a family or individual. The role of the genetic counselor is to help the individual and the family to (a) comprehend the medical facts, including diagnosis, probable course of the disorder, and available medical management; (b) appreciate the way heredity contributes to the disorder and the risk of recurrence in specified relatives; (c) understand the alternatives for dealing with the risk of recurrence; (d) choose the course of action that is appropriate in view of their risk, family goals, and ethical and religious standards, and to act in accordance with that decision; and (e) make the best possible adjustment to the disorder in an affected family member and/or to the risk of recurrence of that disorder (7).

The genetic counseling process involves interactions among many individuals, including clinical geneticists, genetic counselors, cytogeneticists, oncologists, neurosurgeons, biochemical and molecular geneticists, and genetic support groups. The major difference between the genetic counseling approach and more traditional medical approaches involves the decision-making process. That is, when the family chooses a course of action, many different aspects are taken into account. This nondirective approach stresses the family's autonomy and leaves the decision-making process to the individual and his or her family. Therefore the information regarding risks, treatment options, and natural history must be presented in a thorough and unbiased manner, allowing the family members to decide how to proceed based on their own situation.

A key component to genetic counseling is to make an accurate diagnosis. To help arrive at that diagnosis the construction of a family pedigree is vital. The pedigree serves as a graphic representation of the family's history. Both sides of the family history, generally at least through second-degree relatives, are obtained. The specific questions asked depend on the disease in question. In cancer genetic counseling the questions would include, for each affected family member, the age at diagnosis, specific type of cancer, primary site of the tumor, bilaterality/unilaterality, and age at death. In obtaining the family history, the genetic counselor looks for specific patterns that may suggest a genetic etiology to the disease. A physical examination of the individual is imperative to distinguish between a genetic syndrome and an isolated finding. The consequences of not diagnosing a genetic syndrome include an undetermined cancer etiology, uncertain prognosis, empiric rather than specific recurrence risks, unlikely chance for prenatal diagnosis, and inappropriate treatment.

The following is an example of a typical genetic counseling session: A 5-year-old boy was referred with his parents to the Genetics Clinic for counseling about his recent diagnosis of an optic glioma. Optic gliomas can oc-

TABLE 1. *Genetic conditions associated with low-grade brain tumors*

Syndrome	Inheritance	Benign tumor type	Reference
Aicardi	X-linked	Choroid plexus papilloma	22
Ataxia telangiectasia	AR	Glioma; medulloblastoma	11,12,16,39
Hypomelanosis of Ito	AD; mosaic chromosome	Choroid plexus papilloma	14,30,41
Melanoma/astrocytoma	AD	Astrocytoma; possibly glioblastoma multiforme; acoustic neurilemmoma; meningioma	2,23
Cowden (multiple hamartoma)	AD	Cerebellar gangliocytoma; meningioma	19,28,35,38
Papilloma of the choroid plexus	AR	Choroid plexus papilloma	9
Neurofibromatosis type 1	AD	Meningioma; pheochromocytoma; schwannoma; acoustic neuroma	16,40
Neurofibromatosis type 2	AD	Acoustic schwannoma; meningioma	12,33
Tuberous sclerosis	AD	Astrocytoma; ependymoma; hamartoma	7,19,22
Von Hippel Lindau	AD	Cerebellar or spinal cord hemangioblastoma; pheochromocytoma	4,8,24,29,40

AR, autosomal recessive; AD, autosomal dominant.

cur as isolated tumors (36) but can be familial (1), and represent the most common type of central nervous system tumor seen in patients with neurofibromatosis type 1 (21,23). In the patient's family history, his father was noted to have had multiple moles removed from his face. Physical examination of the patient revealed axillary and inguinal freckling. Physical examination of the father revealed multiple cafe-au-lait spots and several skin tumors suggestive of neurofibromas. Based on the family history and physical examination, the patient was diagnosed with neurofibromatosis type 1.

This example shows the significance of obtaining family and medical histories along with performing a physical examination on the index case and other at-risk family members. In this situation a genetic syndrome was identified (versus an isolated optic glioma) and a second affected family member was identified, appropriately evaluated, and counseled regarding the specific medical and genetic risks associated with the diagnosis.

GENETIC ETIOLOGY OF BRAIN TUMORS

To begin a discussion of genetics, several key concepts must be described. Every cell nucleus in the human body, except for the gametes, contains 23 pairs of chromosomes. The autosomes constitute 22 pairs of chromosomes and are the same in both sexes. The 23rd pair are the sex chromosomes, XX in a female and XY in a male. The chromosomes contain the DNA, which encodes the genetic information for human development. There are estimated to be between 50,000 and 100,000 genes. A mutation in a gene can disrupt or alter its function and lead to genetic disease. A locus is the chromosomal location of a specific gene. The various forms of a gene at a particular locus are called alleles. A person who carries two identical alleles at a specific locus is termed *homozygous*, whereas one who carries two different alleles (one normal and one mutant) at a specific locus is termed *heterozygous*. The genetic constitution

of a particular genetic locus is termed the *genotype*. The observable characteristics of an individual are termed the *phenotype*. There are three classic patterns of genetic transmission: autosomal recessive, autosomal dominant, and X-linked.

Autosomal Recessive

Autosomal recessive traits are expressed only if an individual carries two mutant alleles. Both parents of an affected individual are usually heterozygous for the disease gene and are termed *carriers*. Carriers usually do not display any phenotypic features of the disease. Each carrier parent has a one in two (50%) risk of passing on the mutant gene to each child. Therefore the risk that a couple who carries the same mutant gene will have an affected child is one in four (25%). Unaffected siblings of an affected individual have a two in three risk of carrying the mutant gene. Characteristic features of autosomal recessive inheritance include the following: usually only siblings are affected; affected members in multiple generations are usually *not* observed; and males and females are equally likely to be affected (see Fig. 1A). Some autosomal recessive conditions are more frequent in specific racial or ethnic groups, representing the expression of a mutation that was present in one or a few of the founding members of a group (founder effect). Rare autosomal recessive traits tend to be more common in consanguineous relationships (inbreeding), because related individuals are likely to share many of the same genes. Because it has been estimated that everyone carries at least five nonfunctioning (mutated) genes, some of the nonfunctioning genes may be among those shared.

An example of an autosomal recessive condition is papilloma of the choroid plexus. Several families have been described with two affected siblings (5,20), and in one case the parents were first cousins (41). Another example of an autosomal recessive condition associated with low-grade brain tumors is ataxia telangiectasia (AT). AT is characterized by

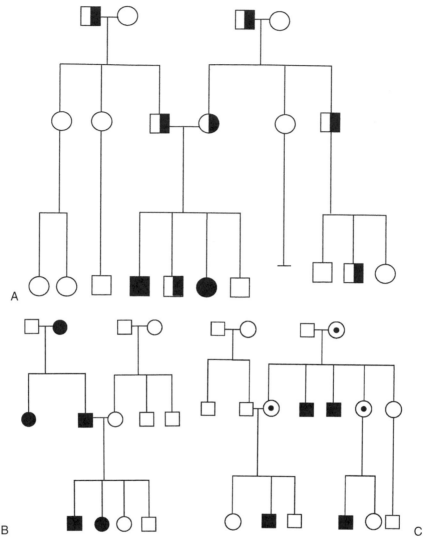

FIG. 1. Pedigrees illustrating (**A**) recessive, (**B**) dominant, and (**C**) X-linked inheritance. Males are indicated by square symbols and females by circles. Filled-in symbols represent people affected with the trait. Half-filled symbols represent carriers of an autosomal recessive trait; dots represent carriers of an X-linked trait.

presentation in early childhood of progressive cerebellar ataxia with later onset of conjunctival telangiectases. This condition is sometimes misdiagnosed because the early ataxia presents similarly to ataxic cerebral palsy. Often it is not until the appearance of oculocutaneous telangiectases that the diagnosis is made. Additional characteristics of the disorder include cellular and humoral immunode-ficiency; thymic and ovarian degeneration; growth retardation; oculomotor apraxia, which is progressive; choreoathetosis and/or dystonia; and neurologic dysfunction (12,39). Patients with AT have a strong predisposition to malignancy, specifically lymphocytic leukemia (16). However, other solid tumors, including medulloblastomas and mixed low-grade gliomas, also occur (11,32).

Autosomal Dominant Inheritance

Unlike autosomal recessive traits that are expressed only when both alleles are non-functioning, autosomal dominant traits are expressed in heterozygotes. Therefore individuals who are heterozygous for an autosomal dominant trait have a one in two (50%) risk of passing on the mutant gene to their offspring. Features of autosomal dominant inheritance include the following: successive generations are affected; males and females are equally likely to be affected; and male-to-male transmission does occur (see Fig. 1B). In an individual noted to be affected with an autosomal dominant condition, evaluation of all first-degree relatives for mild features (variable expressivity) of the disease is warranted. Expressivity of a disease is defined as the range of phenotypic variability of a genetic trait in a population. If neither parent is affected, the recurrence risk depends on the rate of penetrance of the disorder. Penetrance refers to the proportion of individuals possessing a disease-causing genotype who express the disease phenotype. When this proportion is less than 100%, there is said to be incomplete or reduced penetrance. Careful examination of parents and siblings is recommended to determine the recurrence risk. If the disease is due to a new autosomal dominant mutation (in the child), the recurrence risk for the parents would be low, keeping in mind the risk of gonadal mosaicism. Gonadal (germline) mosaicism is defined as the occurrence of two or more cell lines derived from a single fertilization event but differing by the presence or absence of a mutant allele. Gonadal mosaicism can occur during the embryonic development of one of the parents. A mutation can occur that affects all or part of the germline but none of the somatic cells. In such a case, the parent is not affected with the disease but carries the mutation in the germline and can transmit the disease gene to his/her offspring. The recurrence risk, if one of the parents carries a germline mutation, is known for some diseases, but for others an empiric risk of 5% would be given (15). This

would be the recurrence risk given after a thorough genetic evaluation of both parents.

Tuberous sclerosis is an example of an autosomal dominant condition that contains many of the features described above. Tuberous sclerosis affects 1 in 12,000 children under age 10. The condition affects many organ systems, including the brain, kidneys, heart, eyes, lungs, and skin. Approximately 15% of patients with tuberous sclerosis have a parent who is affected. The other 85% presumably represent new autosomal dominant mutations. The condition is characterized by variable expression with approximately 80% to 90% of patients experiencing seizures, 96% of patients having four skin lesions (such as hypomelanotic macules), and 43% of patients having a cardiac rhabdomyoma (13). Other physical features include white ash leaf-shaped macules, pit-shaped enamel defects, fibromatous plaques on the forehead and lumbosacral regions, subungual fibromata, mental deficiency, and other tumors (e.g., astrocytomas, ependymomas, and retinal, optic, cardiac, and olfactory hamartomas). Because of the variable expression of the disease, a physical examination not only of the index case but also of the parents and siblings is warranted. If physical examination of the parents and siblings is negative and the recommended imaging studies are negative, the parents' recurrence risk would be approximately 5% (13). This includes the possibility of gonadal mosaicism. Two gene loci have been identified thus far for tuberous sclerosis. The loci reside at band 9q32-q34 on chromosome 9 and at band 16p13.3 on chromosome 16. Laboratory testing by linkage analysis, protein truncation, and mutation analysis is currently available (3,14,18).

Two other autosomal dominant conditions associated with low-grade brain tumors are neurofibromatosis type 1 (NF-1) and type 2 (NF-2). NF-1, also known as von Recklinghausen disease, is a common heritable disease that predisposes to brain tumors. NF-1 has significant variable expression (even within families), with most affected individuals having numerous cafe-au-lait spots and neurofibromata. Other physical features include lisch nodules (iris hamartomas), axillary/inguinal freckling, and sphenoid dysplasia. Various tumor types are associated with NF-1, including pheochromocytoma, meningioma, glioma, rhabdomyosarcoma, schwannoma, hypothalamic tumor, and neurofibrosarcoma. The NF-1 gene has been localized to chromosome 17q11.2 and encodes a very large messenger RNA. Currently, molecular testing is available by protein truncation assay, which detects 70% of individuals with NF-1. In other families, fluorescent *in situ* hybridization (FISH) for large deletions or linkage analysis can be performed (10,29,33).

NF-2 is characterized by bilateral acoustic neuromata (26), with a median age of onset of diagnosis of 22 years resulting from hearing loss. Other features include spinal tumors, acoustic schwannoma, and cataracts. The gene has been localized to chromosome 22 and the gene product (schwannomin) appears to be a tumor suppressor gene (31). Mutation analysis for NF-2 is available.

Other autosomal dominant conditions associated with low-grade brain tumors are listed in Table 1.

X-Linked Inheritance

Traits expressed by genes on the X or Y chromosome are referred to as sex-linked. Most human sex-linked traits involve the X chromosome. Key features of X-linked recessive inheritance include the following: a much higher incidence in males than females, and absence of male-to-male transmission because an affected father can only transmit his X chromosome to a daughter, who would then be a carrier of the X-linked trait (see Fig. 1C). A woman who carries an X-linked recessive trait has a one in two (50%) risk of passing that gene to her son, who would be affected. She also has a one in two (50%) risk of passing on the gene to her daughter, who would be a carrier. Female carriers are heterozygous and usually do not manifest the disorder. In females, only one X chromosome is genetically active in each cell, as a form of dosage compensation. Inactivation of one X chromosome occurs randomly in each cell early in embryogenesis, which results in approximately half of the cells in a carrier expressing the normal allele and half expressing the mutant gene. We are not aware of any X-linked recessive diseases that are associated with low-grade brain tumors.

X-linked dominant traits can be expressed in both males and females. In some cases the effects in the male are so severe that they are lethal during embryogenesis. One example of an X-linked dominant condition is Aicardi syndrome, which is seen almost exclusively in females. One case was reported of a male affected with Aicardi syndrome, but he also had Klinefelter syndrome (47,XXY). Aicardi syndrome is characterized by infantile spasms, chorioretinal abnormality in the form of lacunae (lakes), and choroid plexus papillomas. There have been some reported cases of cleft lip and palate. Donnenfeld et al. (6) found complete agenesis of the corpus callosum in 72% and partial agenesis in 28% of patients with Aicardi syndrome. Costovertebral defects—including hemivertebrae, scoliosis, and absent or malformed ribs—were present in 39%. Again, because of the variability of expression, a complete genetic evaluation is warranted. Of particular interest in the family history would be early infant deaths or stillbirths involving a male fetus. Presently there is no available molecular testing for Aicardi syndrome; however, cytogenetic analysis for X chromosome rearrangements would be warranted.

PRENATAL DIAGNOSIS AND PRESYMPTOMATIC TESTING

During counseling for a family with a known genetic disease, many individuals are primarily concerned with the risks to their offspring. In some cases where the gene has been identified, prenatal diagnosis may be available to determine if the fetus has inherited the disease gene. However, prenatal diagnosis presently cannot determine the severity or the age of onset of the disease. This raises many ethical questions about testing a fetus for an adult-onset disease that may not manifest for decades. Other ethical considerations include the concepts of autonomy, beneficence, nonmaleficence, and justice. Autonomy is the principle of being one's own person and choosing one's own course of action. Beneficence is the duty to confer benefits and to prevent and remove harm. Nonmaleficence is a duty not to inflict evil or harm. Justice is defined as identical cases being treated in the same manner. These principles are in obvious conflict in prenatal diagnosis. For example, if a diagnosis of tuberous sclerosis is confirmed during a pregnancy and the couple chooses to terminate the pregnancy, there is conflict between maternal and fetal autonomy.

For many genetic conditions the disease gene has not yet been identified; therefore direct DNA testing is not available for prenatal diagnosis. However, for some diseases, linkage analysis may be available. Linkage analysis involves following genetic markers (genetically variable sites on a chromosome near where the disease gene is thought to reside) in a family to determine if an at-risk pregnancy has inherited the chromosome thought to carry the disease gene. Linkage analysis requires DNA samples from multiple affected and unaffected family members. This testing is not as accurate as direct DNA analysis, but it can reassure a family that a fetus has inherited the chromosome that probably carries the normal gene. Alternative options may include artificial insemination by donor sperm or egg donation, depending on the disease and mode of inheritance. Another available option is adopting a child to avoid having an affected child. During prenatal counseling many such issues must be addressed. The views of the family must always be respected and their decision supported.

Another concern often voiced by parents and family members is the availability of predisposition testing. Predisposition testing involves testing asymptomatic individuals who are at-risk for a specific genetic disease. Generally, predisposition testing is not per-formed on minors unless the condition is expected to manifest in childhood or treatment is available. Although predisposition testing is not practical for low-grade brain tumors, there are some cancer families where early-onset cancers are common and predisposition testing would be warranted. For example, in Li-Fraumeni syndrome, 50% of the cancers occur prior to age 30. The most common childhood cancers are soft-tissue sarcomas prior to age 5, and osteosarcomas in adolescence. Acute leukemia and brain tumors can also occur during childhood and early adulthood (22). In 1990, five families with Li-Fraumeni syndrome were found to have an identifiable germline mutation in the p53 gene (25). The identification of this gene allows for direct or linkage analysis in some families with Li-Fraumeni syndrome. Subsequently, predisposition testing can be performed on at-risk family members if a mutation is identified to allow for early detection and prevention. In this situation, testing minors is recommended (22) with the goal of reducing cancer mortality and morbidity. Predisposition testing can determine whether an individual has inherited the disease gene and is at increased risk to develop cancer. It does not determine whether an individual will definitely develop cancer. This differs from presymptomatic testing, such as in Huntington disease, where an individual who inherits the disease gene will be affected with Huntington disease. In counseling a family regarding predisposition testing, the ethical principles of autonomy, beneficence, confidentiality, and justice need to be considered. Confidentiality requires attention to avoid inadvertent disclosure of information to third parties. This is important, especially when counseling large families so that privacy is maintained. Because of the many issues involved in predictive testing and because of the constant new advances in the area of genetics, it is often too great a challenge for most physicians to keep abreast of the tests available. The patient should be referred to a clinical geneticist and/or genetic counselor to provide the most up-to-date information.

GENETIC CONDITIONS ASSOCIATED WITH BRAIN TUMORS

For the clinical work-up of any patient with cancer and birth defects or mental deficiency, it is vital to involve a clinical geneticist who is familiar with such conditions and who can order the specific molecular or cytogenetic tests that will establish the correct diagnosis and lead to appropriate genetic counseling for the family.

At least 10 mendelian conditions predispose to the development of low-grade brain tumors (see Table 1). These and thousands of other heritable conditions can be accessed using McKusick's OnLine Mendelian Inheritance in Man (OMIM) resource, which is available on CDROM, through NetScape (www.ncbi.nlm.nih.gov/omim/), or in standard format (27). Although these resources are readily available, a proper genetic evaluation and formal genetic counseling regarding the additional issues are imperative in providing comprehensive medical care.

CONCLUSION

The value of a genetic evaluation when an apparently isolated brain tumor is involved is multifold. It is of utmost importance to establish whether this is an isolated finding with no risk to other family members and no other risks to the patient, as opposed to a component of a genetic syndrome. If a diagnosis of a syndrome is made, other organ systems may need to be evaluated. Also, because many genetic diseases have variable expression, other family members may unknowingly be at-risk and may need to be evaluated and/or monitored. A genetics clinic can provide service to all family members by referring them to other specialists, providing patient literature, and placing the patient in touch with support groups. Many genetic diseases have national organizations available to help answer questions, put patients in touch with other families, and provide additional literature on the specific disease. Therefore, although the diagnosis of a genetic disease can sometimes be devastating to a family, support groups can help them through a difficult time.

The dramatic and wide-ranging advances in our understanding of human genetics allow ever more precise diagnosis of hundreds of disorders. The possibility of recurrence should be addressed in the care of any medical disorder by analysis of the family history and knowledge of the medical literature. Molecular diagnostic tools and the products of the Human Genome Project increasingly allow the diagnosis of inherited disorders before the appearance of symptoms. This also allows for prenatal diagnosis. As knowledge of pathogenesis is gained, it is clear that many genetic disorders will be amenable to therapy, either medically or through novel means of gene replacement.

ACKNOWLEDGMENTS

The authors thank Drs. G. L. Feldman and E. V. Bawle for a critical reading of the manuscript.

This was supported in part by U.S. Public Health Service NIH grant CA70093 to D.L.V.D.

REFERENCES

1. Abellan P, George JL, Bracard S, Berchet T. Family cases of optic nerve glioma with normal visual acuity. *Ann Med Nancy* 1986;25:27–28.
2. Broca PP. Traité des tumeurs. Paris: Asselin, 1866.
3. Cassidy SB, Pagon RA, Pepin M, Blumhagen JD. Family studies in tuberous sclerosis: evaluation of apparently unaffected parents. *JAMA* 1983;249:1302–1304.
4. Chen F, Kishida T, Yao M, et al. Germline mutations in the von Hippel-Lindau disease tumor suppressor gene: correlations with phenotype. *Hum Mutation* 1995;5: 66–75.
5. Coons S, Johnson PC, Dickman CA, Rekate H. Choroid plexus carcinoma in siblings: a study by light and electron microscopy with KI-67 immunocytochemistry. *J Neuropathol Exp Neurol* 1989;48:483–493.
6. Donnenfeld AD, Packer RJ, Zackai EH, et al. Clinical, cytogenetic, and pedigree findings in 18 cases of Aicardi syndrome. *Am J Med Genet* 1989; 32:461–467.
7. Epstein CJ. Genetic counseling. *Am J Hum Genet* 1975; 27:240–242.
8. Evans DGR, Huson SM, Donnai D, et al. A genetic study of type 2 neurofibromatosis in the United Kingdom. I. Prevalence, mutation rate, fitness, and confirmation of maternal transmission effect on severity. *J Med Genet* 1992;29:841–846.

9. Flannery DB. Pigmentary dysplasias, hypomelanosis of Ito, and genetic mosaicism. *Am J Med Genet* 1990;35: 18–21.

10. Friedman JM, Birch PH. Type 1 neurofibromatosis: a descriptive analysis of the disorder in 1,728 patients. *Am J Med Genet* 1997;70:138–143.

11. Gatti RA, Boder E, Vinters HV, Sparkes RS, et al. Ataxia-telangiectasia: an interdisciplinary approach to pathogenesis. *Medicine* 1991,70.99–117.

12. Gilad S, Khosravi R, Shkedy D, et al. Predominance of null mutations in ataxia-telangiectasia. *Hum Mol Genet* 1996;5:433–439.

13. Gomez MR. *Neurocutaneous diseases: a practical approach.* Boston: Butterworths Publishers, 1987.

14. Gorlin RJ, Cohen MM, Levin LS. *Syndromes of the head and neck.* New York: Oxford University Press, 1990.

15. Hall JG. Review and hypothesis: somatic mosaicism—observations related to clinical genetics. *Am J Hum Genet* 1988;43:355–363.

16. Hecht F, Koler RD, Rigas DA, et al. Leukemia and lymphocytes in ataxia-telangiectasia. *Lancet* 1966;11:1193.

17. Ikizler Y, van Meyel DJ, Ramsay DA, et al. Gliomas in families. *Can J Neurol Sci* 1992;19:492–497.

18. Jones KL. *Smith's recognizable patterns of human malformation,* 5th ed. Philadelphia: WB Saunders, 1996.

19. Knudson AG Jr. Mutation and cancer: statistical study of retinoblastoma. *Proc Natl Acad Sci USA* 1971;68. 820–823.

20. Komminoth R, Woringer E, Baumgartner J, et al. Papillome intraventriculaire familial: caractéristiques angiographiques. *Neurochirurgie* 1965;11:267–272.

21. Lewis RA, Riccardi VM, Gerson LP, et al. Von Recklinghausen neurofibromatosis: II. Incidence of optic nerve gliomata. *Ophthalmology* 1984;91:929–935.

22. Li FP, Garber JE, Friend SH et al. Recommendations on predictive testing for germ line p53 mutations among cancer-prone individuals. *J Natl Cancer Inst* 1992;84: 1156–1161.

23. Listernick R, Charrow J, Greenwald MJ and Esterly NB. Optic glioma in children with neurofibromatosis type I. *J Pediatr* 1989;114:788–792.

24. Maddock IR, Moran A, Maher ER, et al. A genetic register for von Hippel-Lindau disease. *J Med Genet* 1996; 33:120–127.

25. Malkin D, Li FP, Strong LC, et al. Germ line p53 mutations in a familial syndrome of breast cancer, sarcomas, and other neoplasms. *Science* 1990; 250:1233–1238.

26. Martuza RL, Eldridge R. Neurofibromatosis 2 (bilateral acoustic neurofibromatosis). *N Engl J Med* 1988;318: 684–688.

27. McKusick V. *Mendelian inheritance in man,* 11th ed. Baltimore: Johns Hopkins University Press, 1994.

28. Nelen MR, Padber GW, Peeters EAJ, et al. Localization of the gene for Cowden disease to chromosome 10q22–23. *Nature Genet* 1996;13:114 116.

29. Riccardi VM. *Neurofibromatosis phenotype, natural history, and pathogenesis,* 2nd ed. Baltimore: Johns Hopkins University Press, 1992.

30. Ritter CL, Steele MW, Wenger SL, Cohen BA. Chromosome mosaicism in hypomelanosis of Ito. *Am J Med Genet* 1990;35:14–17.

31. Sainz J, Huynh DP, Figueroa K, Ragge NK, Baser ME, Pulst SM. Mutations in the neurofibromatosis type 2 gene and lack of the gene product in vestibular schwannomas. *Hum Molec Genet* 1994;3:885–891.

32. Scully RE, McNeely BU. Case records of the Massachusetts General Hospital: case 22–1975. *N Engl J Med* 1975;292:1231–1237.

33. Shen MH, Harper PS, Upadhyaya M. Molecular genetics of neurofibromatosis type 1 (NF1). *J Med Genet* 1996;33:2–17.

34. Side L, Taylor B, Cayouette M, et al. Homozygous inactivation of the NF1 gene in bone marrow cells from children with neurofibromatosis type I and malignant myeloid disorders. *N Engl J Med* 1997;336:1713–1720.

35. Starink TM, van der Veen JPW, Arwert F, et al. The Cowden syndrome: a clinical and genetic study in 21 patients. *Clin Genet* 1986;29:222–233.

36. Stern JD, Jakobiec FA, Housepian EM. The architecture of optic nerve glioma with and without neurofibromatosis. *Arch Ophthalmol* 1990;98:6506–511.

37. Thomson A. *On neuroma and neurofibromatosis.* Edinburgh: Turnbull & Spears, 1900.

38. Watkins DJG. A family tree bearing upon the question of the inheritance of cancer. *Br Med J* 1904;I:190.

39. Woods CF, Taylor AMR. Ataxia telangiectasia in the British Isles: the clinical and laboratory features of 70 affected individuals. *Q J Med* 1992; 82:169–179.

40. Zbar B, Kishida T, Chen F, et al. Germline mutations in the von Hippel-Lindau disease (VHL) gene in families from North America, Europe, and Japan. *Hum Mutation* 1996;8:348–357.

41. Zwetsloot CP, Kros JM, Paz y Geuze HD. Familial occurrence of tumours of the choroid plexus. *J Med Genet* 1991;28:492–494.

The Practical Management of Low-Grade Primary Brain
Tumors, edited by Jack P. Rock, Mark L. Rosenblum,
Edward G. Shaw, and J. Gregory Cairncross.
Lippincott Williams & Wilkins, Philadelphia, © 1999

12

Practical Case Scenarios

Tom Mikkelsen, Edward G. Shaw, Mark Bernstein, J. Gregory Cairncross, Jae Ho
Kim, Mark L. Rosenblum, and Jack P. Rock

*T. Mikkelsen: Departments of Neurology and Neurosurgery, Henry Ford Hospital,
Detroit, Michigan 48202*
*E. G. Shaw: Department of Radiation Oncology, Wake Forest University School of Medicine,
Winston-Salem, North Carolina 27157*
*M. Bernstein: Division of Neurosurgery, The Toronto Hospital, Western Division,
University of Toronto, Toronto, Ontario M5T 2S8 Canada*
*J. G. Cairncross: Departments of Clinical Neurological Sciences and Oncology,
University of Western Ontario and London Regional Cancer Centre, London,
Ontario N6A 4L6 Canada*
J. H. Kim: Department of Radiation Oncology, Henry Ford Hospital, Detroit, Michigan 48202
*M. L. Rosenblum and Jack P. Rock: Department of Neurosurgery, Henry Ford Hospital,
Detroit, Michigan 48202*

The following discussion on four case presentations of patients with low-grade gliomas reveals the varying opinions on treatment according to experts in neuro-oncology, radiation oncology, and neurosurgery. These six clinicians, all of whom are known for their clinical and research experience, based their opinions on a brief case history and a series of radiographs. The radiographs presented here are selected examples of the full set of films that the clinicians reviewed. Each case discussion is followed by a presentation of the actual treatment method and outcome.

CASE 1

Case Scenario

A 47-year-old right-handed white male factory employee without prior medical illness was noted to have a left-sided focal motor seizure involving the face and hand. Initial episodes lasted approximately 30 seconds and occurred two or three times per day. Two weeks before neurosurgical evaluation the pa-

tient experienced a major motor seizure. Dilantin was started but focal fits persisted. The medical history was otherwise unremarkable and the patient was taking no medications. General physical and neurologic exams were normal. Magnetic resonance imaging (MRI) examination revealed two lesions in the right parietal and temporal lobes with similar characteristics: low intensity on T1, high intensity on T2, and no enhancement after gadolinium injection (Fig. 1A,B,C).

Discussion

Dr. Mikkelsen: This patient has intractable partial motor seizures and a probable secondarily generalized event. Right parietal and temporal lesions on MRI showed T1 hypointensity and T2 hyperintensity, with no gadolinium enhancement, a pattern consistent with low-grade glioma. Because of the location of the temporal lesion at the temporal tip, resection for diagnosis and possibly for improved seizure management would be desirable. The parietal lesion, however, located adjacent to and perhaps in the motor cortex, is more problematic. Focal resection or local radiation by radiosurgery threatens to cause motor

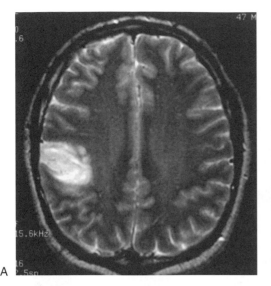
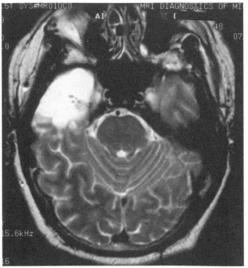
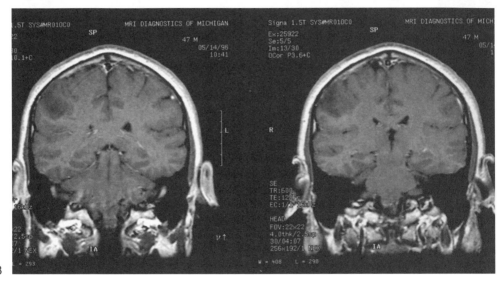

FIG. 1.

deficits in this intact patient. In this circumstance, either fractionated stereotactic radiation or even chemotherapy, which has a low risk of inducing motor deficit in the short term, could be used. Radiation could be reserved for use if and when radiologic or clinical progression is identified.

Dr. Shaw: I would favor an initial surgical approach in this patient—at the least, biopsy of both lesions, with the consideration of maximal resection of one or both. The patient is older than the average low-grade glioma patient, and he has two lesions, putting him at-risk for having higher-grade glioma. Also, the cortical

location suggests at least a component of oligodendroglioma, which, if documented, could affect the recommendation for chemotherapy. Assuming tissue is obtained and it shows a low-grade astrocytoma, oligoastrocytoma, or oligodendroglioma, I would recommend radiation therapy to the two lesions as defined by a treatment planning MRI scan, with a 2-cm margin. Total dose would be 54 Gy in 30 fractions, using a two-and-a-half- or three-dimensional treatment plan that would spare the left (uninvolved) hemisphere from any significant dose of radiation. My justification for using early radiation is based on the patient's age and the presence of persistent seizures despite (presumably optimal) medical therapy.

Dr. Bernstein: This patient has presented with focal seizures and, on imaging, has a multifocal intra-axial process most likely to be a glioma. The individual lesions are fairly typical of low-grade glioma on T1-enhanced and T2-weighted images, but multifocality is relatively uncommon (at least on imaging) in true low-grade gliomas in adults. This factor alone is worrisome and probably portends a more aggressive biology and possibly more aggressive histology (i.e., anaplastic astrocytoma or anaplastic mixed glioma). Furthermore, this patient has another widely accepted risk factor, suggesting more aggressive biology (i.e., age > 40 years). Therefore this patient is not a candidate for a course of observation (i.e., deferral of treatment). I would recommend a course of treatment commencing with an image-guided stereotactic biopsy. This could be done either with a frame-based or a frameless system, but for this case I would likely use the BRW frame and access the right parietal lesion. Cytoreductive surgery is not indicated for control of symptoms and/or signs in this case, and the risk would not justify the potential benefit. Following the likely confirmation of an astrocytoma or oligoastrocytoma (with or without aggressive pathologic features such as the presence of gemistocytic astrocytes), I would recommend a course of fractionated external radiation (at least 50 Gy in 25 fractions) to a field including the two lesions, the intervening brain, and a margin. If there were definite features of anaplasia in the specimen, I would likely also recommend consideration of systemic chemotherapy. Aggressive pharmacologic management of the seizures would be pursued. Follow-up of the patient would consist of evaluation by a multidisciplinary team (neurosurgeon, medical oncologist, and radiation oncologist) along with imaging every 3 months.

Treatment and Outcome

Dr. Rock: Two issues were of concern in this patient: the presumed need for diagnostic certainty in a 47-year-old whose lesion may not have been a low-grade tumor, and multifocality, which is thought to be less common in low-grade lesions. We decided that the temporal lesion could be safely removed but that resection of the parietal lesion would require cortical mapping to limit the likelihood of producing neurologic deficit. The temporal lesion would be approached first and, if malignant, the parietal lesion would not be biopsied because it would be assumed to have the same or less clinically relevant histology. If,

however, the temporal lesion was low grade and gross totally removed, resection of the parietal lesion would be attempted.

The temporal lesion appeared to be an oligodendroglioma on frozen-section with a relatively distinct boundary, and therefore the parietal motor cortex was mapped with excellent responses. Most of the lesion was in the sensory region with slight extension into the motor gyrus. Approximately 90% of the lesion was resected, but the boundary was less distinct than that noted with the temporal lesion. The patient sustained a proprioceptive deficit in the left-upper extremity with paresthesias in the left face that resolved completely 3 weeks postoperatively. Both lesions were documented to be oligodendroglioma grade B with a MIB-1 index of 4%. Regional radiation therapy incorporating both lesions and the tissue in between was recommended and administered. Seizures came under control with anticonvulsant monotherapy and the lesion has demonstrated no growth after 3 years.

CASE 2

Case Scenario

A 36-year-old right-handed white housewife presented to the emergency department after one grand mal seizure. Past medical history and neurologic examination were normal except for bilateral papilledema. She was treated with dilantin, and MRI revealed a large left frontal lesion that was low intensity on T1, high intensity on T2, and nonenhancing (Fig. 2A,B).

Discussion

Dr. Cairncross: The MRI reveals a large, well-circumscribed, nonenhancing, left inferior frontal mass that compresses the ipsilateral ventricle from below, distorting the foramina of Monro and causing contralateral ventricular dilatation. The imaging characteristics of this lesion are consistent with those of a low-grade glioma. Hydrocephalus probably explains the sole abnormal physical finding, papilledema. The patient's acute symptoms may have been a grand mal seizure as reported, or, alternatively, may have been a pressure wave, an underrecognized cause of intermittent seizurelike symptoms in patients with raised intracranial pressure. In addition to dilantin, I would have prescribed dexamethasone (e.g., 4 mg orally

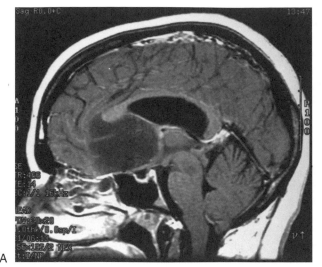 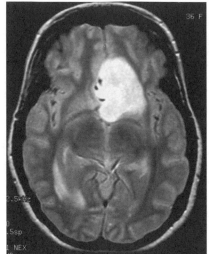

FIG. 2.

twice daily). For patients with pressure waves I have found acetazolamide (e.g., 250 mg orally three times daily) particularly helpful. The tumor is likely an oligodendroglioma, mixed glioma, or fibrillary astrocytoma, less likely an indolent astrocytoma variant. Whatever its histology, the wait-and-see management option that I sometimes prefer for patients with suspected low-grade glioma would be unwise in this case. Initial management will be dictated by the degree to which this tumor can be removed safely and by its histology. Bulk resection, restoring cerebrospinal fluid flow in the process, would be the ideal therapy for this patient. However, I do not know whether a mass in this location can be removed and would defer to an experienced neurosurgical colleague in this regard. Generally speaking, following a major resection, particularly in a young patient, I discourage immediate radiotherapy unless the tumor is anaplastic histologically. If the tumor cannot be removed, I suggest a stereotactic biopsy to establish a tissue diagnosis and recognize that in this case a shunt procedure may also be necessary. Again, generally speaking, following a biopsy or minor resection of a large mass I favor radiotherapy (e.g., 54 Gy in 1.8 Gy fractions over 6 weeks) for patients with fibrillary astrocytomas, whereas I suggest four cycles of standard-dose PCV chemotherapy prior to radiotherapy for those with oligodendrogliomas. PCV occasionally shrinks a low-grade oligodendroglioma substantially, and this might allow the radiation oncologist to treat a smaller volume, reducing the risk of delayed neurotoxicity.

Dr. Kim: This nonenhancing large left frontal mass is located in the frontal lobe extending into the frontal horn of the left lateral ventricle. It appears that the corpus callosum is not involved, based on the MRI scan. I would recommend complete resection of the mass. If complete resection of the lesion is verified by the postoperative MRI scan and the histopathology shows a low-grade glioma, no additional adjuvant therapy would be recommended. Even if there is any suspicion of residual lesion on the postoperative MRI scan, I feel that a regular follow-up MRI scan would be needed to determine the status of the lesion.

Dr. Rosenblum: This 36-year-old woman presented with a seizure and increased intracranial pressure as inferred by the presence of bilateral papilledema. The MRI demonstrates a predominantly left inferior frontal lobe lesion that appears to originate just above the optic chiasm and more likely causes posterior displacement of hypothalamic structures than invasion of that eloquent brain region. The lesion has grown superiorly and posteriorly to the extent that it appears to be blocking the foramen of Monro on the right side, resulting in an enlarged, loculated right ventricular system. This ventriculomegaly is undoubtedly contributing to the patient's increased intracranial pressure. The imaging study suggests that the patient harbors a low-grade glioma probably of astrocytic, oligodendrocytic, or a mixed type. The fact that ventricular blockage and papilledema are present suggests that the tumor is growing and has the potential to produce even more profound hydrocephalus and subsequent increased intracranial pressure. The lesion's location close to, but not presently involving, Broca's area suggests that the patient's language function could be affected in the future. I believe this tumor should be removed surgically to obtain an accurate diagnosis, to obtain an indication of its growth potential by performing a MIB labeling index, to decrease the intracranial pressure and obviate the need for a ventriculoperitoneal shunt at this time. Removing most of the tumor mass should decrease the potential for language dysfunction due to compression of Broca's cortex and reduce the chance of the tumor becoming malignant. The chance for malignant transformation is directly proportional to the number of tumor cells present. The need for additional therapy such as irradiation would depend on the diagnosis and the tumor's potential growth rate. It must be remembered that as many as 25% of nonenhancing gliomas are histologically confirmed as anaplastic.

Surgically, I would use a far-frontal approach on the left side by way of an inferiorly and medially placed frontal lobe resection. In this manner the tumor can be approached along its longitudinal axis. During the tumor-debulking procedure I would use a three-dimensional imaging system and localizing device such as the Viewing Wand to predict the location of, and minimize damage to, the anterior cerebral artery, the middle cerebral artery complex, and the midline structures such as the fornix and the foramen of Monro. The posterior and posterolateral extent of resection should be carefully monitored by the Viewing Wand and real-time intraoperative ultrasound to avoid damage to the critically important fornix, hypothalamic, and thalamic structures. This tumor should be readily separable from the vessels, which should be protected carefully to avoid any trauma-induced vasospasm. It is likely the ventricular system would be entered using this approach and the foramen of Monro opened with decompression of the ventricular system. I would place a catheter into the ventricles for drainage, which would also be used to monitor the intracranial pressure for 1–2 days postoperatively and then removed. This patient is unlikely to need a permanent ventricular diversion procedure. Using modern techniques, more than 90% of the lesion should be able to be removed safely without causing significant neurologic deficit.

Treatment and Outcome

Dr. Rock: It was our impression that the intracranial pressure elevation as evidenced by papilledema was secondary to both the ventriculomegaly and the mass of the tumor, which we presumed to be low-grade based on imaging characteristics typical of either astrocytoma, oligodendroglioma, or mixed glioma. We also felt that the size and location of the lesion justified resection and that resection would be associated with a low risk of deficit. We did not feel that we would necessarily obtain a complete removal of tumor and would be content with 90% lesion resection. Postoperative MRI revealed greater than 90% resection of this oligodendroglioma with a MIB-1 of 0.5%. The patient was neurologically intact and adjuvant therapy was deferred. The lesion has not demonstrated change after 2 years.

CASE 3

Case Scenario

A 27-year-old right-handed white female social worker was evaluated for demyelinating disease after 1 year of frequent enuresis. Complete neurologic work-up failed to document evidence of demyelination, and an MRI was performed. The patient had a history of migraine but was otherwise normal. Physical examination was unremarkable. MRI revealed a 2-cm lesion in the medial left temporal lobe that was cystic, predominantly low intensity on T1, high intensity on T2, and focally contrast enhancing (Fig. 3A,B).

Discussion

Dr. Mikkelsen: This young patient with a history of nocturnal enuresis was probably having nocturnal seizures with postictal incontinence. Imaging studies revealed a medial temporal lesion with cystic features and a focus of contrast enhancement. Because of its location and the contrast enhancement, resection with complete pathologic examination would be important. Although focal contrast enhancement is described in pilocytic astrocytomas and even in hamartomas, one must be concerned about the malignant transformation of a preexisting low-grade astrocytoma toward a more aggressive lesion. With wide local resection of the lesion and surrounding T2 signal abnormality, unless there were pathologic features of malignancy, one would likely monitor her by neuroimaging for radiologic progression before instituting further treatment, by either local radiation or chemotherapy.

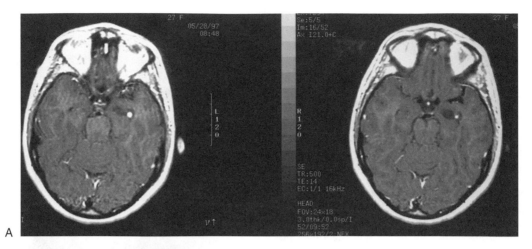

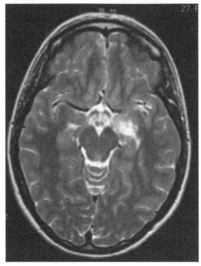

FIG. 3.

Dr. Shaw: I would favor an initial stereotactic biopsy in this patient. The imaging characteristics of this lesion—fairly well-circumscribed and cystic with a small contrast-enhancing nodule—suggest pilocytic astrocytoma for which gross total resection (and no radiation) would be curative. If the biopsy showed a more infiltrative histologic subtype of low-grade glioma (astrocytoma, oligoastrocytoma, or oligodendroglioma), either early or delayed radiation would be appropriate. If radiation therapy were to be given, MRI-based three-dimensional treatment planning utilizing treatment fields that limit dose to the adjacent critical normal tissues—including the brain stem, optic chiasm, and pituitary gland—would be necessary.

Dr. Bernstein: This young woman has presented with symptoms that may well be a relatively unusual type of complex partial seizure and imaging demonstrating a medial dominant temporal lobe lesion characterized by a nodule of enhancement within a cyst, relatively typical of an indolent neuroepithelial neoplasm such as a pilocytic astrocytoma or ganglioma.

There are two issues here: (a) controlling a significant clinical symptom and (b) addressing the neuro-oncological lesion itself. This patient requires a work-up consisting of, as best as possible, identification of the symptom as a seizure disorder, and then aggressive pharmacologic management of the seizure disorder to control the symptom of episodic enuresis. If this can be achieved, then there is no necessity to biopsy or resect this lesion, which is likely to have a very indolent biologic behavior and can be safely observed with regular MRI. This course of observation would defer the risk, albeit relatively small, attendant on resection of this lesion. If new neurologic symptoms or signs and/or growth of the lesion on imaging were found during the course of observation, then I would proceed at that time to do an aggressive removal of the lesion using an image-guided navigation device and awake craniotomy with cortical mapping to minimize the risk.

If satisfactory symptom control cannot be obtained with drugs, then resection of the lesion for symptom control as described earlier with or without a formal epilepsy operation with electrocorticography would be indicated. In this case, if surgery was done and a gross total resection of a low-grade glioma or ganglioglioma was performed, postoperative radiation might well be deferred because of her young age and the likelihood that gross total resection of this lesion could be achieved. The patient would be followed with regular monitoring with imaging (probably every 6 months), and radiation would be given at time of recurrence.

Treatment and Outcome

Dr. Rock: It was felt that the seizure problem might be controlled with anticonvulsants, but the contrast enhancement was worrisome and whether this lesion was a contrast-enhancing low-grade tumor or higher-grade malignancy was unknown. We performed a gross total resection of this oligoastrocytoma with a MIB-1 of 0.5%. The patient awoke with a hemiparesis and dysphasia that after review of the postoperative MRI was suggestive of an anterior choroidal infarct. Because the operative dissection did not extend beyond the pia of the anterior temporal lobe, we concluded that instead of the blood supply to this region occurring as a branch of the anterior choroidal artery as is usually the case, the anterior choroidal artery must have passed through the tip of the temporal horn on its way to its standard supply territory, as has been commented on by Yasargil (1).

Given the extent of resection and the low-grade nature of the lesion, radiation therapy was deferred, and follow-up MRI after 1 year has not demonstrated recurrence.

CASE 4

Case Scenario

This 32-year-old right-handed white male engineer had a 2-month history of stuttering and eventual focal motor seizures involving the right face and tongue. Medical history was unremarkable. Neurologic examination revealed dysarthria with otherwise intact cognitive and linguistic function. MRI demonstrated a lesion in the left frontal region that was low intensity on T1, high intensity on T2, and nonenhancing (Fig. 4A,B,C).

Discussion

Dr. Cairncross: The MRI demonstrates a small, well-circumscribed, nonenhancing, cortically based, left posterior frontal lesion with mass effect. The imaging characteristics are consistent with a low-grade glioma, probably an oligodendroglioma or dysembryoplastic neuroepithelial tumor (DNET). There is a fluid-filled left maxillary sinus, in all likelihood an incidental finding. As I see it, the initial management of this patient will be dictated by the ease of seizure control. If the seizures can be controlled successfully with nontoxic doses of anticonvulsants (e.g., carbamazepine, dilantin), I would initiate surveillance imaging by MRI (e.g., every 3 months the first year, every 4 months the second year, every 6 months the third year, and then yearly, or as dictated by symptoms) and forego a stereotactic biopsy, tumor resection, or other intervention. If, as I suspect, the seizures prove to be refractory to medical management, I would refer this patient to our multidisciplinary epilepsy service for consideration of surgical resection of the epileptic focus and nearby tumor. This should be curative therapy for a DNET and sufficient initial therapy for a low-grade oligodendroglioma. It is most unlikely that we are dealing with a high-grade glioma masquerading as an indolent neoplasm, but careful clinical follow-up with reimaging assessing symptoms, signs, size, and enhancement should guard against this possibility. If surgery is required for seizure control, tissue for precise tumor diagnosis will be an added benefit. Finally, I am intrigued by the possibility that stereotactic fractionated radiotherapy might prove to be a highly satisfactory and low-risk treatment for both the seizure disorder and the neoplasm when small, discrete tumors, such as this one, are deemed to be unresectable.

Dr. Kim: This nonenhancing, moderate-sized mass is located in the left posterior frontal lobe, anterior to the central sulcus, superior to the Sylvian fissure, and posterior to the Broca's area. Because of the location of the lesion, a functional MRI scan might be useful to further delineate the location of the lesion, relative to the motor strip. Although a complete resection might

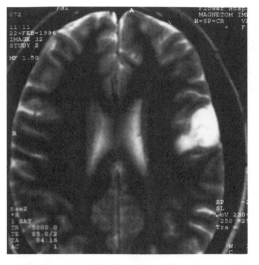

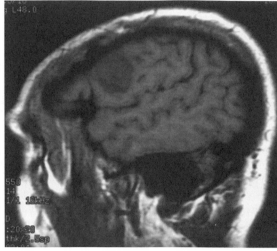

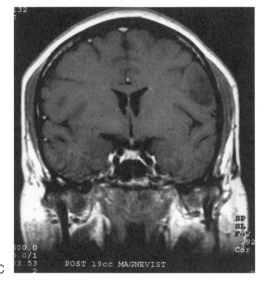

FIG. 4.

be attempted, the postoperative MRI scan would most likely reveal some residual lesion. If the histopathology of the tumor shows low-grade glioma without evidence of any biologic aggressive features—such as increased cellularity, anaplasia, vascularity, and/or labeling index—I would not recommend postoperative radiation therapy. However, if there is any suggestion of aggressive features, postoperative radiation therapy should be seriously considered.

Dr. Rosenblum: This 32-year-old right-handed male with a 2-month history of stuttering and eventual focal motor seizures involving the right face and tongue had dysarthria as his only neurologic symptom. MRI demonstrates an approximately 2- × 2-cm left-sided inferior frontal lobe superficial lesion in what appears to be the frontal operculum close to Broca's area. The lesion has mass qualities and appears to be localized predominantly in one expanded gyrus. There does not appear to be a significant amount of MRI-evident invasion and therefore the lesion remains predominantly a localized disease at this time. The differential diagnosis includes a low-grade astrocytoma, a low-grade oligodendroglioma, or a mixed tumor. Of course there is always the possibility that this is an anaplastic astrocytoma in an early stage of evolution. The presence of dysarthria suggests the involvement or compression of a critical motor speech brain region.

I believe this is a surgically removable lesion with minimal morbidity when modern techniques are used. Approximately 95% to 99% of the tumor can be removed safely as long as the patient has the lesion removed under local anesthesia with language and motor mapping. The surgical approach would be a lateral frontal craniotomy utilizing a regional scalp local anesthetic block and sedation performed with the assistance of an experienced anesthesiology team. A neuropsychologist or speech therapist should assist in testing of language function intraoperatively with cortical stimulation precisely delivered using a bipolar stimulating electrode. Neurologists with experience in electrocorticography could provide assistance in some cases. Ultrasound would be useful as well to help guide and determine the extent of tumor resection. If the tumor has a distinct appearance or consistency that is different from the surrounding brain tissue, resection could proceed to the border of the abnormal tissue–normal tissue interface as long as cortex within 1–2 cm of the localized speech center remained undisturbed. It would be important to map the motor function both cortically and subcortically to avoid resecting important corticospinal tract connections. The most difficult part of the procedure is determining the appropriate depth of the resection to remove as much of the lesion as possible and avoid causing a deficit. This is usually accomplished with the combination of the techniques mentioned previously as well as the experience of the surgeon to distinguish normal from abnormal-appearing tissue. Although some additional speech defect might be present immediately after the operation, most of the new deficit should resolve over the course of the subsequent month. The pathologic diagnosis and its proliferative potential would help determine the need for postoperative radiation therapy and other treatments.

Treatment and Outcome

Dr. Rock: This patient was initially managed for seizures but these proved to be intractable. Surgical resection with language mapping was performed on the awake patient. The lesion, a fibrillary astrocytoma with a MIB-1 of 1%, was gross totally resected without producing a deficit. Postoperative MRI demonstrated residual T2 signal adjacent to the resection cavity. The seizure disorder came under excellent control with monotherapy. Radiation therapy was deferred. MRI at 1 year demonstrated no change in the lesion characteristics. Unfortunately, the patient's seizures recurred 18 months after surgery and follow-up MRI demonstrated regrowth of the tumor to the original volume. Re-resection is being considered and follow-up with radiation therapy will most likely occur.

REFERENCE

1. Yasargil MG, Wieser HG, Valvanis A, von Ammon K, Roth P. Surgery and results of selective amygdala-hippocampectomy in one hundred patients with nonlesional limbic epilepsy. *Epilepsy* 1993;4:243–259.

Research and Future Directions

The Practical Management of Low-Grade Primary Brain
Tumors, edited by Jack P. Rock, Mark L. Rosenblum,
Edward G. Shaw, and J. Gregory Cairncross.
Lippincott Williams & Wilkins, Philadelphia, © 1999

13

Development, Molecular Genetics, and Gene Therapy of Glial Tumors

Steven P. Dudas and Sandra A. Rempel

Department of Neurosurgery, Henry Ford Hospital, Detroit, Michigan 48202

Which brain cells give rise to brain tumors? Which genes are altered in brain tumors? Can gene therapy treatments be devised based on the altered genes? These questions are the focus of neuro-oncologic research, and their answers not only will greatly advance our understanding of the pathogenetic mechanisms that give rise to glial tumors but, it is hoped, also will facilitate the advancement of effective treatment.

This chapter provides an overview of normal brain cell development; the theories regarding cells of tumor origin; the mechanisms and genetic alterations presently characterized for the initiation and progression of astrocytomas, oligodendrogliomas, and ependymomas; and potential gene therapy strategies based on the specific genetic alterations in the low-grade glial tumors. Because of the broad scope of this chapter, it is our intent not to provide an exhaustive review on each topic but to present a comprehensive overview built upon previous reviews and recent observations.

DEVELOPMENT OF THE BRAIN

Multipotent Stem Cells of the Mammalian Fetal Brain

The mature brain is composed of neurons and glial cells, including astrocytes, oligodendrocytes, and ependymal cells. The undifferentiated cell of origin giving rise to these differentiated cells and the characterization of the cell/cell relationships throughout the central nervous system (CNS) development have been described through the study of cell lineages that uses cell-type-specific antigens and developmental stage-specific characteristics (reviewed in ref. 74). Such studies have implicated a neuroectodermal, multipotent stem cell originating in the ventricular zone of the fetal brain and spinal cord as the common precursor for all neuronal and glial cell types (Fig. 1). *In vitro* evidence in support of this multipotent stem cell has been obtained from the study of rat optic nerve and brain neurospheres. The rat optic nerve is the simplest CNS model because it contains only astrocytes and oligodendrocytes, and most of our knowledge about gliogenesis is derived from this model (reviewed in refs. 90, 96). More recently, neurospheres have been used to study fetal and adult brain development (38,104, 118). Neurospheres are generated in culture from cells derived from dissociated fetal or adult brain tissues. The illustration presented in Fig. 2 combines observations from both models and represents mammalian neuronal and glial cell commitment and differentiation pathways and the signals/environmental cues that determine these pathways.

When neurospheres are grown in the presence of epidermal growth factor (EGF) (104, 118) or fibrillary growth factor (FGF) (38),

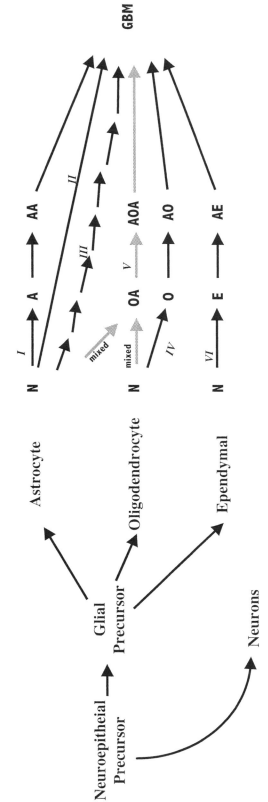

FIG. 1. Proposed development of normal brain and brain tumors. A neuroepithelial cell develops into both neurons and glial precursor cells. The glial precursor cell would ultimately give rise to the differentiated astrocytes, oligodendrocytes, and ependymal cells. Genetic alterations in the normal cells of origin (N) would allow the formation of grade II gliomas (A, astrocytoma; OA, oligoastrocytomas; O, oligodendroglioma; E, ependymoma). Further alterations would permit progression into the grade III anaplastic (A) gliomas, AA, AOA, AO, and AE, respectively. And finally, further aberrations would permit the progression of all tumors into the heterogeneous malignant grade IV glioblastoma multiforme (GBM). Pathways I–III represent alternate pathways for astrocytoma progression based on molecular variants. Pathways IV–VI represent progression of oligodendrogliomas, mixed oligoastrocytomas, and ependymomas, respectively.

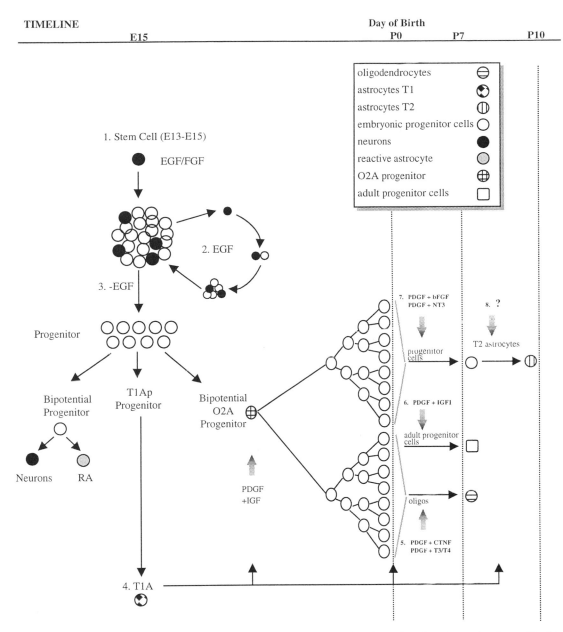

FIG. 2. Proposed development of the mammalian brain. (1) Dissociated embryonic days 13–15 (E13–E15) brain cells aggregate in culture to form neurospheres in the presence of epidermal growth factor (EGF) or fibroblast growth factor (FGF). (2) Neurosphere-derived stem cells can divide, giving rise to stem cells and progenitor cells upon reexposure to EGF. (3) Upon removal of EGF, progenitor cells give rise to neurons, reactive astrocytes (RA), type 1 (T1) astrocytes, and O-2A progenitor cells under the appropriate conditions/stimuli. (4) The T1As secrete PDGF+IGF, which induces the O-2A progenitor cells to divide. (5) At day equivalent P0, T1As secrete CNTF, which induces the differentiation of oligodendrocytes. Thyroid hormones also influence the differentiation of embryonic progenitor cells into oligodendrocytes. (6) The expression of PDGF and IGF-1 promotes the differentiation of adult progenitor cells. (7) The expression of PDGF and bFGF or PDGF and NT3 promotes the division of the progenitor cells. (8) At day equivalent P7, the T1As secrete an as yet unidentified factor that promotes the differentiation of progenitor cells into T2As. By day equivalent P10, adult progenitor cells and differentiated oligodendrocytes, astrocytes, and neurons are present. (Adapted from Reynolds and Weiss [104] and Ibarrola et al. [47].)

growth factor–responsive stem cells can be isolated that divide asymmetrically, giving rise to both secondary stem cells and progenitor cells (see Fig. 2). When these secondary stem cells are isolated and replated, they also generate secondary neurospheres capable of generating stem cells and progenitor cells. When EGF is removed, the progenitor cells proliferate and differentiate into neurons, astrocytes, and oligodendrocytes in the presence of the appropriate signals. These results indicate that the stem cells contain the information necessary for the ultimate differentiation of all CNS cell types through the intermediary progenitor cells.

Multipotent Precursor Cells of the Mammalian Fetal Brain

Recent efforts have focused on determining whether these intermediate progenitor cells represent identical multipotent cells that give rise to all cell types under the appropriate signaling conditions or whether subsets of progenitor cells are generated that are predetermined to undergo limited differentiation into a specific cell type(s) (see Fig. 2). There is evidence for the existence of both bipotential and unipotential neuroprogenitor cells. Using a neurosphere model of astrogliosis, studies were performed comparing primary E13 mouse brain cultures (days 3 or 7 cultures) and long-term E13 EGF-generated progenitor cells passaged for 3–6 months. When the long-term progenitor cells were differentiated into astrocytes by the removal of EGF and the addition of 10% fetal bovine serum (FBS) (118), they found that nascent astrocytes transiently expressed the neuronal antigens Tau, MAP2, and GABA. As expected, mature astrocytes derived from primary brain cultures did not express these antigens. In light of their results, as well as the fact that reactive astrocytes have been shown to express neuronal antigens in response to CNS trauma, the authors suggest that at least a subpopulation of the EGF-generated progenitor cells remained bipotential and could give rise to either neurons or astrocytes, indicating that these differentiated cells shared a common progenitor cell.

The *in vitro* rat optic nerve model reproduces *in vivo* cell differentiation along the *in vivo* time line and has been used to study both the development and the environmental inducers of cell lineages during embryogenesis and after birth (see Fig. 2) (47,90,96). These studies support the existence of both bipotential and unipotential precursor cells. Both T1 astrocyte progenitor (T1Ap) and O-2A progenitor cells exist during embryogenesis (E15) (47). At the equivalent time of embryonic day 16 (E16), the T1A precursors develop only into mature T1A protoplasmic astrocytes that synthesize and secrete platelet-derived growth factor (PDGF). This factor induces the proliferation of the bipotential O-2A progenitor cells. This proliferative phase regenerates and expands the population of O-2A cells. The population of cells gives rise to both oligodendrocytes from days P0 to P7 and mature T2A astrocytes from days P7 to P10 when exposed to the appropriate inducers (see Fig. 2). At time equivalent of birth (P0), the influence of ciliary neurotrophic factor (CNTF) (potentially secreted from the T1As; 78) and the hormones T3/T4 (47) induce differentiation of most progenitor cells into mature oligodendrocytes. Alternatively, the presence of both PDGF and basic fibroblast growth factor (bFGF) (12) or both PDGF and neurotrophin-3 (NT3) tips the balance in favor of fewer differentiated mature oligodendrocytes and more dividing progenitor cells (47). At equivalent day P7, the T1A cells are believed to influence the differentiation of the remaining O-2A progenitor cells into T2A cells by secreting CNTF, which initiates differentiation, and a second as yet unknown protein that is required to ensure differentiation into mature T2A cells (74). By equivalent days P10–P15, the development of mature neurons, astrocytes, and oligodendrocytes is achieved. Thus the rat optic nerve model provides evidence in support of both unipotential and bipotential progenitor cells.

However, because these experiments have been performed *in vitro*, it cannot be conclusively demonstrated whether the developmental potential observed in these cells in culture reflects the developmental fate dictated by the *in vivo* environment in which these cells differentiate. To address the question of developmental fate, lineage-tracing experiments have been performed where individual neuroepithelial cells in embryonic and postnatal rodent brain are marked and their progeny followed. For example, injection of retroviral vectors carrying the beta-galactosidase gene marker into retinas of day of birth and postnatal days 2, 4, and 7 indicates that the four retinal cell types—including the rods, bipolar cells, amacrine cells, and Müller glial cells—share a common lineage that persists late in development (141). These experiments support the *in vivo* observations of multipotential progenitor cells. Similar marking experiments have been used to examine embryonic cerebral cortex development (39). When retrovirus was injected on day E14 and the marked clones were analyzed on postnatal day P14, most marked clusters were composed of a single cell type (39). Exceptions included clusters composed of neurons and oligodendrocytes. The results were interpreted to indicate that the different cortical cell types were generated from separate populations of predetermined precursor cells, suggesting that by E16, VZ cells are developmentally specified. Attempts to mark cells earlier in embryogenesis *in vivo* have been unsuccessful (95). Therefore the determination of the cells giving rise to these predetermined VZ cells has required cell culture approaches. When embryonic day E13–E18 precursor cells are cultured, most precursor cells gave rise to single cell types. However, under optimal culture conditions, 50% of embryonic precursor cells could be induced to give rise to clones of mixed cell types, including neurons, astrocytes, and oligodendrocytes. Thus the authors suggest a model in which multipotential neuroepithelial cells dominate early cortical development. By E16 these cells have disappeared, to be replaced by specified precursors that give rise to a single cell type (95). Thus *in vitro* and *in vivo* experimentation supports the concept of multipotent precursor cells that directly or

through intermediary precursor cells of increasingly diminished potency give rise to the fetal CNS cell types. The major difference lies in the timing of the developmental events.

Multipotent Cells in the Mammalian Adult Brain

It has long been supposed that the mature adult brain is static and that there is little, if any, new cell development. However, an interesting cellular behavior has been described by several studies of the *in vitro* rat optic nerve experiments mentioned previously (see Fig. 2). The O-2A progenitor cell possesses a cell-intrinsic biologic clock driven by PDGF that controls the mitotic lifespan such that cells differentiate into oligodendrocytes. It was found that, even under conditions where self-renewal was promoted by the exposure of cells to PDGF and bFGF, the intrinsic clock in O-2A progenitor cells continued to function (12–14). Therefore this clock is also available to signal the transition of perinatal O-2A progenitors to adult O-2A progenitors (47).

Evidence for the existence of dormant multipotent stem cells in the adult CNS was provided by experiments in which neurospheres derived from adult murine striatal cells were induced to proliferate in the presence of bFGF. These authors (38) found adult cells that could undergo a proliferative response to bFGF, resulting in self-renewal and increased number, and that were multipotent and capable of generating neurons, astrocytes, and oligodendroglial cells. In another study (35), neuronal progenitor cells were isolated from adult rat hippocampus and maintained through multiple passages in cell culture. These cells were transfected with an adenovirus-beta-galactosidase construct and then reimplanted into the hippocampus of adult rats. After 2 months, differentiated, beta-galactosidase-expressing neuronal cells were detected in the granule layer of the dentate gyrus. This experiment indicated that adult neuronal progenitor cells retained the capacity to generate mature neurons when reintroduced into the adult rat brain.

That the fate of progenitor cells might change over time or be dictated by environmental influences was described in a model using 3-month-old, nonpassage EGF-derived neurospheres. Chiang et al. (18) were able to induce three morphologically distinct differentiated astrocytes by varying the inducing agent (Fig. 3). When the neurospheres were withdrawn from EGF, fibrous astrocytes (type 2) were differentiated in the presence of bFGF, protoplasmic astrocytes (type 1) were derived in FCS-containing medium, and spindle-shaped astrocytes were observed in the presence of retinol. Similar results were obtained with neurospheres generated from striatum, cerebral cortex, and mesencephalon cells, suggesting that multipotential stem cells could be found throughout the brain. Because these results differ from those obtained using the optic nerve model, the authors suggest that cell age, culture method, and environmental factors influence the fate of progenitor cell differentiation.

Evidence for Multipotent Progenitor Cells in Human Adult Brain

The study of gliogenesis in humans has been restricted by the lack of access of human fetal tissues. However, existing limited data on human gliogenesis suggest that there are no significant differences between primate and nonprimate mammal CNS development (74). Bipotential glial cells have been confirmed in cultures of human corpus collosa taken at autopsy (56); stem cells have been isolated from white matter resected from adult human epileptic temporal lobe surgical specimens (4); and O-2A progenitor cells have been isolated from human fetal optic nerves from fetal abortions (55).

In summary, multipotential neuroepithelial stem cells give rise to both unipotential and bipotential neuronal and glial progenitor cells that differentiate under the appropriate environmental cues into neurons, astrocytes, and oligodendrocytes. Although little research has been directed to the development of ependymal cells, it is believed that they too are derived from an early glial precursor cell (74). Therefore the human adult brain consists of mature, differentiated cells as well as a small population of adult stem/progenitor cells with self-renewing capabilities. It is in this population of both mature and undifferentiated cells that glial brain tumors develop and give rise to astrocytomas, oligodendrogliomas, and ependymomas.

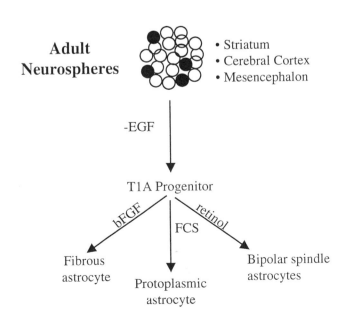

FIG. 3. Factor-specific differentiation of adult neurospheres. Three-month-old, nonpassage adult rat brain–derived neurospheres were maintained *in vitro*. Upon withdrawal of EGF, the T1A progenitor cells differentiated into fibrous astrocytes in the presence of bFGF, protoplasmic astrocytes in the presence of fetal calf serum (FCS), and bipolar spindle cells in the presence of retinol. Similar results were obtained using neurospheres derived from striatum, cerebral cortex, or mesencephalon.

GLIAL TUMORIGENESIS

Clonal Evolution of Tumors

According to Nowell's theory of clonal evolution (92, Fig. 4), tumors of clonal origin arise from a single normal cell that suffered a genetic alteration that conferred a growth advantage on that cell. Subsequent mutations in cells from this parental clone would result in the outgrowth of a tumor with increasingly anaplastic changes and increasing clonal complexity. Further mutations would result in the clonal outgrowth of a fully malignant heterogeneous tumor that may show regions that morphologically reflect the cell of origin. The acquired mutations are associated with imbalances in the normal regulation of cell division and cell death (apoptosis) such that increased cell growth would be favored. This model explains how a tumor can be both histologically and genetically heterogeneous and yet clonally derived. But what is the proposed normal cell from which the tumor is initiated (Fig. 1)? Is it the mature differentiated glial cells that give rise to tumors, or do tumors arise from an adult progenitor cell? The answer to these questions could have profound implications on the research of these tumors and eventual treatment strategies.

The Dedifferentiation Hypothesis

Because of the long-standing association between morphology and tumor classification (see Chapter 3 in this volume for a detailed discussion on glial tumor classification and grading), it has been assumed that the normal cell undergoing mutation is a terminally differentiated astrocyte, oligodendrocyte, or ependymal cell (see Fig. 4). In this hypothesis the differentiated normal cell acquiring the first mutation would appear morphologically differentiated but have increased growth potential, resulting in a tumor of low-grade (grade II). Subsequent, additional mutations would cause the tumor cells to acquire a less differentiated morphologic appearance (grade III). Further mutations would result in a tumor that bears little resemblance to the differenti-

ated cell of origin (accompanied by a loss of expression of cell-specific markers; grade IV). Evidence for this progression model comes from patients who clinically present with a low-grade tumor and who inevitably develop a tumor recurrence of higher grade and eventually die from glioblastoma multiforme (GBM).

The Misdifferentiation Hypothesis

Another hypothesis, which has recently been proposed as a result of the previously described studies of gliogenesis, suggests that there is likely a pool of multipotential adult stem/progenitor cells that can be induced to undergo proliferation by the appropriate stimuli. Such an adult precursor cell, when induced to proliferate inappropriately, may be particularly vulnerable to neoplastic transformation (57). A mutation in such a cell would undergo misdifferentiation, resulting in a cell in a state of limited or blocked differentiation but accompanied by uncontrolled cell proliferation. Thus this concept may explain how progenitor cells that can differentiate along several pathways could give rise to the heterogeneity observed in glial tumors. The histomorphologic features of such a tumor would reflect the stage at which development was halted (57), such that the more undifferentiated-looking the tumor, the earlier in development the mutation was acquired (Fig. 5). Therefore mutations in progenitor cells that are capable of differentiating into both oligodendrocytes or astrocytes could give rise to the heterogeneous GBMs, which have either oligodendro-, astro-, or mixed oligoastrocytic features. Mutations in the progenitor cells further along the differentiation pathway may give rise to either anaplastic oligodendrogliomas or anaplastic astrocytomas. Finally, mutations in cells furthest along the differentiation pathway would result in oligodendrogliomas or astrocytomas having the most differentiated histomorphologic features most resembling oligodendrocytes or astrocytes. This model would explain, for example, the lack of glial fibrillary acidic protein (GFAP)

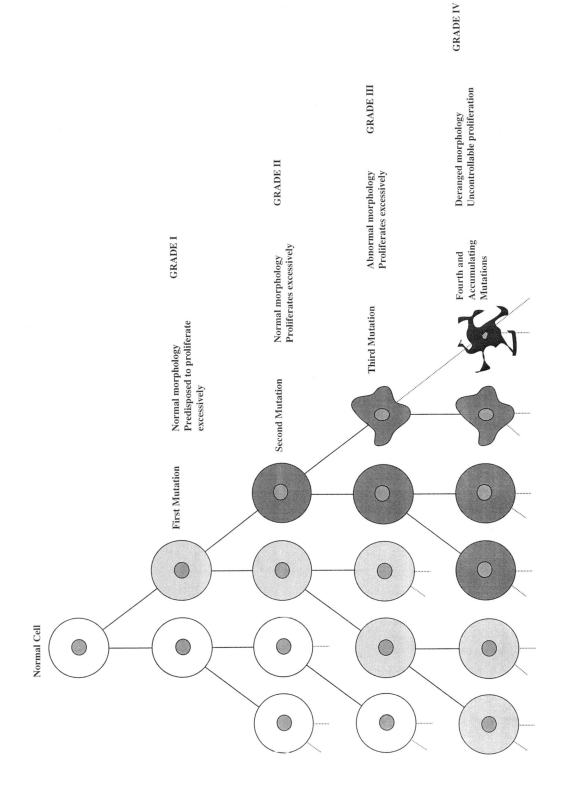

Normal Cell

First Mutation

Second Mutation

Third Mutation

Fourth and
Accumulating
Mutations

GRADE I

Normal morphology
Predisposed to proliferate
excessively

GRADE II

Normal morphology
Proliferates excessively

GRADE III

Abnormal morphology
Proliferates excessively

GRADE IV

Deranged morphology
Uncontrollable proliferation

staining in many GBMs because GFAP expression occurs later in the differentiation of the mature astrocyte. As well, this model may explain the *de novo* GBMs that present without a previously diagnosed lower-grade tumor.

If tumors derived by this mechanism existed, then the most malignant undifferentiated glial tumor should have cells that express the same antigens as their progenitor cells. Recently, a human cell line, Hu-O-2A/Gb-1, has been derived from a glioblastoma that expresses antigens characteristic of the O-2A lineage of the rat (88,89). Like O-2A cells, these tumor cells can be induced to divide by both PDGF and bFGF, simultaneous exposure to both mitogens suppresses differentiation along the oligodendrocyte pathway, and they can generate more progenitor-like cells, oligodendrocytes, or astrocytes in the appropriate conditions. These cells express an H-NMR spectrum identical to perinatal O-2A progenitors derived from rat tissue. These results strongly support the hypothesis that multipotential stem cells in the adult brain may undergo neoplastic transformation, resulting in glial tumors (88–90).

Because glial tumors could develop by either of these two pathways, it is important to identify markers that allow us to discriminate between the origins of the tumors. Treatment therapies may be different, depending on the pathogenesis of a particular tumor. For example, tumor cells derived from human O-2A lineage may have biologic clocks dictated by the cell of origin. Temporarily disrupting the immortalizing mutations in the tumor cells may cause the tumor cells to rapidly undergo terminal differentiation, leading to cessation of the tumor growth (90). However, it may be difficult to determine pathogenesis in malig-

nant tumors in which the continued accumulation of cellular alterations/mutations transforms the neoplastic cell further away from its original phenotype toward an undifferentiated, unresponsive tumor cell, perhaps maintaining only some of its original characteristics (57). Despite this, the continued study of gliogenesis and development will undoubtedly contribute to our understanding of brain tumor pathogenesis. The identification and characterization of cell type–specific, developmental stage–specific, and biochemical pathway–specific proteins will provide not only improved diagnostic markers but also potential therapeutic targets.

Regulators of Cell Growth

Regardless of the mechanism by which these tumors arise, they are all characterized by acquiring mutations that lead to uncontrollable cell growth. This abnormal growth is due to genetic alterations that influence the balance between the growth-promoting genes, such as proto-oncogenes and the growth factors and their receptors, and/or growth-inhibiting genes, such as the tumor suppressor genes (reviewed in ref. 16).

As illustrated in Fig. 6, chromosomes/genes are inherited in matching pairs, one from the mother and the other from the father. When a mutation occurs in a gene that produces too much abnormal or normal protein, the result is described as an activating mutation. When such a mutation happens to an oncogene (which promotes cell division), the up-regulation of the function causes a cell to divide excessively. An inactivating mutation occurs when a mutation happens in a gene that results in no protein or an inactive protein but that produces sufficient product by the normal

---

FIG. 4. Clonal evolution of tumors and the dedifferentiation theory. The accumulation of mutations results in the outgrowth of clonal tumors. Tumor heterogeneity results as a tumor increases in malignancy, having regions associated with higher and lower grade. The tumors are graded on their histomorphologic appearance, which becomes more deranged as the tumor increases in malignancy. According to the dedifferentiation theory, the more malignant the tumor cell, the more deranged the morphology, the less differentiated the tumor. See text for details. (Adapted from Cavenee [16].)

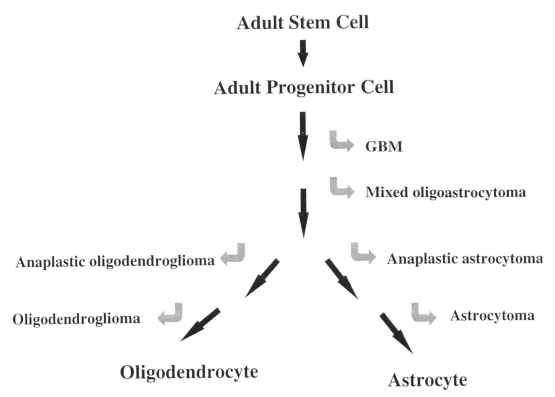

FIG. 5. Misdifferentiation hypothesis. Stem cells proliferate, eventually giving rise to adult progenitor cells. A mutation early in the developmental pathway to mature astrocytes or oligodendrocytes would give rise to GBMs and mixed oligoastrocytomas. Mutations occurring after the developmental pathway splits, which results in astrocytes or oligodendrocytes, would result in anaplastic astrocytoma or anaplastic oligodendrogliomas. Mutations occurring in cells almost completely differentiated would give rise to the astrocytomas and oligodendrogliomas. Therefore the further along the differentiation pathway that a mutation occurs in a cell, the more histologic resemblance there is to the cell it was intended to become.

gene copy. However, if a mutation occurs in the second gene copy, the result is no protein or a mutated protein that cannot function properly. If such mutations occur in a tumor suppressor gene (which negatively regulates cell proliferation), the outcome also results in excessive cell proliferation. It is generally accepted that mutations in oncogenes and tumor suppressor genes are necessary for the initiation of tumors and that the acquisition of further, similar mutations gives rise to progressively more anaplastic and malignant tumors.

FIG. 6. Oncogenes and tumor suppressor genes. Activating mutations result when one allele of an oncogene is mutated and produces too much or abnormal protein. Enhanced expression of an oncogene (which positively regulates cell growth) leads to excess cell proliferation. Inactivating mutations result when one allele of a tumor suppressor gene (which negatively regulates cell growth) is mutant, producing no or abnormal protein, and the second normal allele is still functional. Subsequent loss or mutation of the normal allele unmasks the mutant allele. The loss of expression of the normal allele also leads to excess proliferation. (Adapted from Cavenee [16].)

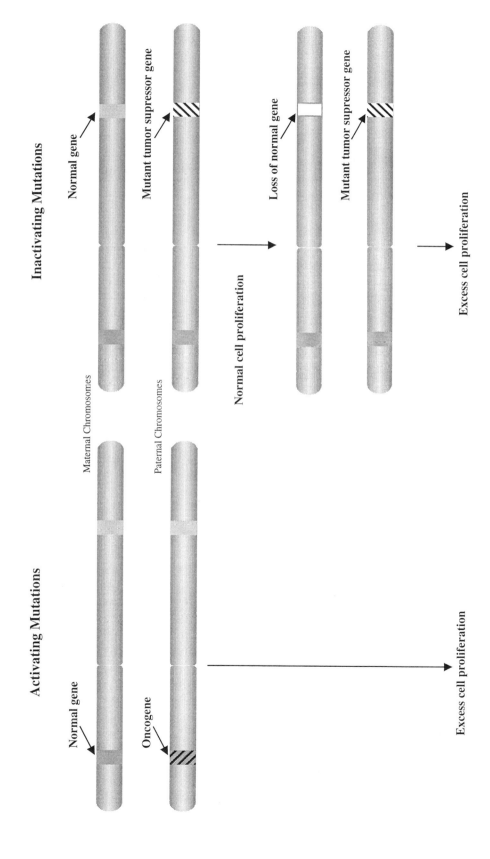

MOLECULAR VARIANTS IN GLIOMA PROGRESSION

Advances in molecular biology and the present characterization of the molecular genetics of gliomas have greatly expanded our knowledge of the progression from the cell of origin (see above) to the heterogeneous GBM (see Fig. 1). GBMs are speculated to arise by the accumulation of specific genetic alterations within three histologically distinct cell lineages: astrocytes, oligodendrocytes, and ependymal cells. These lineage-specific genetic alterations may promote progression through histomorphologically defined grades (see Fig. 1; pathways I, IV, V, and VI), by progression directly to GBM (see Fig. 1; pathway II), or by pathways as yet uncharacterized (see Fig. 1; pathway III). Attempts to better understand the genetic variants will increase our ability to develop gene-specific therapeutic interventions into the disease. This section describes the characteristic genetic oncogene and tumor suppressor gene alterations associated with tumor progression in each of the cell lineages.

Astrocytomas

Astrocytomas comprise approximately 60% to 75% of primary CNS tumors and typically arise in middle-aged patients (37.3 years) (125). The astrocytic tumors are graded from I to IV based on their histologic, biologic, and clinical properties. Because the grade I pilocytic astrocytomas are clinically and biologically distinct from the grades II–IV astrocytomas and usually follow a benign course often curable by surgical intervention, they are not included in the following progression models.

Just as these tumors are graded on their histomorphologic features, attempts have been made to classify the astrocytomas as a result of their genetic mutations. Some controversies still exist in attempting to categorize astrocytomas based on the molecular variants. However, these controversies may often be attributed to the methods of analysis and differences in the original grading of the tumors. Therefore for the purpose of this chapter, we have chosen to present a model based on pathways proposed by von Diemling et al. (149) and Lang et al. (66) incorporating recent observations. The current molecular data combined with clinical observations suggest that the astrocytomas may be allocated into three major progression pathways (see Fig. 1).

Pathway I

Tumors allocated to this pathway (Fig. 7) are proposed to arise through the dedifferentiation mechanism whereby astrocytomas (grade II) would progress to anaplastic astrocytomas (grade III) that would ultimately progress into GBM (grade IV), accumulating mutations through progression.

Astrocytoma

The most common alteration occurs on chromosome 17, which is associated with the tumor suppressor gene TP53 (70). p53 is a multifunctional protein involved in the regulation of cell growth, apoptosis, and both the activation and suppression of gene-specific transcription (reviewed in ref. 69). Deletions or mutations of this gene are the most frequent genetic lesion observed in more than 50% of a wide variety of human malignancies (69), and the reported incidence of TP53 gene mutation in astrocytomas is approximately 30% to 45% (34,61,68,149). Because the incidence does not increase significantly in the higher-grade tumors, the loss of function in this gene is presumed to be an early event in the progression of astrocytomas (149). It is the alteration to this gene that distinguishes tumors in this pathway from tumors allocated to pathways II and III.

Alterations on chromosome 22 occur in approximately 20% to 30% of the low-grade astrocytomas (34) and present as either monosomy 22 (21) or loss on 22q (122,153). The large loss of chromosomal material has impeded the ability to localize the candidate tumor suppressor gene. The neurofibromatosis

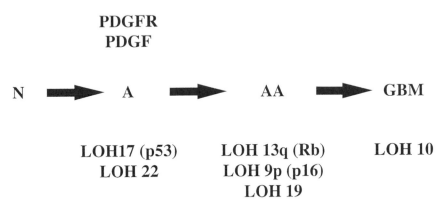

FIG. 7. (See text for details.) Genetic alterations in genes/loci above the progression pathway are overexpressed and/or mutant; genetic alterations below the pathway are lost and/or mutant. Alterations accumulate throughout progression. N, normal cell of origin; A, astrocytoma; AA, anaplastic astrocytoma; GBM, glioblastoma multiforme.

2 (NF2) tumor suppressor gene localized to 22q was excluded as the candidate astrocytoma gene (86), and evidence suggests that it is localized to a more telomeric locus on chromosome 22 (108,152). In a recent study attempting to elucidate the role of this candidate gene in tumorigenesis, a normal copy of the chromosome 22 was reintroduced into a human monocytic leukemia cell line resistant to FAS and p55 TNFR-mediated apoptosis (91). The introduction of a normal chromosome 22 into this cell line was able to reestablish the apoptotic mechanism. It remains to be determined whether the reintroduction of chromosome 22 into glioma cells would have the same effect.

Overexpression of the proliferation-promoting platelet-derived growth factors (PDGF-A and -B) and the PDGFR-α receptor occurs in most astrocytomas (77). The overexpression of these genes at both the mRNA and protein levels has been observed in all grades of malignant astrocytomas but increases with progression with the highest level of expression in GBMs (40,45). Hermanson et al. (45) demonstrated that in all the low-grade astrocytomas tested, none showed an amplification of the PDGFR-α gene, suggesting some other mechanism is responsible for the overexpression of PDGFR-α mRNA.

PDGF and its receptor are speculated to function in an autocrine loop and thereby contribute to unregulated growth (40,155). Elevated levels seen in low-grade astrocytoma suggest that it occurs early in tumor initiation. Furthermore, the association between elevated levels of PDGF-α-receptor mRNA and loss of heterozygosity (LOH) on 17p (45) supports the assignment of these alterations to this pathway.

A number of cytokines and other growth factors have recently been implicated in the modulation of tumors of the CNS. Of all the growth factors studied, bFGF and one of its receptors, FGFR-1 (FLG), are of particular interest. Elevated levels of bFGF protein were observed in 95% of the cases studied (137), and significantly elevated FGFR-1 (FLG) mRNA was also observed (159). Although overexpression was observed in low-grade tumors in comparison with normal brain, both genes demonstrated further increases in expression throughout progression (137,159). In addition, the FGF overexpression was associated with highly vascular tumors (137), which correlated with the overexpression of the FGFR-1 protein in capillary endothelial cells (142). Therefore the elevated expression of bFGF and FGFR-1 in astrocytomas and endothelial cells within the tumors suggests that these genes are also involved in autonomous autocrine growth stimulation and may contribute to angiogenesis as well (142).

Anaplastic Astrocytoma

Mutations to the RB1 gene and LOH of 13q have been implicated in a number of human malignancies (15,139,157). Approximately 30% to 50% of glial tumors present with alterations to the RB1 gene, suggesting it is a major target for alterations in these tumors. Alterations occur as early as anaplastic grade (43) and increase in frequency in GBMs (34,42,43,140). These alterations arise either by a mutation in the RB1 gene or by LOH at 13q14, the locus encoding this gene. RB1 is a critical gene in the control of the cell cycle at the G_1-S-phase transition checkpoint (see next section), and the loss or disruption of its normal function results in the release of this control, resulting in increased proliferation.

The altered expression of the $p16^{INKA4}$ protein has been implicated in a number of other human cancer types, including bladder, colon, small cell lung carcinoma, non–small cell lung carcinoma, and head and neck squamous cell carcinoma (44). Mutations to the CDKN2A (MTS1) gene encoding the $p16^{INKA4}$ are reported in 50% to 59% of the gliomas studied (87,150). The alterations occur as early as anaplastic grade and increase in frequency in GBMs (87,120). This finding indicates that this genetic alteration is significant in the progression and not in the initial phases of the tumorigenesis.

LOH on 19q has been reported, with deletion occurring in both grade III astrocytomas and grade IV GBMs (147). The putative tumor suppressor locus has been mapped to 19q13.3 (161). Although this region is reportedly lost in both astrocytomas and oligodendrogliomas, suggesting a shared tumor suppressor locus, it is lost with greater frequency in oligodendrogliomas (see "Oligodendrogliomas"; 105). In fact, a chromosome 19p13.2 region is more frequently deleted in astrocytomas (105). Therefore it appears as though more than one tumor suppressor gene exists on chromosome 19, one of which predominantly promotes astrocytomas and the other of which promotes oligodendrogliomas.

GBM

Tumors of this grade typically demonstrate whole or partial deletion of a copy of chromosome 10 and occur in 53% to 97% of the reported cases (32,33,146,151,160). Although LOH of 10 occurs occasionally in lower-grade tumors (98), most studies indicate that the loss predominantly occurs in GBMs. Evidence that loss of a gene(s) on this chromosome contributes to hyperproliferation was demonstrated by analyzing the proliferation rate (Ki-67) in tumors with either one or both of monosomy 10, trisomy 7 (131). The results indicated that positive Ki-67 was associated with monosomy 10 and not trisomy 7. Thus the authors suggest that monosomy 10 promotes proliferation, implying that the loss of a tumor suppressor gene(s) provides a selective growth advantage.

It has been difficult to identify putative tumor suppressor genes on chromosome 10 simply because of the large deletions. However, limited deletion mapping studies suggest that there may be up to three candidate tumor suppressor genes on this chromosome. The most frequently lost locus is on the long arm at q25 (33,54,98), with two additional loci implicated on 10p (54,146) and 10q (54). Progress has been made recently with the identification of a candidate gene encoding a protein tyrosine phosphatase (PTEN/MMAC-1) in the region of 10q23 (71,130). This gene appears to be mutated in high-grade gliomas as well as in breast and prostate cancer (71) and Cowden's disease (CD) (72). The protein interacts with actin filaments at focal adhesions and is suggested to act in regulating tumor invasion and metastasis through the loss of the normal interactions at these focal adhesions (71). The study of CD patients suggests that this gene may function developmentally to ensure proper cellular, tissue, and organ organization (72). Liaw et al. postulated that loss of function of PTEN/MMAC-1 could cause proliferation and disorganization that could lead to the formation of hamartomas, which is a hallmark of CD. The critical assay defining the function of PTEN/MMAC-1 as a candidate tumor suppressor gene has not yet been reported.

Pathway II

De Novo *GBM*

Tumors in pathway II (Fig. 8) arise without evidence of progression from a lower-grade tumor. It is arguable that progression did occur but initially went undetected because of the tumor site. However, molecular genetic evidence supports the suggestion that these tumors belong to a separate category and could arise by the misdifferentiation mechanism (see preceding discussion). In common with pathway I tumors, these tumors have LOH on chromosomes 19q, 10, and 9p (p16) (149). However, tumors allocated to this pathway distinctly have some alteration of the epidermal growth factor receptor (EGFR) gene without loss or alteration of the TP53 gene, and it is this distinction that establishes the molecular basis for these variants (103,149).

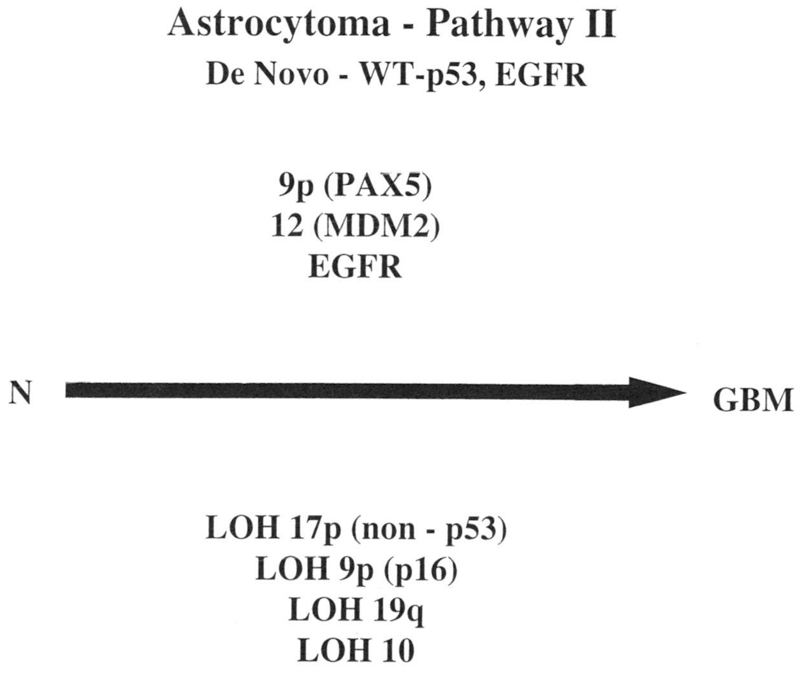

Astrocytoma - Pathway II
De Novo - WT-p53, EGFR

9p (PAX5)
12 (MDM2)
EGFR

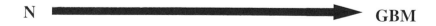

N ➤ **GBM**

LOH 17p (non - p53)
LOH 9p (p16)
LOH 19q
LOH 10

FIG. 8. (See text for details.) Genetic alterations in genes/loci above the progression pathway are overexpressed and/or mutant; genetic alterations below the pathway are lost and/or mutant. Alterations accumulate throughout progression. N, normal cell of origin; GBM, glioblastoma multiforme.

Alterations to the EGFR gene may occur either by the amplification with overexpression of the gene, which occurs in approximately 40% to 50% of all GBMs (25,73,119) and/or by a mutation to a more constitutively active form that causes the increased activity of this transmembrane receptor tyrosine kinase. The most common mutation in the EGFR gene is an in-frame deletion of exons 2–7 within the extracellular domain, resulting in a truncated mutant receptor that is constitutively active. When U87 cells expressing this truncated EGFR mutant were mixed with parental cells and injected into a mouse brain in a mutant-to-parental ratio of 1:50,000, the resultant tumor had a 5:1 ratio, demonstrating the intrinsic growth advantage the mutant EGFR conferred to these cells (85). This remarkable growth rate was due to both increased proliferation and decreased apoptosis. These cells expressing the EGFR mutant had increased Bcl-X_L expression that would protect the cells from the expected apoptotic response elicited by the wild-type p53 present in these cells (see next section). Thus the EGFR alteration was shown to contribute to both cell growth and apoptosis.

The amplification of the MDM2 gene, which is localized to 12q13–14, has been observed in a significant proportion of GBMs (8% to 10%) (99,102). Amplification has been observed in both GBMs and anaplastic astrocytomas. Therefore amplification of this gene is not exclusive to tumors in this pathway. MDM2 happens to be localized to a region that includes the CDK/SAS genes for which the CDK4 gene is also implicated in glioma progression. A close study of this region indicated that the MDM2 gene is in a separate amplicon from the other two genes, which provides further evidence that these genes represent two independent targets of selection (102).

The cytogenetic location of PAX5 is 9p13 (134), a region highly implicated in the progression of gliomas (76). Overexpression of the PAX5 was observed to varying degrees in seven GBMs examined with little or no expression of the transcript in normal brain and lower-grade astrocytomas (134). In the same study, the presence of EGFR protein coincided to the regions highly expressing PAX5 protein, supporting the allocation of the overexpression of this gene to this pathway. However, significantly lower levels of PAX5 protein were observed in five anaplastic tumors, which suggests that elevated expression may not be restricted to this pathway.

Pathway III

All Other Tumors

Tumors designated to pathway III (Fig. 9) may share some, but not all, of the previously described genetic alterations. A significant number of these GBMs manifest themselves without any of the commonly observed chromosomal aberrations and/or gene amplifications observed in tumors allocated to the previous two pathways. Cytogenetic techniques such as LOH, karyotyping, and comparative genome hybridization have been useful for implicating gains (1, 2q, 3p,4, 5q, 6p, 7, 8q, 9, 12, 13q, 17p, 19p, 20p, and 21q) and losses (2q, 3, 4q, 5, 6q, 9p,10, 11p, 12q, 13q, 14q, 15q, 17, 18q, 19q, 22q, and Xp or Y) of chromosomal material (21,53,66,115,122,153, 156,158). Most tumors demonstrate multiple gross changes, making it difficult to determine whether the changes cause or result from tumor progression. Therefore it is helpful when tumors present with only one gross abnormality, such as the report of a low-grade astrocytoma having only an inversion on chromosome 8 (115). The study of this inversion may provide information about the initial neoplastic event in astrocytomas progression.

These alternate genetic losses and amplifications (66) suggest that there are multiple and redundant genetic alterations that may affect common biologic processes that contribute to the development of gliomas. Obviously, future work involving both cytogenetic and molecular *in situ* analyses will be necessary to evaluate the relationship of these chromosomal alterations to neoplastic transformation.

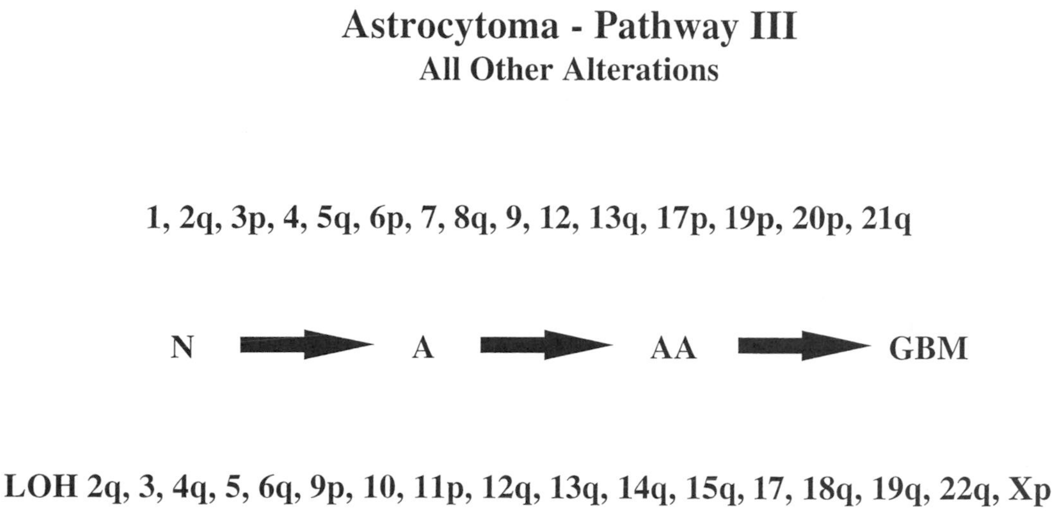

Astrocytoma - Pathway III
All Other Alterations

1, 2q, 3p, 4, 5q, 6p, 7, 8q, 9, 12, 13q, 17p, 19p, 20p, 21q

N ➡ A ➡ AA ➡ GBM

LOH 2q, 3, 4q, 5, 6q, 9p, 10, 11p, 12q, 13q, 14q, 15q, 17, 18q, 19q, 22q, Xp

FIG. 9. (See text for details.) Genetic alterations in genes/loci above the progression pathway are overexpressed and/or mutant; genetic alterations below the pathway are lost and/or mutant. Alterations accumulate throughout progression. N, normal cell of origin; A, astrocytoma; AA, anaplastic astrocytoma; GBM, glioblastoma multiforme.

In summary, the subgrouping of astrocytomas into molecular variants suggests at least three possible pathways to GBM. Pathway I consists of tumors that exhibit a loss of functional p53; pathway II consists of tumors that exhibit an overexpression of the EFGR gene and normal p53; and pathway III represents all the other tumors. Clearly, more studies are needed to elucidate the significance of molecular aberrations in a large number of primary tumors. Such studies will allow us to determine which of the numerous genetic aberrations reflect changes critical to the progression of this disease and enable us to further classify astrocytomas into molecular variants and/or progression pathways.

Oligodendrogliomas

Oligodendrogliomas represent approximately 4% to 15% of primary CNS tumors and typically are diagnosed between the ages of 40 and 45 years. The early genetic events in oligodendroglial oncogenesis are distinct from astrocytic oncogenesis. However, they share later genetic events, suggesting common pathways of progression that culminate in GBMs (see Fig. 1).

Pathway IV

The progression model for the pure oligodendrogliomas consists of one major pathway (Fig 10; pathway IV), where the oligodendroglioma (grade II) progresses into the anaplastic oligodendroglioma (grade III), with ultimate progression to the GBM (grade IV).

Oligodendroglioma

A striking feature of oligodendrogliomas is the particularly high (81%) loss of chromosome 19q13.2–13.4 (7,100,105). Von Deimling et al. (147) have extensively examined the LOH on 19q, originally mapping the candidate region to a 5-Mb region between the APOC2 and HRC loci. They further refined the localization to a 425-kb region between D19S219 and D19S112 (161), in agreement with the localization observed by Ritland et al. (105). A number of potentially interesting genes were previously mapped to this region,

Oligodendroglioma Progression

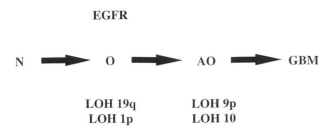

FIG. 10. (See text for details.) Genetic alterations in genes/loci above the progression pathway are overexposed or mutant; alterations below the progression pathway represent lost or mutant expression. Alterations accumulate throughout progression. N, normal cell of origin; O, oligodendroglioma; AO, anaplastic oligodendroglioma; GBM, glioblastoma multiforme.

including the DNA excision and repair genes ERCC1, ECRR2, and XRCC1. However, Yong et al. (161) have scrutinized this region and have excluded these genes, as well as a putative phosphatase and the more centromeric LIG1 (a DNA ligase gene), as the gene necessary for oligodendroglioma tumorigenesis. As previously mentioned, LOH on 19q is common to both astrocytomas and oligodendrogliomas (147,148). It will therefore be interesting to determine whether the oligodendroglial tumor suppressor gene localized to this region is identical to the tumor suppressor gene(s) necessary for astrocytoma progression.

Studies that have critically looked at the LOH on 1p have determined that the smallest deleted region mapped to 1pter-p13 (6,7). In two studies, six of six and 10 of 11 oligodendrogliomas demonstrated LOH on 1p. This was also true of five of six and eight of 10 anaplastic oligodendrogliomas (6,7). However, none of the astrocytomas (6) showed LOH 1p. To date, no known tumor suppressor gene has been identified in this region.

A characteristic and consistent observation is the concurrent LOH on 1p and 19q occurring in 60% to 75% of the low- and high-grade tumors (7,100). These observations suggest that the inactivation of tumor suppressor genes on 1p and 19q represents cooperative alterations occurring in the early stages of oncogenic transformation of these neoplasms. This concurrent loss of 1p and 19q and the absence of p53 gene alterations (100) are changes specific to the oligodendrogliomas. In addition,

other molecular alterations associated with astrocytomas such as CDK4 and MDM2 amplification and alteration of p16 (112) are rarely observed in these tumors.

It was originally thought that the alteration to the EGFR gene was specific to the astrocytomas because the amplification of the EGFR gene is reportedly rare in oligodendrogliomas. However, a recent study of 13 grade II and 20 grade III oligodendrogliomas demonstrated increased expression of this gene at both mRNA and protein levels in six grade II and 10 of 18 grade III tumors (101). Thus the overexpression of this gene due to causes other than gene amplification occurs early in oligodendroglioma progression and is a common alteration shared with the high-grade astrocytomas.

Anaplastic Oligodendroglioma and GBM

There are limited data concerning genetic alterations required in the progression from OII to AOIII to GBM. A few reports indicate a noted occurrence of LOH 9 and LOH 10 (100). The LOH on 9 and 10 may represent the alteration of unknown glial-specific tumor suppressor genes that contribute to a common biologic pathway needed by both oligodendrogliomas and astrocytomas to progress to the malignant grade IV GBM.

Mixed Oligoastrocytomas

The mixed oligoastrocytomas are not well characterized, and therefore the molecular description of this class of tumors is limited. However, the classical dedifferentiation progression pathway has been proposed for these tumors as well (see Fig. 1, pathway V).

Pathway V

The progression model for the oligoastrocytomas consists of one major pathway (Fig. 11), where the oligoastrocytoma (grade II) progresses into the anaplastic oligoastrocytoma (grade III), with ultimate progression to GBM (grade IV). However, the origin of these tumors may be better explained by the misdifferentiation hypothesis (see Fig. 5) than by the dedifferentiation hypothesis (see Fig. 4). Because of the limited research, discussion will be combined for all grades.

All Grades

Most of the studies that deal with the molecular progression of oligoastrocytomas are done as a part of studies that are also investigating pure oligodendrogliomas, which focus primarily on the analysis of LOH on 1p and/or 19q. There appears to be a contradiction in the conclusions from these studies. Two groups have found that in the oligoastrocytomas there is a similar pattern and percentage of LOH on both 1p and 19q as seen in pure oligodendrogliomas (7,142). In contrast, two other groups have found a significantly lower incidence of LOH of 1p (100) and/or LOH on 19q (100,105), which more closely approximates

the level of occurrence observed in pure astrocytomas. This disagreement could be the result of a number of technical difficulties encountered when working with heterogeneic tumors that result in an unintentional sample bias.

To more closely examine the relationship between mixed oligoastrocytomas and oligodendroglioma, the astrocytic and oligodendroglioma regions of three mixed oligoastrocytomas were examined for the LOH of 1p and 19q. In all three tumors, both regions demonstrated LOH for both chromosomes (63), suggesting that the oligodendroglioma and astrocytoma components were probably of clonal origin. Because both histomorphologic cell types exhibited identical chromosomal alterations on 1p and 19q, a subsequent branching event may have occurred that permits the two histomorphologically distinct oligodendroglial and astrocytic components within the tumor, which could each then undergo specific mutations.

For example, in a study of c-*myc* expression in low-grade and high-grade oligoastrocytomas, the elevated c-*myc* expression was restricted to the astrocytic areas of the high-grade tumors (5). These observations suggest that alteration to c-*myc* expression would presumably have had to occur after chromosome 1p and 19q alterations.

Ependymomas

Ependymomas are a rare class of brain tumors that comprise approximately 5% of CNS

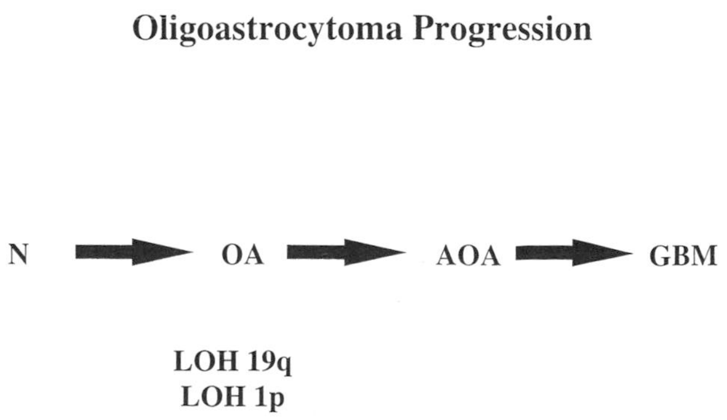

Oligoastrocytoma Progression

N ➡ OA ➡ AOA ➡ GBM

LOH 19q
LOH 1p

FIG. 11. (See text for details.) Alterations below the pathway represent lost or mutant expression. Alterations accumulate throughout progression. N, normal cell of origin; OA, oligoastrocytoma; AOA, anaplastic oligoastrocytoma; GBM, glioblastoma multiforme.

tumors and are the least studied on a molecular level. A limited number of primary tumors and cell lines have been described for which only a few genetic alterations have been implicated in these tumors. Therefore minimal data are available to confirm the progression model illustrated in Figure 1 (pathway VI).

Pathway VI

It is proposed that ependymomas would also progress from ependymoma (grade II) to anaplastic ependymoma (grade III) to GBM (grade IV) (Fig. 12). Because of the limited data regarding these tumors, discussion will be combined for all grades.

All Grades

Studies of small numbers of tumors have implicated an overexpression of growth factors and receptors in ependymomas. Transforming growth factor (TGF)β 1 and TGFβ 2 are suggested as growth promoters (52). Both PDGF-A and -B growth factor and the PDGF receptor are up-regulated in these tumors (11), suggesting that ependymomas share this autocrine loop mechanism with the astroglial tumors.

The loss of a candidate tumor suppressor gene on 1p has been reported (114). However, in a larger study, no loss of chromosome 1p or 16 q was observed in 17 tumors (9). Other alterations in these 17 tumors included loss of 22q (in three of 17), loss of 10 (in two of 17), loss of 17p (in two of 17), and loss of 6q, 9p, 13q, and 19q (in one of 17 each). None of the tumors had EGFR amplification. The authors

conclude that, in general, ependymomas resemble the other glial tumors with regard to the type of chromosomal changes present; however, changes occur at a low frequency.

The most consistent change in these tumors is an early genetic alteration resulting in full or partial monosomy of chromosome 22 (94,97,154). The tumor suppressor gene neurofibromatosis 2 on 22q was studied in eight ependymal tumors and only one NF-2 mutation was detected, which presented as a single base deletion in exon 7 (108). This observation has been supported by other studies (20,128). The low occurrence of detectable mutations in this gene led to the suggestion that it is not the critical ependymoma tumor suppressor gene. Presently, there is no known tumor suppressor gene localized to chromosome 22 that is attributed to ependymal progression.

Fink et al. (27) investigated the possible role that the tumor suppressor gene, TP53, may have in ependymal progression. In this study of 31 ependymomas and anaplastic ependymomas, only a single silent mutation was found in exon 6 of the TP53 gene. In addition, Lee et al. (68) examined three ependymomas for LOH out of 17 and found no alteration on this chromosome. These few studies suggest that neither a deletion nor a mutation of the p53 gene is involved in the progression of this disease. The infrequently observed alteration in the TP53 gene in these tumors establishes a molecular distinction that separates this lineage from the astrocytic pathway I in the progression model.

In a small study of three ependymomas, it was indicated that the initiation of this disease

Ependymoma Progression

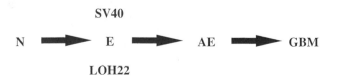

FIG. 12. (See text for details.) Alterations below the pathway represent lost or mutant expression. N, normal cell of origin; E, ependymoma; AE, anaplastic ependymoma; GBM, glioblastoma multiforme.

may be attributed to a viral agent, simian virus 40 (SV40). The viral sequence was PCR amplified and sequenced and found to be authentic SV40 in all the samples (67). This discovery segregates the epidemiologic onset of this cancer from the other gliomas. The SV40 virus is known for its tumorigenic properties (67) and can induce this tumor type experimentally. The SV40 proteins are known to inhibit the function of both p53 and Rb proteins and is postulated to exert their transforming effects through the disruption of these proteins' functions and thereby to inhibit growth control (see below). Clearly, a larger study is needed to elucidate the extent that this virus initiates ependymal tumorigenesis.

In summary, the three different glial tumors have shared and lineage-specific genetic alterations that contribute to the initiation and progression of these neoplasms. A review of these genetic alterations reinforces the fact that one of the early events required for tumorigenesis is a disruption of normal growth control and that several mechanisms exist by which a cell can disrupt cell division and/or apoptosis to affect this goal. The next section reviews these two biochemical pathways and emphasizes the alterations currently observed in the gliomas.

THE CELL CYCLE CONTROL AND GLIAL TUMORS

Cell Cycle

The direct evidence for the involvement of alterations affecting the normal cell cycle control and cancer has been well established (reviewed in ref. 126), and a number of cell cycle control genes have been implicated in the initiation and progression of the glial tumors to more malignant grades (48,140). As described in the previous section, a number of gene alterations in gliomas appear to affect tumor cell growth. The objective of this section is to integrate the molecular alterations that affect the increased cellular proliferation observed in gliomas into the context of the cell cycle.

The decision for the cell to divide is directed by positive or negative external signals conveyed through signal transduction pathways that initiate a cascade of events involving positive or negative signaling molecules that either promote or halt cell division. If the decision is made to divide, the cell passes from G_1 through the S-phase (DNA synthesis phase), through a second gap phase (G_2), and then through mitosis (M), resulting in the two daughter cells (see Fig. 12). Each of these phases of the cell cycle requires the expression and activation of distinctive sets of proteins that direct the cell through division.

To facilitate the proper regulation of the cell through the cell cycle, the cell possesses an intricate series of control complexes that consist of the cyclin-dependent kinases (CDKs) and the cyclins. These complexes have a central role in the progression of the cell cycle through the activation of other key proteins via phosphorylation. The growth-promoting regulation of these complexes is balanced by a number of cyclin-dependent kinases inhibitors (CKIs) that negatively modulate the activity of the CDKs.

In the event that the cell divides, a positive signal is relayed to affect the phosphorylation of Rb, which results in the dissociation of the Rb/E2F complex releasing E2F, which is essential for the cell to cross the restriction point. Therefore this restriction point represents a critical juncture where the decision is made to either divide or enter growth arrest.

The remaining part of this section will describe the mutations observed in gliomas and the effect these mutations have on the cell's ability to regulate division. Gene alterations have been associated with several genes required for cell cycle control, including the Rb, p16, p53, MDM2, and PAX5 genes.

Genetic Alterations of Cell Cycle Genes in Gliomas

RB

The retinoblastoma protein (Rb1) functions as the critical protein at the restriction point that monitors the cellular conditions to determine whether the cell will progress through the G_1 to S-phase or remain in a resting G_0 phase. The Rb1 protein functions as a transcriptional regulator having both negative and positive modulating effects over genes whose functions are required for progression of the cell cycle. The Rb1 protein is activated via phosphorylation at multiple sites by the CDK4/cyclin D and CDK2/cyclin E complexes. Rb1 in the unphosphorylated state is bound to the transcriptional factor E2F. Sequestering E2F by binding to Rb1 during the G_1 phase ensures that S-phase cannot be initiated. Genes whose products are essential for S-phase are transcriptionally repressed by the Rb1/E2F complex itself or transcriptionally inactivated because of the lack of free E2F. Upon activation of Rb1, the E2F protein is released, which results in the transcriptional activation of the genes required for S-phase and the cell proceeds through the cell cycle.

Studies to determine the sites of mutations within the 200-kb, 27-exon gene found a large spectrum of deletions, rearrangements, and point mutations within both intron and exons (43). All effectively produce no or nonfunctional protein. The loss of function of the Rb1 protein would thus disrupt the cellular decision to undergo growth arrest at the end of the G_1 phase. This disruption would be facilitated by the loss of the repression of genes whose activities are required for S-phase. Therefore the loss of Rb1 normal function eliminates the cell's ability to inhibit proliferation.

p16-CDK4/cyclinD-Rb1 Axis

The Rb protein is the terminal protein of the signaling pathway known as the p16-CDK4/cyclinD-Rb1 axis. The CDK4/cyclinD complex monitors incoming positive signals from growth factors and proto-oncogenes and balances them against negative signals from the CKIs (p16, p18/p19, and p15). In gliomas, genetic alterations have been documented in p16 and CDK4 members of this pathway.

p16

The INK family of CKIs includes the p15, p16, p18, and p19 proteins that inhibit cyclin D binding with CDK4 and CDK6, thereby inducing G_1 growth arrest. p16 specifically competes with cyclin D for the binding of the CDK4 protein, inhibiting the formation of the cyclin D/CDK4 complex (124) and thereby inhibiting the activation of Rb1 via phosphorylation. In turn, p16 is negatively regulated by phosphorylated Rb1. Therefore the expression of both proteins is regulated by a feedback loop. Thus the loss of functions of p16 disrupts the proper regulation of cellular growth arrest at the end G_1 phase of the cell cycle.

That the loss of function of the tumor suppressor gene, p16 (MTS-1,CDKN2A), contributes to astrocytoma progression was demonstrated by the reexpression of this gene into p16-null glioblastoma cell lines, with resultant growth suppression (3). Furthermore, there may be an advantage to the tumors harboring p16 deletion rather than alterations to RB and CDK4 genes. Proliferative indices were shown to be higher in tumors that had a homozygous deletion of p16 than those without deletion, suggesting that alterations to p16 may have a more deleterious effect on cell cycle than mutations to RB or amplification of CDK4 (93).

The loss of function of the p16 can occur by several mechanisms—including homozygous deletion of 9q (51,140,150), mutation (140), and altered methylation of the gene (19,81), resulting in the absolute inhibition of transcription (transcriptional silencing) (37)—or perhaps by perturbations in upstream p16 regulatory proteins (87). The prevalence of methylation as a mechanism in p16 gene inactivation depends on whether primary glial tumors or cell lines were used for the studies. Merlo et al. (81) examined the occurrence of DNA methylation in glioma cell lines and found aberrant methylation of the 5′ CpG island within the first exon of the CDKN2A genes in 30% of the samples having no detectable mutation or deletion in the p16 gene. Alternatively, Schmidt et al. (121) studied the hypermethylation patterns of the CDKN2A gene in 21 primary gliomas and found only three cases of aberrant methylation patterns. Of these three cases, only one exhibited a loss of the gene's expression. These observations suggest that aberrant methylation is not a predominant cause of disruption of the p16 gene in primary glial tumors. Whether the gene is silenced by methylation or functionally inactivated by other mechanisms, the final consequence is a loss of inhibition of the CDK4/cyclin D complex formation that results in the release of cellular growth arrest at the G_1-S-phase checkpoint.

CDK4

The amplification of the 12q13–14 chromosomal region is observed in a significant portion of gliomas (15%), and it is the cytogenetic location of a number of potentially oncogenic genes, including the CDK4 gene (38). The overexpression of the CDK4 gene has been observed in gliomas and is suggested to function as an alternate mechanism to the deletion of the CDKN2A (p16 encoding) gene (42,120). The overexpression of the CDK4 protein would overwhelm the negative regulation by p16, ensuring sufficient protein to complex with cyclin D and thereby promoting Rb phosphorylation and cell division. This would have a result analogous to a p16 deletion whereby the cell is released from cellular growth arrest at the G_1-S-phase checkpoint.

Because mutations in any one of these genes should be sufficient to override negative growth regulation, studies were performed to determine whether these disruptions were exclusive of each other. If they were, then gliomas might utilize redundant progression pathways, which suggests that gliomas could be subtyped on the basis of which alteration was present in a particular tumor (42,48,143). Ichmura et al. (48) determined that 64% of the glioblastomas in their study had distinct genetic aberrations of the p16-CDK4/cyclin D-Rb1 axis, with either no

wild-type p16 (40%), amplified CDK4 (12%), or no wild-type Rb1 (14%). He et al. (42) reached a similar conclusion from data demonstrating that the highest incidence of disruptions in the p16-CDK4/cyclin D-Rb1 axis involved the loss of p16 expression (28%) followed by an amplification of the CDK4 gene (11%) and loss of Rb1 protein (15%). These studies strongly support the notion of redundant pathways to malignant progression and suggest that tumors can be subtyped based on their molecular genetic profiles, as described previously.

p53

p53 is a multifunctional transcription factor that monitors cellular responses to DNA damage. The protein is a potent tumor suppressor with the ability to halt cell division until genetic damage is corrected, thereby ensuring genetic stability, or, if DNA damage is too great, it can commit the cell to suicide by inducing the apoptotic pathway. When normal cells are induced to divide, low p53 expression permits the cell cycle to proceed. These responsibilities place this gene in the position of being the guardian of the cell and make it a target that must be overcome or subverted if a cell is to become neoplastic. As described in the section on molecular progression, the overall observed alteration of the TP53 gene in astrocytomas is appropriately 60% to 65%. Mutations in this gene are one of the earliest observed in astrocytomas. The resultant lack of DNA damage monitoring most likely contributes to the short time to tumor recurrence and increased malignant progression observed in these tumors.

p21-p53-MDM2/PAX5 Axis

With regard to the cell cycle, p53 is also a member of a biochemical pathway that ultimately impacts upon the same cyclin D/CDK4 complex as the p16 pathway, thereby indirectly regulating RB gene phosphorylation. A signaling response to DNA damage induces the accumulation of p53 protein, which in turn modulates the cyclin/ CDK4 complex via the transcriptional activation of p21$^{WAF1/CIP1}$ gene.

p21

The p21 family of CKIs includes p21$^{WAF1/CIP1}$, p27^{Kip1}, and p57^{Kip2}. The p21$^{WAF1/CIP1}$ CKI binds to the cyclin D/CDK4 and cyclin E/CDK2 complexes and inhibits their abilities to activate Rb1 by phosphorylation (126). Mutations/deletions of the p21 gene are rare in glial tumors, suggesting that a reduction in expression levels of normal p21 could alter cell cycle regulation. A study of seven malignant glioma cell lines indicated that p21 expression was decreased in all but that reduced expression did not correlate with the p53 mutational status, thus implicating other unknown regulators of p21 (23).

MDM2

It has been shown in Hela cells that the mdm2 oncoprotein binds to the p53 protein, inhibiting its DNA binding domain (and p21 transcriptional activation) by concealing it and then inducing the rapid degradation of the p53 protein (41,64). The transforming capability of MDM2 was demonstrated by the overexpression of the gene in neonatal rat astrocytes (60). MDM2 overexpression promoted DNA synthesis and abrogated the transcriptional activity of p53. In addition, the astrocytes were transformed and demonstrated invasive capability *in vivo*. These results indicate that enhanced MDM2 overexpression may promote astrocytoma progression.

In a study examining the correlation between p53 expression and MDM2 overexpression in 15 GBMs overexpressing MDM2, only one tumor was found to have both mutations (8). Therefore the amplified expression of MDM2 in gliomas could exert its effects by eliminating the accumulation of active p53 in response to DNA damage or hypoxia. Thus an overexpression of MDM2 would be functionally analogous to an inactivating p53 mutation.

PAX5

PAX5 (reviewed in ref. 132) represses the transcriptional activation of the TP53 gene (133) by binding to a 5' regulatory region that is absolutely necessary for TP53 promoter activity. Stuart et al. (134) demonstrated an increased expression of PAX5 with increased malignancy in human astrocytomas and found the highest levels of expression in grade IV glioblastomas with little or no expression in normal brain and low-grade astrocytomas. The late occurrence of an alteration in the PAX5 gene in the progression of astrocytomas suggests that it may not function by repressing apoptotic abilities of p53 but by inhibiting cell cycle arrest. Furthermore, p53 may be only one of a set of genes that are the target of PAX5 transcriptional regulation. The activation or inhibition of this set of genes may confer a selective growth advantage in the tumor cell. High expression of the PAX5 genes was also correlated with areas of the tumor that exhibited an increased expression of the EFGR gene, suggesting that these two genes may be intricately connected in the progression to increased malignancy (134). Therefore the neoplastic effects of the overexpression of the PAX5 gene would be analogous to the overexpression of the mdm2 protein. Overexpression of either gene would function to eliminate the p53 signal to inhibit cellular growth.

In summary, a number of cell cycle control genes have been implicated in tumor progression by directly or indirectly disrupting a crucial restriction checkpoint at the end of the G_1. All these alterations influence the CDK4/ cyclin complex and downstream Rb phosphorylation and entry into S-phase of the cell cycle. It is interesting to consider the diversity of genetic alterations at different cytogenetic locations that can affect a singular cellular biochemical pathway and result in a similar outcome. It is this commonality that connects them in their ability to disrupt cellular growth arrest at a particular point in the cell cycle even though most of these genes have multiple functions in the cell and may individually exert other neoplastic influences. The alteration of the cell cycle regulatory machinery appears to be a process that is common in a high proportion of gliomas and may represent a critical target for therapeutic intervention.

APOPTOSIS AND GLIAL TUMORS

Apoptosis

Because the overall growth rate of a tumor is regulated both by promoting cell proliferation and by inhibiting cell death, an extensive amount of work has recently focused on understanding the molecular biology of programmed cell death, or apoptosis. A number of external and internal stimuli—such as the withdrawal of growth factors, metabolic or cell cycle perturbations, activation of death receptors, DNA damage (reviewed in ref. 138), and administration of glucocorticoids (106)—are inducers of apoptosis (Fig. 13). Studies of FAS/TNF ligand-mediated (reviewed in ref. 29), p53-mediated (31), and glucocorticoid-induced (106) apoptosis indicate that they, and presumably all apoptotic stimuli, induce pathways that culminate in a common signaling pathway triggering the activation of a family of cysteine proteases called caspases. The caspase cascade of protease activation activates the proteolytic elements that functionally carry out the death of the cell, which is characterized by nuclear condensation and degradation of genomic and cytoskeletal changes with accompanying cell surface blebbing. The cells eventually break up into smaller membrane-bound fragments referred to as apoptotic bodies that are engulfed by neighboring phagocytic cells (138).

Fas Ligand and TNF-Induced Pathway

One pathway of apoptosis results from a death signal received at the cell surface by the death receptors Fas/APO-1 or TNF-R (Fig. 14; reviewed in ref. 29). Following ligand binding to these receptors, the death signal is conveyed through the formation of CD95-FADD or TNFR1-TRADD-FADD/receptor complexes. The complexes are able to proteolytically activate FLICE/MACH1, an initial protease in the signaling cascade. FLICE/MACH1 proteolytically activates the IL-1B-converting enzyme (ICE), which is suggested to act as an intermediate event that conveys the signal to downstream proteases and which eventually results in the activation of caspase-3 (also known as CPP32/Yama/Apopain), which normally exists in the cell as an inactive precursor. A direct demonstration of the role of caspase-3 in the later stages of apoptotic induction was performed by using cell extracts from thymocytes of ICE-null mice in a cell-free system. When these cell extracts, which are incapable of inducing the apoptotic response, were supplemented with activated caspase-3, the apoptotic response was induced as measured by induction of the characteristic DNA fragmentation (26). These observations suggest that caspase-3 is a necessary factor and functions in the final stages of the apoptotic response.

A number of substrates have been identified for caspase-3, including the recently characterized DNA fragmentation factor (DFF) (75) and the p21-activated kinase 2 (PAK2) (109). Liu et al. (75) identified DFF as an important factor in conveying the death signal from the cytosol into the nucleus, which triggered the enodonuclease DNA fragmentation. Rudel et al. (109) correlated the proteolytic activation of PAK2 with the regulation of cell membrane blebbing. Therefore the activation of these substrates by caspase-3 induces the molecular and morphologic changes characteristic of apoptotic cells.

p53-Mediated Pathway

The activation of caspase-3 appears to be crucial not only for FAS ligand- and TNF-mediated apoptosis but also for p53-mediated apoptosis (31). In a normal cell, wild-type p53 balances the signal between cell death and division (69). In response to certain deleterious conditions such as hypoxia or DNA damage, rapid accumulation of p53 promotes

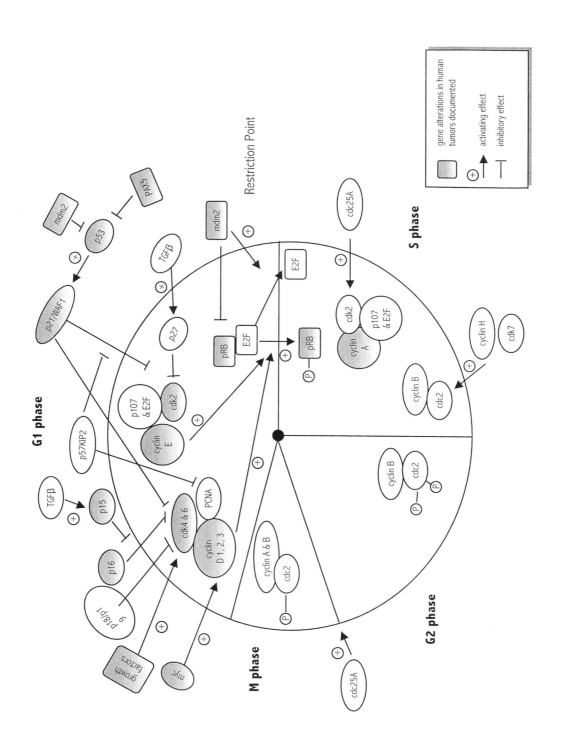

a death signal. The direct mode of action in which p53 induces death of the cell is unclear. However, using temperature-sensitive E1A and p53 BRK transfectants, the caspase enzyme cascade was found to be essential for p53-induced apoptosis (111).

An intermediate event in p53-mediated apoptosis is this collapse of mitochondrial membrane potential and subsequent loss of function. The normal stabilization of the mitochondrial membrane and resultant cell survival are mediated by the Bcl-2 family of proteins (127). This family consists of a growing number of hetero- and homodimeric molecules that can either promote cell survival (antiapoptotic) or enhance cell death (pro-apoptotic), depending on their dimerization profiles.

Antiapoptotic members of the family include Bcl-2 and Bcl-X$_L$, which function as negative regulators by stabilizing the mitochondrial intracellular membrane potential (22,83,116) by forming ion channels that maintain the permeability of the intracellular membranes (83). Thus overexpression of these genes could promote cell survival by maintaining mitochrondrial function and thereby blocking p53-mediated apoptosis.

Hyperexpression of Bcl-2 and Bcl-X$_L$ has also been shown to protect mitochondria from noxious substances such as chemotherapeutic agents. In one study (22), cultured myelomonocytic cells treated with the chemotherapeutic agents doxorubicin, etoposide, and aracytine underwent a disruption of the inner membrane potential preceding nuclear apoptosis that was abrogated by the hyperexpression of Bcl-2 or Bcl-X$_L$. The overexpression of these proteins prevented the release of cytochrome C and the subsequent activation of caspase-3. Therefore a tumor cell could gain a

selective advantage by overexpressing the Bcl-2 or Bcl-X$_L$ genes and offering protection against chemotherapy. These genes present another potential route of therapeutic intervention by the direct inhibition of these genes (by Bax directly) and/or the reintroduction of wild-type p53 expression.

Two of the better-understood pro-apoptotic members of the Bcl-2 family are Bax and Bad. Bad can dimerize with Bcl-2 and Bcl-X$_L$, and the overexpression of Bad can eliminate the survival-promoting effect of either. This suggests that the heterodimer disrupts the ability of Bcl-2 and Bcl-X$_L$ to stabilize the inner membrane potential. Bax can also dimerize with Bcl-2 and Bcl-X$_L$ but with less affinity than Bad (36). Interestingly, Bax is transcriptionally activated by p53 in some cell types (69), suggesting a possible mode in which p53 mediates apoptosis. By increasing Bax and inhibiting Bcl-2 and Bcl-X$_L$, p53 could ensure apoptosis. Thus the balance of the Bcl-2 family members may play a crucial role in the ability of a cell to survive.

Genetic Alterations of Apoptotic Genes in Gliomas

Fas Ligand-Mediated Pathway

To investigate the possible role of Fas in glioma progression, Fas transcript was analyzed in astrocytomas of all grades (I–IV). Increased transcript abundance was detected (from 25% to 100%) during progression (135). The same authors showed immunoreactivity to FAS ligand increasing from 11% in astrocytomas to 87% in glioblastomas (136). In GBMs the immunoreactivity was localized almost exclusively to glioma cells surrounding regions of necrosis. In these same regions

---

FIG. 13. Genetic alterations associated with the cell cycle. The cell cycle is composed of four phases: G$_1$ (gap) phase, S (synthesis) phase, G$_2$ (gap) phase 2, and M (mitosis) phase. The restriction point represents an important juncture in the cell's decision to continue through the cell cycle and divide. Proteins participating in the regulation of this process are indicated. The shading indicates genetic alterations associated with human tumors, including gliomas. (See text for details.) (Adapted from Hunter and Pines [46].)

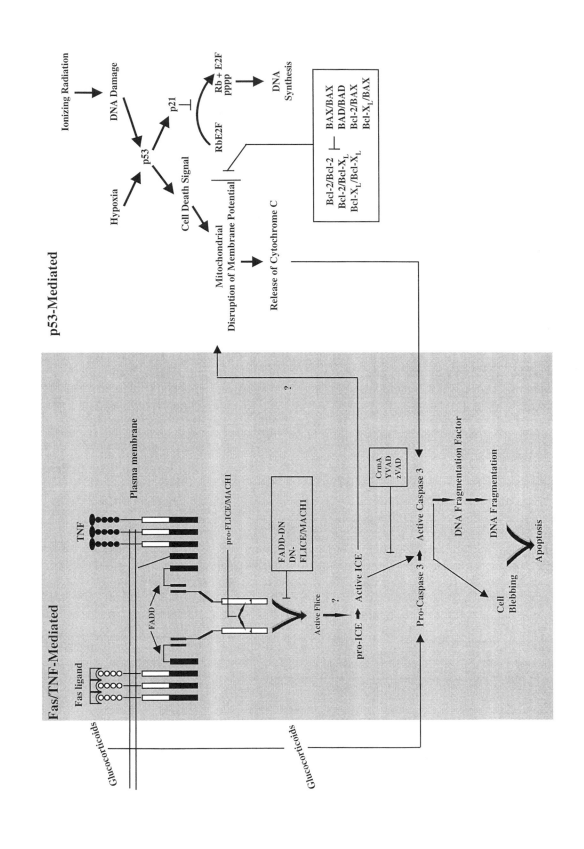

cells were undergoing apoptosis. The authors suggested that FAS-mediated apoptosis may play a role in the pathogenesis of necrosis. Other authors finding FasL expression in astrocytomas further suggest that tumor cell FasL-induced apoptosis may play a role in both immunosuppression and regulation of tumor growth (110).

p53-Mediated Pathway

Besides the obvious results that would arise from the mutations or loss of the p53 gene because of its pivotal role in cell cycle and apoptosis regulation, two other members of this pathway have been implicated in glioma progression. Strong immunohistochemical staining of the Bcl-2 protein was found in astrocytoma and ependymal cells, but minimal staining was observed in oligodendroglial cells (117). Bcl-2 overexpression was associated with tumors having elevated levels of wild-type p53 (7/7) rather than mutant p53 (1/7) (2). In addition, increased expression of Bcl-X_L was observed in astrocytic tumor and correlated with the overexpression of the EGFR gene (85). Therefore overexpression of Bcl-2 or Bcl-XL is a mechanism by which apoptotic resistance could be conferred.

In summary, many of the genetic mutations observed in the glial tumors contribute to cell growth by subverting cell cycle and/or apoptosis control. By characterizing the gene-specific alterations associated with these pathways, tumor-specific, gene-specific therapies could be devised for the treatments of these patients.

GENE THERAPY STRATEGIES IN GLIOMA TREATMENT

Gene therapy is based on the premise that the neoplastic phenotype resulting from a mutated gene can be reversed or halted by replacement with a normal gene in an appropriate delivery vehicle. It was initially expected that gliomas should be ideal candidates for genetic intervention because they rarely metastasize and in theory are accessible to techniques that allow for the direct administration of the gene-specific therapeutic agents (62), which permits the cells to synthesize a cloned gene necessary for either cytotoxic or cytostatic effects. In reality, gene therapy generally has not been as successful as initially anticipated and with regard to low-grade tumors has yet to be considered on any but theoretical grounds. The major impediments have been the inability to deliver genes efficiently and to obtain sustained expression of the introduced gene (145). A particular impediment with regard to solid tumors such as glioblastomas results from tumor heterogeneity. These tumors are composed of cells that are either dividing, nondividing, invading, or undergoing apoptosis. The expectation that single-gene therapy/single-vector delivery will reverse or address complications arising in such a tumor is likely not conceivable. Such impediments, however, can be met using a

---

FIG. 14. Genetic alterations associated with Fas/TNF ligand–associated and p53-mediated apoptosis. Fas and TNF ligands bind to their receptors to induce a cascade of events culminating in the activation of ICE from pro-ICE. Activation of ICE promotes further events and results in the activation of caspase-3 from pro-caspase-3. Active caspase-3 induces cell blebbing and the DNA fragmentation factor, which activates endonucleases that fragment the DNA. The cell ultimately undergoes apoptosis. In p53-mediated apoptosis, p53 induced by ionizing radiation, DNA damage, or hypoxia assesses the extent of DNA damage. Increased p53 may activate p21 and cause cell cycle arrest (see Fig. 13). Alternatively, p53 induction can induce a cell death signal associated with disruption of the mitochondrial membrane potential. Mitochondrial membrane potential is influenced by the balance of expression of the Bcl-2 family members classified as either pro-apoptotic (BAD and BAX) or antiapoptotic (Bcl-2 and Bcl-XL). Disruption of the mitochondria releases cytochrome C, which activates caspase-3 and results in apoptosis. (Adapted from Fraser and Evan [29].)

strategy of combined gene therapies with adjuvant synergistic radiation therapy and/or chemotherapy regimes designed to increase the therapeutic index by targeting tumor cells specifically. One of the most promising aspects of gene therapy is the ability to employ the cell's specific mutations and behavioral characteristics in future therapeutic regimes (59). As demonstrated in the following discussion, strides are being taken in these directions and initial results are promising in their prospects for successful future gene therapy approaches.

Viral Vectors

Initial studies focused on the appropriate gene vector and methods of vector delivery. There are currently several vectors/delivery options, including viruses, liposomes, and even naked DNA, all of which have their pros and cons with regard to efficiency (reviewed in ref. 30). Most of the neuro-oncology-related gene therapy vectors have focused on using viral vectors. The retroviral-based vectors have the advantage of integrating introduced genes into the host chromosomes, which enables long-term stability. However, a drawback is that the integration site is chosen at random and could occur at a site that disrupts host genes, effectively creating an oncogene or a tumor suppressor gene. Adenoviral vectors have been the vector of choice for some researchers because they have the ability to carry large genes and do not integrate into the host DNA, thereby eliminating the worry of integration site effects. However, a major disadvantage is that because they do not integrate, they can only be used for transient treatment. Thus the choice of gene delivery system will ultimately depend on the therapeutic goal and the necessity of long-term expression.

Nonspecific Gene Therapy

Present treatment strategies used in human clinical trials include viral vector constructs that deliver agents locally and thereby prevent the unwanted toxic side-effects when the drug is administered systemically, such as IL-2 (129). Other strategies include viral vectors that deliver suicide genes, which have the capability of metabolizing a systemically given innocuous drug into a tumor cell–specific killing drug within the tumor cell. Examples of clinical trials include the administration of adenovirus-mediated herpes simplex virus–thymidine kinase (HSV-TK) gene delivery followed by ganciclovir treatment (24,50).

Much of the current nonhuman research focuses on enhancing the efficacy of such chemotherapy-based treatments. For example, 9L gliosarcoma cells transduced with a HSV-TK/CD (cytosine deaminase) fusion gene construct followed by treatment with both ganciclovir and 5-fluorocytosine treatment (107) resulted in a slight but significant synergistic toxicity to the cells. In addition, the toxicity was enhanced when the chemotherapy treatment was augmented with radiotherapy. Such treatment strategies are important, but they have limitations, for they affect cell death in any dividing cell, even normal dividing cells. Thus these treatments, although somewhat beneficial, are still not targeting in a tumor-cell or mutation-specific manner.

Cell Cycle and Apoptosis-Directed Gene Therapy

As the genes involved in glioma progression are characterized, gene therapy treatments focusing on a specific gene or a downstream target in a particular biochemical pathway will effectively be produced. In treating low-grade tumors, the most likely gene targets will be involved in the disruption of cell growth (i.e., those that promote excess cell division or inhibit apoptosis [see above]). Depending on the specific mutations, targets for gene therapy could include the inhibition of proto-oncogenes and growth factors, replacement of wild-type tumor suppressor genes involved in cell cycle control, replacement of genes required for the restoration of apoptotic induction, or introduction of genes that induce cell death only in tumor cells carrying a defective gene. Recent endeavors using these strategies *in vitro* and *in vivo* are paving the way for future clinical trials.

TNF

Astrocytoma tumors and cell lines overexpress a number of autocrine growth factors, including PDGF (77), bFGF (84,123), and TNF (65), and the inhibition of the transcription and consequent expression of such growth factors should restore growth control. When synthetic antisense oligodeoxynucleotides to TNF were administered to a TNF-dependent astrocytoma cell line, TNF transcription was specifically inhibited, blocking the growth of these cells (1). The authors suggest that the future administration of viral vectors encoding gene-specific oligodeoxynucleotides against growth factors may prove beneficial for restoring growth control on a long-term basis.

p21

The p21 gene is the downstream effector of the p53 gene. In tumor cells for which this gene has been mutated, reintroduction of the normal gene should reintroduce growth control as well. Using a replication-defective adenovirus p21 construct, Chen et al. (17) tested the effects of reexpressing p21 in glioma cells in culture and *in vivo*. Cell growth *in vitro* and tumor growth *in vivo* were both markedly inhibited by the reexpression of this gene.

p53

The loss of the normal p53 prevents the detection of DNA damage, subverting both apoptosis and cell cycle control (see the preceding section entitled "Cell Cycle") and allowing increased proliferation regardless of the extent of DNA damage. This inability of the cells to sense DNA damage and undergo apoptosis is speculated to underlie the enhanced resistance to chemotherapeutic agents (49) and ionizing radiation seen in tumors that

are deficient in p53 (reviewed in ref. 69). Tumors that possess a wild-type p53 respond well to chemotherapeutic agents such as 5-fluorouracil, etoposide, and adriamycin or ionizing radiation. Thus restoration of the wild-type p53 may provide therapeutic benefit not only in regaining cell cycle control but also in decreasing drug resistance.

Since p53 plays a pivotal role in regulating cell cycle control and apoptosis, the reintroduction of this gene can modulate both of these pathways. Reintroducing the wild-type p53 gene into human glioma cells has been known to suppress neoplastic growth (79,80, 82). Kock et al. (58) utilized an adenovirus to mediate the transfer of the wild-type p53 gene into six human glioblastoma cell lines. The results of this study demonstrated that in the p53-deficient cell lines the reintroduction of the wild-type gene was capable of both inhibiting tumor growth and restoring the normal apoptotic capability. However, it has been demonstrated that tumor cells harboring mutant or null p53 alleles can not only retain a transfected wild-type allele, inducing cell cycle arrest as expected, but also mutate or eliminate the exogenous allele altogether (144), which suggests that the simple reintroduction of the wild-type p53 gene is not a guarantee of tumor growth suppression.

Recently, a novel approach was taken. Rather than reintroduce wild-type p53 into tumor cells to regain apoptotic control, a treatment strategy was devised in which the p53-deficient mutant cells could be targeted specifically. An adenovirus mutant for its E1B protein can replicate in and lyse p53-mutant cells but not wild-type p53 cells. Using *in vitro* and *in vivo* studies, Bischoff et al. (10) demonstrated that the mutant adenovirus killed p53-mutant C33A cells but did not kill p53 wild-type U87 glioblastoma cells. The authors suggest that human tumors could be treated with this same virus, which would be harmless in normal cells and selectively kill p53 mutant cells. These experiments are exciting in their approach to eradicating tumor cells by taking advantage of their mutations.

ICE

Because all pathways that induce apoptosis converge on the caspase cascade (see "Apoptosis"), the ICE (IL-1-converting enzyme) or caspase-3 genes may represent targets that could be manipulated to circumvent the effects of any defective upstream factor such as increased BCL-2 expression. Using the rat glioma model system, Yu et al. (162) employed a tetracycline-inducible system to maintain controlled apoptotic death. The system utilizes a tetracycline-responsive promoter to manipulate the expression of ICE at the transcriptional level. Upon the withdrawal of tetracycline from the system, there is an artificially induced expression of active ICE. In this experiment, expression of the ICE induced the apoptotic response in essentially all the tumor cells. The induction of apoptosis in these gliosarcoma 9L cells that are deficient in wild-type p53 demonstrated that ICE-mediated tumoricidal therapy is possible regardless of the p53 status of the tumor cells (162).

Disappointingly, inhibition of tumor growth with p53- or ICE-expressing vectors (58,162) was not observed on a long-term basis. Tumor growth was observed 7–12 weeks after either infection of the adenovirus or withdrawal of the tetracycline and subsequent expression of active ICE *in vivo*. Tumor growth was speculated to result from cells acquiring the ability to suppress the effects of the introduced gene or from the incomplete expression in the death gene in all cells. The limitations of these systems at their current level of development should not detract from the hope they represent that such approaches may yield useful therapies in the future.

In summary, current gene therapy strategies based on regulating the cell cycle and apoptosis are promising with regard to eventually being able to control cell growth of these tumors. These types of approaches will be useful for the low-grade gliomas. However, gene therapy tactics for the treatment of the higher-grade gliomas will have to include strategies that not only target cell growth but also inhibit tumor cell invasion and angiogen-esis. Strides are being taken with the characterization of the genes involved in these processes as well.

CONCLUSION

Advances in molecular and cellular biology have contributed to a better understanding of cell processes such as brain development, cell cycle control, and apoptosis. The discovery and characterization of oncogenes and tumor suppressor genes have provided insights into the pathogenesis of the glial tumors. The characterization of the glial tumor-specific and cellular process-specific genetic mutations has provided targets for the design of gene-specific therapeutic strategies. Although many questions remain to be answered, these investigations have established the groundwork for rational approaches for the diagnosis, prognosis, and treatment of this devastating disease.

ACKNOWLEDGMENTS

The authors are grateful to Dr. Oliver Bögler for his review of this chapter. Special acknowledgment is made to Devina Khan for the illustrations.

REFERENCES

1. Aggarwal BB, Schwarz L, Hogan ME, Rando RF. Triple helix-forming oligodeoxyribonucleotides targeted to the human tumor necrosis factor (TNF) gene inhibit TNF production and block the TNF-dependent growth of human glioblastoma tumor cells. *Cancer Res* 1996;56:5156–5164.
2. Alderson LM, Castleberg RL, Harsh IV GR, Louis DN, Henson JW. Human gliomas with wild-type p53 express bcl-2. *Cancer Res* 1995;55:999–1001.
3. Arap W, Nishikawa R, Furnari FB, Cavenee WK, Huang H-JS. Replacement of the p16/CDKN2 gene suppresses human glioma cell growth. *Cancer Res* 1995;55:1351–1354.
4. Armstrong RC, Dorn HH, Kufta CV, Friedman E, Dubois-Dalq ME. Pre-oligodendrocytes from adult human CNS. *J Neurosci* 1992;12:1538–1547.
5. Banerjee M, Dinda AK, Sinha S, Sarkar C, Mathur M. c-*myc* oncogene expression and cell proliferation in mixed oligo-astrocytoma. *Int J Cancer* 1996;65:730–733.
6. Bello MJ, Vaquero J, de Campos JM, et al. Molecular analysis of chromosome 1 abnormalities in human

gliomas reveals frequent loss of 1p in oligodendroglial tumors. *Int J Cancer* 1994;57:172–175.

7. Bello MJ, Leone PE, Vaquero J, et al. Allelic loss at 1p and 19q frequently occurs in association and may represent early oncogenic events in oligodendroglial tumors. *Int J Cancer* 1995;64:207–210.

8. Biernat W, Kleihues P, Yonekawa Y, Ohgaki H. Amplification and overexpression of MDM2 in primary (*de novo*) glioblastomas. *J Neuropathol Exp Neurol* 1997; 56:180–185.

9. Bijlsma EK, Voesten AMJ, Bijleveld EH, et al. Molecular analysis of genetic changes in ependymomas. *Gene Chromosome Cancer* 1995;13:272–277.

10. Bischoff JR, Kirn DH, Williams A, et al. An adenovirus mutant that replicates selectively in p53-deficient human tumor cells. *Science* 1996;274:373–376.

11. Black P, Carroll R, Glowacka D. Expression of platelet-derived growth factor transcripts in medulloblastomas and ependymomas. *Pediatr Neurosurg* 1996;24:74–78.

12. Bögler O, Wren D, Barnett SC, Land H, Noble M. Cooperation between two growth factors promotes extended self-renewal and inhibits differentiation of oligodendrocyte-type-2 astrocyte (O-2A) progenitor cells. *Proc Natl Acad Sci* 1990;87:6368–6372.

13. Bögler O, Noble M. Studies relating differentiation to a mechanism that measures time in O-2A progenitor cells. *Ann NY Acad Sci* 1991;633:505–507.

14. Bögler O, Noble M. Measurement of time in oligodendrocyte-type-2astrocyte (O-2A) progenitors is a cellular process distinct from differentiation or division. *Dev Biol* 1994;162:525–538.

15. Cance WG, Brennan MF, Dudas ME, Huang C-M, Cordon-Cardo C. Altered expression of the retinoblastoma gene product in human sarcomas. *N Engl J Med* 1990;323:1457–1462.

16. Cavenee WK, White RL. The genetic basis of cancer. *Sci Am* 1995;272:72–79.

17. Chen J, Willingham T, Shuford M, et al. Effects of ectopic overexpresion of p21[WAF1/CIP1] on aneuploidy and the malignant phenotype of human brain tumor cells. *Oncogene* 1996;13:1395–1403.

18. Chiang YH, Silani V, Zhou FC. Morphological differentiation of astroglial progenitor cells from EGF-responsive neurospheres in response to fetal calf serum, basic fibroblast growth factor, and retinol. *Cell Transplantation* 1996;5:179–189.

19. Costello JF, Berger MS, Huang H-JS, Cavenee WK. Silencing of p16/CDKN2 expression in human gliomas by methylation and chromatin condensation. *Cancer Res* 1996;56:2405–2410.

20. De Vitis LR, Tedde A, Vitelli F, et al. Analysis of the neurofibromatosis type 2 gene in different human tumors of neuroectodermal origin. *Hum Genet* 1996;97: 638–641.

21. Debiec-Rychter M, Alwasiak J, Liberski PP, et al. Accumulation of chromosomal changes in human glioma progression. *Cancer Genet Cytogenet* 1995; 85:61–67.

22. Decaudin D, Geley S, Hirsch T, et al. Bcl-2 and Bcl-X$_L$ antagonize the mitochondrial dysfunction preceding nuclear apoptosis induced by chemotherapeutic agents. *Cancer Res* 1997;57:62–67.

23. Dirks PB, Hubbard SL, Murakami M, Rutka JT. Cyclin and cyclin-dependent kinase expression in human astrocytoma cell lines. *J Neuropathol Exp Neurol* 1997;56:291–300.

24. Eck SL, Alavi JB, Alavi A, et al. Treatment of advanced CNS malignancies with the recombinant adenovirus H5.010RSVTK: a phase I trial. *Human Gene Ther* 1996;7:1465–1482.

25. Ekstrand AJ, James CD, Cavenee WK, Seliger B, Pettersson RF, Collins VP. Genes for epidermal growth factor receptor, transforming growth factor α, and epidermal growth factor and their expression in human gliomas *in vivo*. *Cancer Res* 1991;51:2164–2172.

26. Enari M, Talanian RV, Wong WW, Nagata S. Sequential activation of ICE-like and CPP32-like proteases during Fas-mediated apoptosis. *Nature* 1996;380:723–726.

27. Fink KL, Rushing EJ, Schold SC Jr, Nisen PD. Infrequency of p53 gene mutations in ependymomas. *J Neurooncol* 1996;27:111–115.

28. Fischer U, Meltzer P, Meese E. Twelve amplified and expressed genes localized in a single domain in glioma. *Hum Genet* 1996;98:625–628.

29. Fraser A, Evan G. A license to kill. *Cell* 1996;85: 781–784.

30. Friedmann T. Overcoming the obstacles to gene therapy. *Sci Am* 1997;276:96–101.

31. Fuchs EJ, McKenna KA, Bedi A. p53-dependent DNA damage-induced apoptosis requires Fas/APO-1-independent activation of CPP32. *Cancer Res* 1997;57: 2550–2554.

32. Fujimoto M, Fults DW, Thomas GA, et al. Loss of heterozygosity on chromosome 10 in human glioblastoma multiforme. *Genomics* 1989;4:210–214.

33. Fults D, Pedone C. Deletion mapping of the long arm of chromosome 10 in glioblastoma multiforme. *Genes Chromosome Cancer* 1993;7:173–177.

34. Furnari FB, Huang H-JS, Cavenee WK. Molecular biology of malignant degeneration of astrocytoma. *Pediatr Neurosurg* 1996;24:41–49.

35. Gage FH, Coates PW, Palmer TD, et al. Survival and differentiation of adult neuronal progenitor cells transplanted to the adult brain. *Proc Natl Acad Sci USA* 1995;92:11879–11883.

36. Gajewski TF, Thompson CB. Apoptosis meets signal transduction: elimination of BAD influence. *Cell* 1996;87:589–592.

37. Gonzalez-Zulueta M, Bender CM, Yang AS, et al. Methylation of the 5′ CpG island of the p16/CDKN2 tumor suppressor gene in normal and transformed human tissues correlates with gene silencing. *Cancer Res* 1995;55:4531–4535.

38. Gritti A, Parati EA, Cova L, et al. Multipotential stem cells from the adult mouse brain proliferate and self-renew in response to basic fibroblast growth factor. *J Neurosci* 1996;16:1091–1100.

39. Grove EA, Williams BP, Li D-Q, Hajihosseini M, Friedrich A, Price J. Multiple restricted lineages in the embryonic rat cerebral cortex. *Development* 1993;117: 553–561.

40. Guha A, Dashner K, Black P McL, Wagner JA, Stiles CD. Expression of PDGF and PDGF receptors in human astrocytoma operation specimens supports the existence of an autocrine loop. *Int J Cancer* 1995;60: 168–173.

41. Haupt Y, Maya R, Kazaz A, Oren M. Mdm2 promotes the rapid degradation of p53. *Nature* 1997;387: 296–299.

42. He J, Olson JJ, James CD. Lack of p16^{INK4} or retinoblastoma protein (pRb), or amplification-associated overexpression of CDK4 is observed in distinct subsets of malignant glial tumors and cell lines. *Cancer Res* 1995;55:4833–4836.

43. Henson JW, Schnitker BL, Correa KM, et al. The retinoblastoma gene is involved in malignant progression of astrocytomas. *Ann Neurol* 1994;36:714–721.

44. Herman JG, Merlo A, Mao L, et al. Inactivation of the CDKN2/p16/MTS1 gene is frequently associated with aberrant DNA methylation in all common human cancers. *Cancer Res* 1995;55:4525–4530.

45. Hermanson M, Funa K, Koopmann J, et al. Association of loss of heterozygosity on chromosome 17p with high platelet-derived growth factor α receptor expression in human malignant gliomas. *Cancer Res* 1996;56:164–171.

46. Hunter T, Pines J. Cyclins and cancer II: cyclin D and CDK inhibitors come of age. *Cell* 1994;79:573–582.

47. Ibarrola N, Mayer-Pröschel M, Rodriguez-Peña A, Noble M. Evidence for the existence of at least two timing mechanisms that contribute to oligodendrocyte generation *in vitro*. *Dev Biol* 1996;180:1–21.

48. Ichimura K, Schmidt EE, Goike HM, Collins VP. Human glioblastomas with no alterations of the CDKN2A (p16^{INK4A}, MTS1) and CDK4 genes have frequent mutations of the retinoblastoma gene. *Oncogene* 1996;13:1065–1072.

49. Iwadate Y, Fujimoto S, Tagawa M, et al. Association of p53 gene mutation with decreased chemosensitivity in human malignant gliomas. *Int J Cancer* 1996;69(3):236–240.

50. Izquierdo M, Martín V, de Felipe P, et al. Human malignant brain tumor response to herpes simplex thymidine kinase (HSVtk)/ganciclovir gene therapy. *Gene Ther* 1996;3:491–495.

51. Jen J, Harper JW, Bigner SH, et al. Deletion on p16 and p15 genes in brain tumors. *Cancer Res* 1994;54:6353–6358.

52. Jennings MT, Kaarianinen IT, Gold L, Maciunas RJ, Commers PA. TGF 1 and TGF 2 are potential growth regulators for medulloblastomas, primitive neuroectodermal tumors, and ependymomas: evidence in support of an autocrine hypothesis. *Hum Pathol* 1994;25:464–475.

53. Joos S, Scherthan H, Speicher MR, Schlegel J, Cremer T, Lichter P. Detection of amplified DNA sequences by reverse chromosome painting using genomic tumor DNA as probe. *Hum Genet* 1993;90:584–589.

54. Karlbom AE, James CD, Boethius J, et al. Loss of heterozygosity in malignant gliomas involves at least three distinct regions on chromosome 10. *Hum Genet* 1993;92(2):169–174.

55. Kennedy PG, Kof-Seang J. Studies on the development, antigenic phenotype and function of human glial cells in tissue culture. *Brain* 1986;109:1261–1277.

56. Kim SU. Antigenic expression by glial cells grown in culture. *J Neuroimmunol* 1985;8:255–282.

57. Kirsch M, Zhu J, Cavenee W. Pathogenetic mechanisms of nervous system tumors. In: Black P McL, Loeffler J, eds. *Cancer of the nervous system*. Cambridge, MA: Blackwell Sciences, 1997:703–743.

58. Köck H, Harris MP, Anderson SC, et al. Adenovirus-mediated p53 gene transfer suppresses growth of human glioblastoma cells *in vitro* and *in vivo*. *Int J Cancer* 1996;67:808–815.

59. Kondo S, Barna BP, Kondo Y, et al. WAF1/CIP1 increases the susceptibility of p53 non-functional malignant glioma cells to cisplatin-induced apoptosis. *Oncogene* 1996;13:1279–1285.

60. Kondo S, Morimura T, Barnett GH, et al. The transforming activities of MDM2 in cultured neonatal rat astrocytes. *Oncogene* 1996;13:1773–1779.

61. Kordek R, Biernat W, Alwasiak J, Maculewicz R, Yanagihara R, Liberski PP. p53 protein and epidermal growth factor receptor expression in human astrocytomas. *J Neurooncol* 1995;26:11–16.

62. Kornblith PK, Welch WC, Bradley MK. The future of therapy for glioblastoma. *Surg Neurol* 1993;39:538–543.

63. Kraus JA, Koopmann J, Kaskel P, et al. Shared allelic losses on chromosomes 1p and 19q suggest a common origin of oligodendroglioma and oligoastrocytoma. *J Neuropathol Exp Neurol* 1995;54:91–95.

64. Kubbutat MHG, Jones SN, Vousden KH. Regulation of p53 stability by Mdm2. *Nature* 1997;387:299–303.

65. Lachman LB, Brown DC, Dinarello CA. Growth-promoting effect of recombinant interleukin 1 and tumor necrosis factor for a human astrocytoma cell line. *J Immunol* 1987;138:2913–2916.

66. Lang FF, Miller DC, Koslow M, Newcomb EW. Pathways leading to glioblastoma multiforme: a molecular analysis of genetic alterations in 65 astrocytic tumors. *J Neurosurg* 1994;81:427–436.

67. Lednicky JA, Garcea RL, Bergsagel DJ, Butel JS. Natural simian virus 40 strains are present in human choroid plexus and ependymoma tumors. *Virology* 1995;212:710–717.

68. Lee S-H, Kim J-H, Rhee C-H, et al. Loss of heterozygosity on chromosome 10, 13q(Rb), 17p, and p53 gene mutations in human brain gliomas. *J Korean Med Sci* 1995;10:442–448.

69. Levine AJ. p53, the cellular gatekeeper for growth and division. *Cell* 1997;88:323–331.

70. Li Y-J, Sanson M, Hoang-Xuan K, et al. Incidence of germ-line p53 mutations in patients with gliomas. *Int J Cancer* 1995;64:383–387.

71. Li J, Yen C, Liaw D, et al. PTEN, a putative tyrosine phosphatase gene mutated in human brain, breast, and prostate cancer. *Science* 1997;275:1943–1947.

72. Liaw D, Marsh DJ, Li J, et al. Germline mutations of the PTEN gene in Cowden disease, an inherited breast and thyroid cancer syndrome. *Nature Genet* 1997;16:64–67.

73. Libermann TA, Nusbaum HR, Razon N, et al. Amplification, enhanced expression and possible rearrangement of EGF receptor gene in primary human brain tumours of glial origin. *Nature* 1985;313:144–147.

74. Linskey ME, Gilbert MR. Glial differentiation: a review with implications for new directions in neuro-oncology. *Neurosurgery* 1995;36:1–22.

75. Liu X, Zou H, Slaughter C, Wang X. DFF, a heterodimeric protein that functions downstream of caspase-3 to trigger DNA fragmentation during apoptosis. *Cell* 1997;89:175–184.

76. Maruno M, Yoshimine T, Muhammad AKMG, Tokiyoshi K, Hayakawa T. Loss of heterozygosity of microsatellite loci on chromosome 9p in astrocytic tu-

mors and its prognostic implications. *J Neurooncol* 1996;30:19–24.

77. Maxwell M, Naber SP, Wolfe HJ, et al. Coexpression of platelet-derived growth factor (PDGF) and PDGF-receptor genes by primary human astrocytomas may contribute to their development and maintenance. *J Clin Invest* 1990;86:131–140.

78. Mayer M, Bhakoo K, Noble M. Ciliary neurotrophic factor and leukemia inhibitory factor promote the generation, maturation and survival of oligodendrocytes *in vitro*. *Development* 1994;120:143–153.

79. Mercer WE, Shields MT, Lin D, Appella E, Ullrich SJ. Growth suppression induced by wild-type p53 protein is accompanied by selective down-regulation of proliferating-cell nuclear antigen expression. *Proc Natl Acad Sci USA* 1991;88:1958–1962.

80. Mercer WE, Shields MT, Amin M, et al. Negative growth regulation in a glioblastoma tumor cell line that conditionally expresses human wild-type p53. *Proc Natl Acad Sci USA* 1990;87:6166–6170.

81. Merlo A, Herman JG, Mao L, et al. 5′ CpG island methylation is associated with transcriptional silencing of the tumor suppressor p16/CDKN2/MTS1 in human cancers. *Nature Med* 1995;1:686–692.

82. Merzak A, Raynal S, Rogers JP, Lawrence D, Pilkington GJ. Human wild type p53 inhibits cell proliferation and elicits dramatic morphological changes in human glioma cell lines *in vitro*. *J Neurol Sci* 1994;127:125–133.

83. Minn AJ, Vélez P, Schendel SL, et al. BCL-X$_L$ forms an ion channel in synthetic lipid membranes. *Nature* 1997;385:353–357.

84. Morrison RS, Yamaguchi F, Saya H, et al. Basic fibroblast growth factor and fibroblast growth factor receptor I are implicated in the growth of human astrocytomas. *J Neurooncol* 1994;18:207–216.

85. Nagane M, Coufal F, Lin H, Bögler O, Cavenee WK, Huang H-JS. A common mutant epidermal growth factor receptor confers enhanced tumorigenicity on human glioblastoma cells by increasing proliferation and reducing apoptosis. *Cancer Res* 1996;56:5079–5086.

86. Ng H-K, Lau K-M, Tse JYM, et al. Combined molecular genetic studies of chromosome 22q and the neurofibromatosis type 2 gene in central nervous system tumors. *Neurosurgery* 1995;37:764–773.

87. Nishikawa R, Furnari FB, Lin H, et al. Loss of P16[INK4] expression is frequent in high grade gliomas. *Cancer Res* 1995;55:1941–1945.

88. Noble M. The O-2A lineage: from rats to humans. *Recent Results Cancer Res* 1994;135:67–75.

89. Noble M, Gutowski N, Bevan K, et al. From rodent glial precursor cell to human glial neoplasia in the oligodendrocyte-type-2 astrocyte lineage. *Glia* 1995; 15(3):222–230.

90. Noble M. Steps toward a cellular biological analysis of human gliomas. In: Raffel C, Harsh G IV, eds. *The molecular basis of neurosurgical disease: concepts in neurosurgery*. Baltimore: Williams & Wilkins, 1996;8:87–97.

91. Noguchi K, Naito M, Kugoh H, et al. Chromosome 22 complements apoptosis in Fas- and TNF-resistant mutant UK110 cells. *Oncogene* 1996;13:39–46.

92. Nowell PC. The clonal evolution of tumor cell population. *Science* 1976;194:23–28.

93. Ono Y, Tamiya T, Ichikawa T, et al. Malignant astrocytomas with homozygous CDKN2/p16 gene deletions have higher Ki-67 proliferation indices. *J Neuropathol Exp Neurol* 1996;55:1026–1031.

94. Park JP, Chaffee S, Noll WW, Rhodes CH. Constitutional *de novo* t(1;22)(p22;q11.2) and ependymoma. *Cancer Genet Cytogenet* 1996;86:150–152.

95. Price J, Williams BP, Götz M. The generation of cellular diversity in the cerebral cortex. In: *Development of the cerebral cortex* (Ciba Foundation Symposium 193). New York: Wiley, 1995;71–84.

96. Raff MC. Glial cell diversification in the rat optic nerve. *Science* 1989;243:1450–1455.

97. Ransom DT, Ritland SR, Kimmel DW, et al. Cytogenetic and loss of heterozygosity studies in ependymomas, pilocytic astrocytomas, and oligodendrogliomas. *Genes Chromosome Cancer* 1992;5:348–356.

98. Rasheed BKA, Fuller GN, Friedman AH, Bigner DD, Bigner SH. Loss of heterozygosity for 10q loci in human gliomas. *Genes Chromosome Cancer* 1992;5:75–82.

99. Reifenberger G, Liu L, Ichimura K, Schmidt EE, Collins VP. Amplification and overexpression of the MDM2 gene in a subset of human malignant gliomas without p53 mutations. *Cancer Res* 1993;53:2736–2739.

100. Reifenberger J, Reifenberger G, Liu L, James CD, Wechsler W, Collins VP. Molecular genetic analysis of oligodendroglial tumors shows preferential allelic deletions on 19q and 1p. *Am J Pathol* 1994;145:1175–1190.

101. Reifenberger J, Reifenberger G, Ichimura K, Schmidt EE, Wechsler W, Collins VP. Epidermal growth factor receptor expression in oligodendroglial tumors. *Am J Pathol* 1996;149:29–35.

102. Reifenberger G, Ichimura K, Reifenberger J, Elkahloun AG, Meltzer PS, Collins VP. Refined mapping of 12q13-q15 amplicons in human malignant gliomas suggests CDK4/SAS and MDM2 as independent amplification targets. *Cancer Res* 1996;56:5141–5145.

103. Reifenberger J, Ring GU, Gies U, et al. Analysis of p53 mutation and epidermal growth factor receptor amplification in recurrent gliomas with malignant progression. *J Neuropathol Exp Neurol* 1996;55:822–831.

104. Reynolds BA, Weiss S. Clonal and population analyses demonstrate that an EGF-responsive mammalian embryonic CNS precursor is a stem cell. *Dev Biol* 1996;175:1–13.

105. Ritland SR, Ganju V, Jenkins RB. Region-specific loss of heterozygosity on chromosome 19 is related to the morphologic type of human glioma. *Genes Chromosome Cancer* 1995;12:277–282.

106. Robertson NM, Zangrilli J, Fernandes-Alnemri T, Friesen PD, Litwack G, Alnemri ES. Baculovirus p35 inhibits the glucocorticoid-mediated pathway of cell death. *Cancer Res* 1997;57:43–47.

107. Rogulski KR, Kim JH, Kim SH, Freytag SO. Glioma cells transduced with an *Escherichia coli* CD/HSV-1 TK fusion gene exhibit enhanced metabolic suicide and radiosensitivity. *Hum Gene Ther* 1997;8:73–85.

108. Rubio M-P, Correa KM, Ramesh V, et al. Analysis of the neurofibromatosis 2 gene in human ependymomas and astrocytomas. *Cancer Res* 1994;54:45–47.

109. Rudel T, Bokoch GM. Membrane and morphological changes in apoptotic cells regulated by caspase-mediated activation of PAK2. *Science* 1997;276: 1571–1574.

110. Saas P, Walker PR, Hahne M, et al. Fas ligand expression by astrocytoma *in vivo*: maintaining immune privilege in the brain? *J Clin Invest* 1997;99:1173–1178.

111. Sabbatini P, Han J, Chiou S-K, Nicholson DW, White E. Interleukin 1 converting enzyme-like proteases are essential for p53-mediated transcriptionally dependent apoptosis. *Cell Growth Differentiation* 1997;8: 643–653.

112. Sato K, Schauble B, Kleihues P, Ohgaki H. Infrequent alterations of the p15, p16, CDK4 and cyclin D1 genes in non-astrocytic human brain tumors. *Int J Cancer* 1996;66:305–308.

114. Sawyer JR, Sammartino G, Husain M, Boop FA, Chadduck WM. Chromosome aberrations in four ependymomas. *Cancer Genet Cytogenet* 1994;74: 132–138.

115. Sawyer JR, Thomas JR, Teo C. Low-grade astrocytoma with a complex four-breakpoint inversion of chromosome 8 as the sole cytogenetic aberration. *Cancer Genet Cytogenet* 1995;83:168–171.

116. Schendel SL, Xie Z, Montal MO, Matsuyama S, Montal M, Reed JC. Channel formation by anti-apoptotic protein BCL-2. *Proc Natl Acad Sci USA* 1997;94: 5113–5118.

117. Schiffer D, Cavalla P, Migheli A, Giordana MT, Chiado-Piat L. Bcl-2 distribution in neuroepithelial tumors: an immunohistochemical study. *J Neurooncol* 1996;27:101–109.

118. Schinstine M, Iacovitti L. Expression of neuronal antigens by astrocytes derived from EGF-generated neuroprogenitor cells. *Exp Neurol* 1996;141:67–78.

119. Schlegel J, Merdes A, Stumm G, et al. Amplification of the epidermal-growth-factor-receptor gene correlates with different growth behaviour in human glioblastoma. *Int J Cancer* 1994;56:72–77.

120. Schmidt EE, Ichimura K, Reifenberger G, Collins VP. CDKN2 (p16/MTS1) gene deletion or CDK4 amplification occurs in the majority of glioblastomas. *Cancer Res* 1994;54:6321–6324.

121. Schmidt EE, Ichimura K, Messerle KR, Goike HM, Collins VP. Infrequent methylation of CDKN2A (MTS1/p16) and rare mutation of both CDKN2A and CDKN2B(MTS2/p15) in primary astrocytic tumours. *Br J Cancer* 1997;75:2–8.

122. Schröck E, Thiel G, Lozanova T, et al. Comparative genomic hybridization of human malignant gliomas reveals multiple amplification sites and nonrandom chromosomal gains and losses. *Am J Pathol* 1994;144: 1203–1218.

123. Segal DH, Germano IM, Bederson JB. Effects of basic fibroblast growth factor on *in vivo* cerebral tumorigenesis in rats. *Neurosurgery* 1997;40:1027–1033.

124. Serrano M, Hannon GJ, Beach D. A new regulatory motif in cell-cycle control causing specific inhibition of cyclin D/CDK4. *Nature* 1993;366:704–707.

125. Shaw EG, Scheithauer BW, Dinapoli RP. Low grade hemispheric astrocytomas. In: Black P, Loeffler J, eds. *Cancer of the nervous system.* Cambridge, MA: Blackwell Sciences, Inc, 1997:441–463.

126. Sherr CJ. Cancer cell cycles. *Science* 1996;274: 1672–1677.

127. Shimizu S, Eguchi Y, Kamiike W, et al. Bcl-2 blocks loss of mitochondrial membrane potential while ICE inhibitors act at a different step during inhibition of death induced by respiratory chain inhibitors. *Oncogene* 1996;13:21–29.

128. Slavc I, MacCollin MM, Dunn M, et al. Exon scanning for mutations of the NF2 gene in pediatric ependymomas, rhabdoid tumors and meningiomas. *Int J Cancer* 1995;64:243–247.

129. Sobol RE, Fakhrai H, Shawler D, et al. Interleukin-2 gene therapy in a patient with glioblastoma. *Gene Ther* 1995;2:164–167.

130. Steck PA, Pershouse MA, Jasser SA, et al. Identification of a candidate tumour suppressor gene, MMAC1, at chromosome 10q23.3 that is mutated in multiple advanced cancers. *Nature Genet* 1997;15:356–362.

131. Steilen-Gimbel H, Henn W, Kolles H, et al. Early proliferation enhancement by monosomy 10 and intratumor heterogeneity in malignant human gliomas as revealed by smear preparations from biopsies. *Genes Chromosome Cancer??* 1996;16:180–184.

132. Stuart ET, Gruss P. PAX: developmental control genes in cell growth and differentiation. *Cell Growth Differentiation??* 1996;7:405–412.

133. Stuart ET, Haffner R, Oren M, Gruss P. Loss of p53 function through PAX-mediated transcriptional repression. *EMBO J* 1995;14:5638–5645.

134. Stuart ET, Kioussi C, Aguzzi A, Gruss P. PAX5 expression correlates with increasing malignancy in human astrocytomas. *Clin Cancer Res* 1995;1:207–214.

135. Tachibana O, Nakazawa H, Lampe J, Watanabe K, Kleihues P, Ohgaki H. Expression of Fas/APO-1 during the progression of astrocytomas. *Cancer Res* 1995;55:5528–5530.

136. Tachibana O, Lampe J, Kleihues P, Ohgaki H. Preferential expression of Fas/APO1 (CD95) and apoptotic cell death in perinecrotic cells of glioblastoma multiforme. *Acta Neuropathol* 1996;92:431–434.

137. Takahashi JA, Fukumoto M, Igarashi K, Oda Y, Kikuchi H, Hatanaka M. Correlation of basic fibroblast growth factor expression levels with the degree of malignancy and vascularity in human gliomas. *J Neurosurg* 1992;76:792–798.

138. Thompson CB. Apoptosis in the pathogenesis and treatment of disease. *Science* 1995;267:1456–1462.

139. Trudel M, Mulligan L, Cavenee W, Margolese R, Côté J, Gariépy G. Retinoblastoma and p53 gene product expression in breast carcinoma: immunohistochemical analysis and clinicopathologic correlation. *Hum Pathol* 1992;23:1388–1394.

140. Tsuzuki T, Tsunoda S, Sakaki T, Konishi N, Hiasa Y, Nakamura M. Alterations of retinoblastoma, p53, p16(CDKN2), and p15 genes in human astrocytomas. *Cancer* 1996;78:287–293.

141. Turner DL, Cepko CL. A common progenitor for neurons and glia persist in rat retina late in development. *Nature* 1987;328:131–136.

142. Ueba T, Takahashi JA, Fukumoto M, et al. Expression of fibroblast growth factor receptor-1 in human glioma and meningioma tissues. *Neurosurgery* 1994;34: 221–226.

143. Ueki K, Ono Y, Henson JW, Efird JT, von Deimling A, Louis DN. CDKN2/p16 or RB alterations occur in the majority of glioblastomas and are inversely correlated. *Cancer Res* 1996;56:150–153.

144. Van Meir EG, Roemer K, Diserens A-C, et al. Single cell growth arrest and morphological changes induced by transfer of wild-type p53 alleles to glioblastoma cells. *Proc Natl Acad Sci USA* 1995;92:1008–1012.

145. Verma IM, Somia N. Gene therapy-promises, problems and prospects. *Nature* 1997;389:239–242.

146. Von Deimling A, Louis DN, von Ammon K, et al. Association of epidermal growth factor receptor gene amplification with loss of chromosome 10 in human glioblastoma multiforme. *J Neurosurg* 1992;77:295–301.

147. Von Deimling A, Louis DN, von Ammon K, Petersen I, Wiestler OD, Seizinger BR. Evidence for a tumor suppressor gene on chromosome 19q associated with human astrocytomas, oligodendrogliomas, and mixed gliomas. *Cancer Res* 1992;52:4277–4279.

148. Von Deimling A, Nagel J, Bender B, et al. Deletion mapping of chromosome 19 in human gliomas. *Int J Cancer* 1994;57:676–680.

149. Von Deimling A, Louis DN, Wiestler OD. Molecular pathways in the formation of gliomas. *Glia* 1995;15: 328–338.

150. Walker DG, Duan W, Popovic EA, Kaye AH, Tomlinson FH, Lavin M. Homozygous deletions of the multiple tumor suppressor gene 1 in the progression of human astrocytomas. *Cancer Res* 1995;55:20–23.

151. Watanabe K, Nagai M, Wakai S, Arai T, Kawashima K. Loss of constitutional heterozygosity in chromosome 10 in human glioblastoma. *Acta Neuropathol* 1990;80: 251–254.

152. Watkins D, Ruttledge MH, Sarrazin J, et al. Loss of heterozygosity on chromosome 22 in human gliomas does not inactivate the neurofibromatosis type 2 gene. *Cancer Genet Cytogenet* 1996;92:73–78.

153. Weber RG, Sabel M, Reifenberger J, et al. Characterization of genomic alterations associated with glioma progression by comparative genomic hybridization. *Oncogene* 1996;13:983–994.

154. Wernicke C, Thiel G, Lozanova T, et al. Involvement of chromosome 22 in ependymomas. *Cancer Genet Cytogenet* 1995;79:173–176.

155. Westermark B, Heldin C-H, Nistér M. Platelet-derived growth factor in human glioma. *Glia* 1995;15: 257–263.

156. Westphal M, Hänsel M, Hamel W, Kunzmann R, Hölzel F. Karyotype analyses of 20 human glioma cell lines. *Acta Neurochir* 1994;126:17–26.

157. Xu H-J, Hu S-X, Cagle PT, Moore GE, Benedict WF. Absence of retinoblastoma protein expression in primary non-small cell lung carcinomas. *Cancer Res* 1991;51:2735–2739.

158. Yamada K, Kasama M, Kondo T, Shinoura N, Yoshioka M. Chromosome studies in 70 brain tumors with special attention to sex chromosome loss and single autosomal trisomy. *Cancer Genet Cytogenet* 1994;73: 46–52.

159. Yamaguchi F, Saya H, Bruner JM, Morrison RS. Differential expression of two fibroblast growth factor-receptor genes is associated with malignant progression in human astrocytomas. *Proc Natl Acad Sci USA* 1994; 91:484–488.

160. Ye Z, Wu JK, Darras BT. Loss of heterozygosity for alleles on chromosome 10 in human brain tumours. *Neurol Res* 1993;15:59–62.

161. Yong WH, Chou D, Ueki K, et al. Chromosome 19q deletions in human gliomas overlap telomeric to D19S219 and may target a 425 kb region centromeric to D19S112. *J Neuropathol Exp Neurol* 1995;54: 622–626.

162. Yu JS, Sena-Esteves M, Paulus W, Breakefield XO, Reeves SA. Retroviral delivery and tetracycline-dependent expression of IL-1-converting enzyme (ICE) in a rat glioma model provides controlled induction of apoptotic death in tumor cells. *Cancer Res* 1996;56: 5423–5427

The Practical Management of Low-Grade Primary Brain
Tumors, edited by Jack P. Rock, Mark L. Rosenblum,
Edward G. Shaw, and J. Gregory Cairncross.
Lippincott Williams & Wilkins, Philadelphia, © 1999

14

Low-Grade Glioma:
Guidelines and Outcomes Analysis

Jack P. Rock, Beverly C. Walters, and Edward G. Shaw

J. P. Rock: Department of Neurosurgery, Henry Ford Hospital, Detroit, Michigan 48202
B. C. Walters: Department of Clinical Neurosciences, Brown University School of Medicine,
Providence, Rhode Island 02912
E. G. Shaw: Department of Radiation Oncology, Wake Forest University School of Medicine,
Winston-Salem, North Carolina 27157

PRACTICE PARAMETERS OR GUIDELINES

Practice parameters (or guidelines) are patient management strategies that are developed to enable physicians to base treatment upon some recommended criteria. They may be used in varying ways, depending upon the perspective of the user. Physicians may use a guideline to help direct patient diagnosis and management (their usual intent), whereas corporations and insurance companies may use a guideline as a benchmark for reimbursement schemes. Two major approaches have been utilized to establish guidelines that include consensus and evidence-based methods. The simplest method involves the consensus-derived approach in which experienced clinicians record their estimate of the most effective steps with which to take a patient's presenting symptoms and signs or other pertinent information and arrive at a diagnosis and proposed management strategy. Because this method is based on clinical experience, it is limited by the clinical biases of the involved clinicians. Therefore, despite these clinicians' experience and conscientious intent, the recommendations from these guidelines may remain controversial. Currently, the least con-

troversial approach for developing guidelines is one that is evidence-based; that is, the team of clinicians relies on information from studies in the literature that not only are well-designed but are also carried out and interpreted with the utmost attention to scientific objectivity. Unfortunately, relatively few studies of the highest quality are found in the literature. This results from difficulties encountered in attempting to carry out appropriate studies using true human experimentation, including the common limitations related to adequate patient numbers, follow-up, and disease dissimilarities. Established methodology allows the team to quantitatively evaluate the quality of the literature (i.e., evidence) and generate guidelines for which the certainty is related to evidence quality.

The process used in developing the guidelines described herein began under the auspices of the American Association of Neurological Surgeons and the Congress of Neurological Surgeons Guidelines and Outcomes Committee as a response to the widely variable recommendations for treatment of low-grade brain tumors. The group assembled to work on these recommendations involved representatives from several disciplines, including neurosurgery, neurology, and radiation oncology, and included some of the most widely quoted authors on the treatment of brain tumors (2). Since low-grade brain tumors represent a diverse group of pathologic entities, the group decided to focus on low-grade gliomas (astrocytoma, oligodendroglioma, and mixed oligoastrocytoma) because these were the most frequently encountered histologic subtypes and represent a relatively common problem that most involved clinicians would have to manage.

As a starting point for an evidence-based approach to the development of guidelines, the team developed a consensus-derived decision tree reflecting management possibilities in the treatment of these tumors (Fig. 1). Answers for the questions derived from branch points in the decision tree were searched for in the literature through Medline and scientific citation routes. The key words used were *adult, supratentorial, low-grade glioma, astrocytoma, oligodendroglioma, computed tomography, magnetic resonance imaging, surgery, radiation therapy,* and *chemotherapy.* The resulting literature was selected for English-language, peer-reviewed publications after 1975, direct or indirect attention to natural history, survival, tumor recurrence, and quality of life in patients managed with observation,

biopsy, resection, or radiation therapy. Sixty citations were selected, and consideration of the quality of the evidence was based on the following criteria (3):

Class I—evidence provided by one or more well-designed randomized, controlled clinical trials, reflecting a high degree of clinical certainty, and from which treatment *standards* could be derived.

Class II—evidence provided by one or more well-designed nonrandomized comparative studies such as case control and cohort studies, reflecting a moderate degree of clinical certainty and from which treatment *guidelines* could be derived.

Class III—evidence provided by expert opinion, nonrandomized historical controls, or case reports, reflecting unclear clinical certainty and from which treatment *options* could be derived.

Fifteen key citations were chosen to support the text of the results section, 14 of which were designated as class III evidence and one of which was class II evidence.

Based on the preceding criteria, recommendations for the management of patients with low-grade gliomas were divided into either standards, guidelines, or options. Realiz-

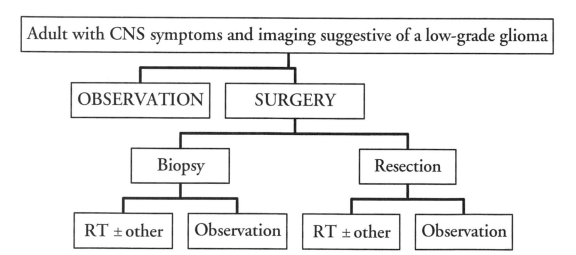

FIG. 1. Consensus-derived algorithm for adults with a supratentorial lesion suggestive of a low-grade glioma.

ing that conclusions generated from most of the relevant English literature reflect inherent clinical biases, the following summarizes the evidence table found in that document and represents the current state of knowledge relating to the four key questions regarding the management of adult patients with an imaging diagnosis suggestive of a supratentorial nonoptic pathway low-grade glioma:

1. *Is biopsy (i.e., tissue diagnosis) required in all patients?* In two series, 35% of patients with an imaging diagnosis of low-grade glioma had histopathology other than low-grade glioma. Therefore because imaging studies cannot predict histology with complete accuracy, the gold standard for histologic verification is tissue diagnosis obtained through biopsy. The quality of the evidence was class III.

   The first approach supported in the literature is to obtain histologic verification of the lesion by biopsy and/or resection if, based on physician and/or patient preference, treatment—usually radiation therapy—is to be administered. Because the patient is to have a therapy with potentially adverse side-effects and because the patient may have another diagnosis for which radiation is not recommended (e.g., infection), it is mandatory that the pathologic entity be verified histologically with biopsy-obtained tissue. This recommendation is considered a *standard*. The literature, however, also supports as a treatment *option* a second recommendation based on an imaging diagnosis of low-grade glioma—one may observe the patient with scheduled follow-up magnetic resonance imaging assessments and without intervention (i.e., biopsy) until the patient's symptoms and/or signs or the imaging characteristics of the lesion change. Following the latter approach, the physician and patient must remain aware that the diagnosis is uncertain and that the patient may have an alternative diagnosis.

2. *Can patients be observed without treatment?* In two case series (class III evidence), patients observed following tissue diagnosis had survival rates comparable to those of patients from other series receiving early radiation therapy. Therefore, as the literature is considered insufficient to determine a standard or guideline regarding whether or not to recommend observation following biopsy, the recommendation remains an *option*. Thus patients may be observed without treatment after biopsy as long as careful and frequent follow-up is assured.

3. *What is the role of surgical resection?* This question pertains to non-life-threatening mass lesions. Seven case series reported improved survival for patients undergoing resection. In four the survival differences were significant, and survival was proportional to the extent of resection. Again, the quality of evidence is class III and therefore the literature is considered insufficient to establish a standard or guideline regarding whether or not to recommend surgical resection. Therefore, based on the available literature, it remains an *option* to recommend resection.

4. *What is the role of radiation therapy?* Two of six case series reported significantly longer survival for patients undergoing radiation therapy. In three of the other four series reported, the survival was not significantly improved when compared with survival of nonirradiated patients. All the literature regarding this issue is class III evidence and is considered insufficient to establish either a standard or a guideline. The *option* remains to follow the patient with or without radiation therapy.

The conclusions of this guidelines effort will not be surprising to most clinicians involved in the management of these patients, but the effort makes clear the relative lack of definitive information available in the literature and sets the foundation and tone for future clinical research.

TREATMENT OUTCOMES

Measuring treatment success in terms of specific outcomes is integral to clinical research and practice. Modern outcome studies have originated from the desire to gauge the overall effectiveness of medical treatments, to provide improved treatments to physicians for patients, and to develop improved guidelines for practice. Such studies in the past have presented specifically clinical outcomes, but current concepts of outcome studies are concerned not only with physician-oriented assessments (e.g., numerical survival), but also with outcomes relating to patient functional status, patient health-related quality of life, patient satisfaction, as well as economic analyses (e.g., cost-effectiveness for patients, employers, and third-party payers, including government). Therefore, there has been a shift from the perspective of the clinician and the clinical recommendation to the patient and the patient's perspective. In addition, with the escalating cost of high-technology care, efforts to determine cost/benefit have become equally important. Cost containment has been promoted by the increase in managed and capitated health care organizations as well as governmental concerns over hospital certification based on reliable-outcomes information. In the best scenario, these diverse interests coincide; in the worst, they conflict, and choices must sometimes be made in which one or more of the vested parties must be disappointed.

Notwithstanding ongoing studies, which have yet to be reported in the literature, currently no outcomes studies are organized for the evaluation of patients with low-grade brain tumors.

Recently under way is the GO (Glioma Outcomes) project cosponsored by the American Association of Neurological Surgeons and Rhone Poulenc Rorer, a pharmaceutical company (1). This effort requires written responses to questionnaires from neurosurgeons in academic or private group and individual practices, as well as from patients and families regarding the management of these same patients with malignant glioma. The objectives of the project are to improve quality of care for patients with glioma, describe diagnostic and treatment strategies and patient outcomes, provide physicians with data to evaluate and improve their practices, publish objective data on temporal trends and regional differences in the care of patients with glioma, and develop hypotheses for future clinical trials.

The first step toward accomplishing these objectives is to establish a national cooperative database. The feasibility of this type of project will be assessed, and it is hoped that analysis of the data will provide important insights necessary for paving the way for future outcome studies. It is intended that projects of this nature will be developed for the management of patients with low-grade brain tumors.

REFERENCES

1. Anderson FA Jr. The Glioma Outcomes Project: a resource for measuring and improving glioma outcomes. *Neurosurg Focus* 1998;4(6).
2. Low Grade Glioma Guidelines Team. Practice parameters in adults with suspected or known supratentorial non-optic pathway low-grade glioma. *Neurosurg Focus* 1998;4(6).
3. Rosenberg J, Greenberg MK. Practice parameters: strategies for survival into the nineties. *Neurology* 1992; 42:1110–1115.

Subject Index

Entries followed by a t indicate a table;
entries followed by an f indicate a figure.

A

Age
distribution of ependymomas related to, 48
as outcome predictor
in diffuse astrocytomas, 35
in low-grade gliomas, 135, 137–138, 142
in oligodendrogliomas, 46
and survival after radiation therapy, 84
tendency toward malignant evolution of gliomas in, 140
Aicardi syndrome
brain tumors associated with, 172t
X-linked inheritance in, 176
Angiogenesis inhibitors, 100
Angiostatin, 100
Antibiotic therapy, perioperative, for cerebellar astrocytoma, 106, 108
Antiepileptics, 159t, 159–161
Apoptosis, 217–221
Fas ligand and TNF-induced pathway in, 217, 220f–221f
in gene therapy strategy, 222–224
genetic alterations in, 219, 221
in Fas ligand-mediated pathway, 219, 221
in p53-mediated pathway, 221
induction of, 217
caspase cascade in, 217
genetic alterations in, 218f–219f
p53-mediated pathway in, 217, 219
Armed Forces Institute of Pathology Ringertz classification system, 34
Arteriovenous malformations, risk of seizure with, 151
Astroblastoma
incidence and clinical presentation of, 111
management of, 111–112
Astrocytomas, 34–43
anaplastic
gemistocytic astrocytomas vs., 37
genetic mutations in, 206
seizure risk in, 151
brain stem gliomas, 43
CCNU chemotherapy of, 99
cerebellar
classification and pathobiology of, 42
management of, in children, 103–109
circumscribed
classification and pathobiology of, 37–42
desmoplastic cerebral, of infancy, 41–42
pilocytic, 39–41
pleomorphic xanthoastrocytoma, 37–38
subependymal giant cell, 38–39
classification and pathobiology of, 34–43
classification systems in, 34, 136, 137
histologic grade in, 35–36, 137, 137t

diffuse, 34–37
cellular proliferation of, 35–36
classification and pathobiology of, 34–37
grading systems for, 34, 35
microscopy of, 34–35
molecular genetics of, 36
pilocytic astrocytomas vs., 42
survival in, 36
types of, 35
ultrastructure of, 35
fibrillary
pathology of, 35
prognosis in, 136
seizures in, case study of, 187–189, 188f
gemistocytic, 35, 37, 137, 138
genetic mutations in progression of, 204–209
pathway I, 204–207, 205f
pathway II, 207–208, 207f
pathway III, 208–209, 209f
imaging studies of, 5–13, 6f–13f
optic pathway gliomas, 7f, 43
pilocytic. See Pilocytic astrocytomas
pleomorphic. See Pleomorphic xanthoastrocytomas
protoplasmic, 35, 36–37
radiation therapy, of low grade, 82–83
radiation necrosis of, recurrent neoplasm vs., 8
regional, 42–43
seizure risk in, 151
spinal cord, 42–43
subependymal giant cell, 18, 38–39, 92, 122
supratentorial, 7, 9f, 42, 138
Ataxia telangiectasia syndrome
autosomal recessive inheritance in, 173–174
brain tumors associated with, 172t
Autonomy principal, in genetic counseling, 177
Autosomal dominant inheritance, 174f, 175–176
Autosomal recessive inheritance, 173–174, 174f

B

Bad gene, in apoptosis, 219
Basic fibroblast growth factor. See Fibroblast growth factor (bFGF)
Bax gene, in apoptosis, 219
Bcl-2 and Bcl-X$_L$ genes, in apoptosis, 219, 221
Beneficence principal, in genetic counseling, 177
Biopsy
practice parameters for, 233
proposed classification scheme based on, 73
stereotactic, 33–34, 71–72, 143, 145, 145f
Brachytherapy
for epilepsy, 164
for supratentorial low-grade gliomas, 92
Brain
Broca and Wernicke areas in, presurgical localization of, 75

Brain (*contd.*)
    eloquent areas/speech centers of, presurgical
        localization of, 74–76, 75f
    motor strip in, presurgical localization of, 74–75, 75f
Brain development, 193–198
    adult brain, multipotent cells in, 197–198, 198f
        evidence for, 198
    fetal, multipotent precursor cells of, 196–197
    multipotent stem cells in, 193, 194f–195f, 196
    of normal brain cells and tumor cells, 194f
Brain edema
    reduction of, by surgical debulking, 144
    surgical morbidity related to, 74
Brain stem gliomas, 43
Broca's area, presurgical localization of, 75
Bromodeoxyuridine (BUdR) labeling index, 140

C

Carbamazepine (Tegretol), 160
Carboxyamido-triazole (CAI), antitumor activity of, 100
Carriers, in autosomal recessive inheritance, 173
Caspase cascade, in apoptosis induction, 217, 219
Caspase-3 (CPP32/Yama/Apopain)
    in apoptosis induction
        in Fas ligand/TNF-induced pathway, 217
        in p53-induced pathway, 217, 219
    in gene therapy, 224
Cavernous angiomas, risk of seizure with, 151
CCNU chemotherapy, 99
CDK4 gene, cell cycle effects of, 215
CDKN2A (MTS1) gene, in progression of
        anaplastic astrocytomas, 206
Cell cycle control, 213–217. See also Apoptosis
    in gene therapy strategy, 222–224
    genetic alterations in, 213–217
        CDK4, 215
        MDM2, 216
        p16, 214–215
        p16-CDK4/cyclinD-Rb1 axis, 214–215
        p21, 216
        p21-p53-MDM2/PAX5 axis, 215–217
        p53, 215
        PAX5, 216–217
        RB gene, 213–214
    phases of cell cycle, 213
Cell proliferation, activating and inactivating gene
        mutations in, 201–202, 202f–203f
Central neurocytomas
    characteristics of, 117–118
    classification and pathobiology of, 55–57
    clinical presentation of, 118
    differential diagnosis of, 26
    imaging studies of, 24–26, 25f–26f, 118
    immunohistochemistry of, 55–56
    incidence of, 55, 118
    management of, 118
    microscopic features of, 55
    nature and origin of, 56–57
    prognosis in, 56
    radiation therapy of, 92, 118
    recurrence of
        follow-up imaging for, 26
        management of, 118
Cerebellar astrocytomas
    in children, 103–109

clinical presentation of, 103–104
    histopathology of, 105
    long-term outcome of, 108
    radiological and preoperative studies of,
        104–105, 104f–105f
    recurrence rate in, 108
    surgical management of, 105–108, 107f
    classification and pathobiology of, 42
Cerebellar dysplastic gangliocytomas
    association with Cowden's disease, 54
    classification and pathobiology of, 54–55
    imaging studies of, 22–23, 23f
Cerebrospinal fluid
    dissemination of ependymomas via, 50, 123
    risk of uncontrolled drainage, through
        ventricular peritoneal shunt, 106
Chemotherapy
    combined with radiation therapy, for
        oligodendrogliomas, 99–100
    cytostatic agents in, 100
    of ependymomas, 124
    of ganglioglioma, 117
    of glial neoplasms, 99–101
    of pilocytic astrocytomas, 120
Children
    cerebellar astrocytomas of
        classification and pathobiology of, 42
        management of, 103–109
    desmoplastic cerebral astrocytoma of infancy in, 41–42
    desmoplastic infantile ganglioglioma of, 59
    dysembryoplastic neuroepithelial tumors of, 60
    ependymomas of, 48, 50, 123
    gangliogliomas of, 57
    Lhermitte-Duclos disease of, 115
    pilocytic astrocytomas of, 39
Choroid plexus papillomas, 112–113
    autosomal recessive inheritance in, 173
    brain tumors associated with, 172t
    imaging studies of, 18–19, 19f, 112
    incidence and clinical presentation of, 112
    management of, 113
Chromic phosphate (^{32}P), in radiation therapy, 92
Chromosome abnormalities. See also Loss of
        heterozygosity; Molecular genetics
    of central neurocytomas, 56
    in diffuse astrocytomas, 36
    of ependymomas, 51
    in malignant progression
        of anaplastic astrocytomas, 206
        of astrocytomas, 204–205, 208, 209f
        of ependymomas, 212, 212f
        of oligoastrocytomas, 211, 211f
        of oligodendrogliomas, 209–210, 210f
    of myxopapillary ependymoma, 51
    in oligodendrogliomas, 47
    of pilocytic astrocytomas, 41
    in tuberous sclerosis, 175
Ciliary neurotrophic factor (CNTF), in brain
        development, 195f, 196
Circumscribed astrocytomas
    classification and pathobiology of, 37–42
    desmoplastic cerebral, of infancy, 41–42
    pilocytic, 39–41
    pleomorphic xanthoastrocytoma, 37–38
    subependymal giant cell, 38–39

Classification and pathobiology, 33 61
  advances in, 33–34
  astrocytomas, 34–43
    brain stem gliomas, 43
    cerebellar, 42
    circumscribed, 37–42
    desmoplastic cerebral, of infancy, 41–42
    diffuse, 34–37
    gemistocytic, 37, 137
    optic pathway gliomas, 43
    pilocytic, 39–41
    pleomorphic xanthoastrocytoma, 37–38
    protoplasmic, 36–37
    regional, 42–43
    spinal cord, 42–43
    subependymal giant cell, 38–39
    supratentorial, 42
  central neurocytomas, 55–57
  cerebellar dysplastic gangliocytomas, 54–55
  desmoplastic infantile gangliogliomas, 59
  dysembryoplastic neuroepithelial tumor (DNET),
    59–60
  ependymomas, 48–52
    myxopapillary, 51
    subependymomas, 51–52
  gangliocytomas, 53–54
  gangliogliomas, 57–59
  glial neoplasms, 34–53
  Kernohan classification, 5
  mixed gliomas, 52–53
  mixed neuronal and glial tumors, 57 60
  morphology-based, 33
  neuronal cell tumors, 53–57
  oligodendrogliomas, 43–48
  operative classification system, based on biopsy
    materials, 73
  St. Anne-Mayo Clinic grading system, 34, 137, 140
  stereotactic biopsy in, 33–34
  World Health Organization classification, 5, 34,
    136–137, 140
Clonal evolution of tumors, 199, 200f–201f
Cognitive effects, of radiation therapy, 92, 93
Computed tomography (CT). See also Imaging studies
  of astroblastomas, 111
  of astrocytomas, 5, 6f, 7, 8
  of central neurocytomas, 24, 118
  of cerebellar astrocytomas, 104–105
  of cerebellar dysplastic gangliocytomas, 22, 23f
  of choroid plexus papillomas, 19, 19f, 112
  of desmoplastic infantile gangliogliomas, 24
  of dysembryoplastic neuroepithelial tumors, 20, 114
  of gangliocytomas, 22, 114
  of gangliogliomas, 21, 116
  of Lhermitte-Duclos disease, 115
  of oligodendrogliomas and oligoastrocytomas, 14–15,
    15f
  of pleomorphic xanthoastrocytomas, 121
  of radionecrosis, 95f
  with stereotactic biopsy, 72
  of subependymal giant cell astrocytomas, 18, 122
  of subependymomas, 16–18, 17f
Confidentiality, in genetic counseling, 177
Conformal radiation, 86, 87f 90f
Cortical dysplasia, dysembryoplastic neuroepithelial
  tumors related to, 113

Cortical motor mapping. See also Electrocorticography
  in ganglioglioma surgery, 117
  presurgical, 76
Cowden's disease
  brain tumors associated with, 172t
  cerebellar dysplastic gangliocytoma related to, 54
  characteristics of, 115
  Lhermitte-Duclos disease related to, 115
  PTEN/MMAC-1 gene mutation in, 207
Cyclin-dependent kinase inhibitors, 213
Cyclin-dependent kinases, 213
Cytostatic agents, for arresting tumor progression, 100

D
Dedifferentiation hypothesis of tumorigenesis, 199,
  200f–201f
Deferred treatment
  delayed radiation therapy in, 81–82, 82t
  of low-grade gliomas, 141–142, 143f
  practice parameters for, 233
Desmoplastic cerebral astrocytomas
  classification and pathobiology of, 41–42
  differential diagnosis of, 41–42
Desmoplastic infantile gangliogliomas
  classification and pathobiology of, 59
  imaging studies of, 23–24
  prognosis in, 136
Dexamethasone, for intracranial hypertension, 105
Diagnostic imaging. See Imaging studies
Diffuse astrocytomas. See Astrocytomas, diffuse
Dilantin (diphenylhydantoin), 159–160
DNA methylation, and p16 gene disruption, 214–215
Dysembryoplastic neuroepithelial tumors (DNET)
  classification and pathobiology of, 59 60
  imaging studies of, 19–20, 114
  incidence and clinical presentation of, 113–114
  management of, 114
  prognosis in, 136
  radiation therapy of, 91–92
  recurrence of, 114
Dysplastic cerebellar gangliocytomas. See Cerebellar
  dysplastic gangliocytomas

E
Edema
  reduction of, by surgical debulking, 144
  surgical morbidity related to, 74
EGF (epidermal growth factor), in brain development,
  193, 195f, 196
EGFR gene
  in apoptosis, 221
  in glioblastoma multiforme development, 207–208,
    207f, 216
Electrocorticography. See also Cortical motor mapping
  of epilepsy, 161–162, 158 (see insert)
  of gangliogliomas, 117
  preoperative, 76
Eloquent areas of brain, presurgical localization of,
  74–76, 75f
Endostatin, as angiogenesis inhibitor, 100
Ependymomas. See also subependymomas
  anaplastic, 50
  chemotherapy of, 124
  classification and pathobiology of, 48–52
  CSF seeding of, 123

Ependymomas (*contd.*)
  genetic abnormalities in, 51, 211–213, 212f
  grading system for, 49
  immunoreactivity of, 50
  incidence and clinical presentation of, 123
  intramedullary, 48
  lateral type of, 48
  management of, 123–124
  microscopic features of, 49
  midfloor type of, 48
  MR imaging of, 123
  myxopapillary, 51
  papillary, 49
  prognostic factors in, 49
  proliferative activity of, 50
  roof type of, 48
  spinal and intraspinal, 48
Epidermal growth factor (EGF), in brain development,
      193, 195f, 196
Epilepsy and seizures, 149–164
  associated with low-grade gliomas, 149
  basic mechanisms of, 149–151, 150f, 150t
  case studies of
      in fibrillary astrocytoma, 187–189, 188f
      in oligoastrocytoma, 185–187, 186f
      in oligodendroglioma, 181–185, 182f, 184f
  characteristics of, 152–158, 152t
      in frontal lobe, 152–155, 152f–153f
      in occipital lobe, 157–158
      in parietal lobe, 157, 157f
      in temporal lobe, 155–157, 155f–156f
  in dysembryoplastic neuroepithelial tumors, 60,
      113
  in gangliogliomas, 21, 116
      surgical treatment of, 117
  medical treatment of, 158–161
      common medications in, 159, 159t
      Dilantin (diphenylhydantoin) in, 159–160
      duration of, 159
      Lamictal (lamotrigine) in, 160–161
      for postoperative seizures, 158
      prophylactic, 158–159
      Tegretol (carbamazepine) in, 160
  preoperative evaluation of, in gangliocytoma, 115
  radiation therapy of, 84, 86, 163–164
  risk of developing, 151–152, 151t
  surgical treatment of, 161–163
      electrocorticography in, 161–162, 158 (see insert)
      for intractable seizures, 144
      results of, 161–162
  tumor pathology and, 163
Ethics of genetic counseling, 177

F
Fas ligand/TNF-induced apoptosis, 217, 220f–221f
  genetic alterations in, 219, 220f–221f, 221
Fibrillary astrocytomas
  pathology of, 35
  prognosis in, 136
  seizures in, case study of, 187–189, 188f
Fibrillary growth factor (FGF), in brain development,
      193, 195f
Fibroblast growth factor (bFGF)
  in brain development, 195f, 196, 197
  in progression of astrocytomas, 205–206

F-fluoro-2-deoxyuridine (FudR), in radionuclide
      imaging, 9
Fluorodeoxyglucose (FDG)
  ^{18}F FDG, in PET tumor uptake study, 141
  in radionuclide imaging, 8
Frontal lobes
  operability of, 73, 73t
  seizures in, 152–155, 152f–153f
Functional magnetic resonance imaging (fMRI)
  for metabolic activity of brain abnormalities, 8
  for presurgical brain mapping, 76

G
GABA (gamma aminobutyric acid), in glioma-related
      epilepsy, 149, 150, 150t
Gangliocytomas, 114–115
  cerebellar dysplastic
      associated with Cowden's disease, 54
      classification and pathobiology of, 54–55
      imaging studies of, 22–23, 23f
  classification and pathobiology of, 53–54
  clinical presentation of, 114
  imaging studies of, 21–22, 114
  management of, 114–115
Gangliogliomas, 57–59, 115–117
  anaplastic features of, 58–59
  chemotherapy of, 117
  classification and pathobiology of, 57–59
  clinical presentation of, 116
  desmoplastic infantile
      classification and pathobiology of, 59
      imaging studies of, 23–24
      prognosis in, 136
  imaging studies of, 21, 116
  management of, 116–117
  microscopic features of, 57–58
  prognostic factors in, 58–59
  radiation therapy of, 91, 117
  seizure risk in, 151, 151t
  surgical treatment of, 116–117
Gap junction communication, in glioma-related
      epilepsy, 150–151, 150f, 150t
Gemistocytic astrocytomas
  anaplastic astrocytomas vs., 37
  classification and pathobiology of, 35, 37
  malignant transformation of, 37
  oligodendrogliomas vs., 37
  prognosis in, 137, 138
Gender, as prognostic indicator, 139
Gene therapy strategies, 221–224
  cell cycle and apoptosis-directed, 222–224
      ICE in, 224
      p21 in, 223
      p53 in, 223
      TNF in, 223
  nonspecific, 222
  viral vectors in, 222
Genetic counseling, 171–173
  confidentiality in, 177
  ethics of, 177
  family pedigree construction for, 172–173
  linkage analysis in, 177
  prenatal diagnosis and presymptomatic
      testing in, 176–177
  process and purpose of, 171–172

Genetics. See also Molecular genetics, Heredity
  autosomal dominant inheritance, 174f, 175–176
  autosomal recessive inheritance, 173–174, 174f
  basic concepts in, 173
  of brain tumors, 171, 173–176
    conditions associated with, 171, 172t, 176
    McKusick's OnLine Mendelian Inheritance in Man
      resource, 178
    X-linked inheritance, 174f, 176
Genotype, 173
Germline (gonadal) mosaicism, 175
Glia
  GABA uptake in, 149
  role in epilepsy, 149–151
Glial neoplasms
  chemotherapy of, 99–101
  classification and pathobiology of, 34–53
  gene therapy strategies in, 221–224
  mixed neuronal and glial tumors, 57 60
  molecular genetics of, 199–202
    apoptosis in, 217–221
    cell cycle control in, 213–217
    tumorigenesis of, 199–202
      cell growth regulation and, 201–202, 202f–203f
      clonal evolution in, 199, 200f–201f
      dedifferentiation hypothesis in, 199, 200f–201f
      misdifferentiation hypothesis in, 199, 201, 202f
Glioblastoma multiforme
  contrast enhancement in, 139
  development of
    dedifferentiation hypothesis of, 199
    loss of heterozygosity in, 206, 207, 207f
    misdifferentiation hypothesis of, 200–201
  genetic alteration in progression of
    from astrocytomas, 207–208, 207f
    from oligodendrogliomas, 210, 210f
Gliomas (low-grade)
  benign tumors vs., 3
  brain stem, 43
  classification and pathobiology of, 34–53
    astrocytomas, 34–43
    ependymomas, 48–52
    mixed gliomas, 52–53
    oligodendrogliomas, 43–48
  epilepsy in, 149–150, 150t, 163. See also Epilepsy and
    seizures
  gene therapy strategies for, 221–224
  general perspectives on, 3–4
  incidence of, 3
  limbic and neocortical, epilepsy in, 163
  management of, 141–144
    algorithm for, 145, 145f
    controversies in, 135
    deferred treatment in, 141–142, 143f
    EORTC trial and, 135
    timing of surgery in, 142–144
  mixed, 52–53
  molecular variants in progression of, 204–213
    in apoptosis, 219, 221
    in astrocytomas, 204–209, 205f, 207f, 209f
    developmental pathways in, 194f, 204
    in ependymomas, 211–213, 212f
    in mixed oligodendrogliomas, 210–211, 211f
    in oligodendrogliomas, 209–210, 210f
    redundant pathways in, 215

natural history and prognostic factors in, 136–141
  age in, 135, 137–138, 142
  clinical presentation and, 139, 139t
  detection of malignant evolution in, 140–141
  diagnostic imaging in, 138–141
  gender in, 139
  histology in, 136–137, 137t
  proliferation markers in, 140
  tumor volume in, 139–140
optic pathway, 7f, 43
practice parameters for, 231–233, 232f
radiation therapy of
  early vs. delayed therapy in, 81–82, 82t
  for favorable low-grade variants, 91–92
  postoperative, 82, 83t, 84
surgical treatment of. See Surgical treatment
Glutamine, in glioma-related epilepsy, 150, 150t
Gonadal (germline) mosaicism, 175
Growth factors, in brain development, 193, 195f, 196
Guidelines for glioma therapy. See Practice parameters
  (guidelines), for glioma therapy

H
Headache
  in cerebellar astrocytomas, 103
  in dysembryoplastic neuroepithelial tumors, 113
Heredity. See Genetics
Herpes simplex virus thymidine kinase (HSV-TK)
  gene delivery system, 222
Heterozygosity, 173
  loss of. See Loss of heterozygosity
Hippocampus, resection of, for epilepsy
  management, 163
Homozygosity, 173
HSV-TK gene delivery system, 222
Hydrocephalus. See also Intracranial hypertension
  in cerebellar astrocytomas
    diagnosis of, 104
    emergency ventriculostomy for, 105–106
    postoperative ventriculostomy management in,
      107–108
  in choroid plexus papillomas, 112–113
  in Lhermitte-Duclos disease, 115
  in oligodendroglioma, case study of, 183–185, 184f

I
ICE (IL-1-converting enzyme), in gene therapy, 224
Imaging studies, 5–26. See also Computed tomography
  (CT); Magnetic resonance imaging (MRI)
  of astroblastoma, 111
  of astrocytomas, 5–13, 6f–13f
  of central neurocytomas, 24–26, 25f–26f, 118
  of cerebellar astrocytomas, 104–105, 104f–105f
  of choroid plexus papillomas, 18–19, 19f, 112
  contrast enhancement in
    as indicator for surgical treatment, 144
    as prognostic indicator, 138–139
  of desmoplastic infantile ganglioglioma, 23–24
  of dysembryoplastic neuroepithelial tumors,
    19–20, 114
  of dysplastic cerebellar gangliocytomas, 22–23, 23f
  of ependymomas, 123
  of gangliocytomas, 21–22, 114
  of gangliogliomas, 21, 116
  of ganglion cell tumors, 20–23, 23f

Imaging studies (*contd.*)
of Lhermitte-Duclos disease, 115
of low-grade gliomas, 138–139
of neurocytomas, 24–26, 25f–26f, 118
for observation of nontreated patients, 142, 143f
of oligodendroglioma and mixed oligoastrocytomas,
14–16, 15f–16f
of pleomorphic xanthoastrocytomas, 13–14, 14f, 121
with stereotactic biopsy, 72
of subependymal giant cell astrocytomas, 18, 122
of subependymomas, 16–18, 17f, 124
Imaging systems, three-dimensional
in cerebellar astrocytoma surgery, 107
for surgical therapy, 74, 76 78, 78f
Infants
desmoplastic cerebral astrocytoma of, 41–42
desmoplastic ganglioglioma of, 59
INK family of cyclin-dependent kinase inhibitors, 214
Interleukin-1-converting enzyme (ICE),
in gene therapy, 224
Intracranial hypertension. See also
Hydrocephalus
in cerebellar astrocytomas, dexamethasone
for controlling, 105
in Lhermitte-Duclos disease, 115
in oligodendroglioma, 184, 185
pressure wave due to, 183–184

J

Juvenile pilocytic astrocytomas. See Pilocytic
astrocytomas

K

Kernohan classification, 5

L

Lamictal (lamotrigine), 160–161
Language centers, presurgical localization of, 74, 75 76
Lhermitte-Duclos disease
associated with Cowden's disease, 115
clinical presentation of, 115
management of, 115
recurrence of, 115
Li-Fraumeni syndrome, 177
Linkage analysis, in genetic counseling, 177
Loss of heterozygosity
in anaplastic astrocytomas, 206
in diffuse astrocytomas, 36
in glioblastoma multiforme, 206, 207, 207f
in oligoastrocytomas, 211, 211f
in oligodendrogliomas, 47, 206, 210, 210f
Low-grade gliomas. See Gliomas (low-grade)

M

Magnetic resonance imaging (MRI). See also Imaging
studies
of astroblastoma, 111
of astrocytomas, 5, 6f–7f, 7
of central neurocytomas, 24–26, 25f–26f, 118
of cerebellar astrocytomas, 104–105, 104f–105f
of cerebellar dysplastic gangliocytomas, 22, 23f
of choroid plexus papillomas, 19, 112
of desmoplastic infantile gangliogliomas, 24
of dysembryoplastic neuroepithelial tumors, 20, 114
of ependymomas, 123

of fibrillary astrocytoma, 187, 188f
functional (fMRI), 8, 76
of gangliocytomas, 22, 114
of gangliogliomas, 21, 116
intraoperative, 77 78
of Lhermitte-Duclos disease, 115
of oligoastrocytomas, 15–16, 16f, 185, 186f
of oligodendrogliomas, 15–16, 16f
in case studies, 181, 182f, 183, 184f
of pleomorphic xanthoastrocytomas, 13–14, 14f, 121
of radionecrosis, 94f
with stereotactic biopsy, 72
of subependymal giant cell astrocytomas, 18, 122
of subependymomas, 18, 124
Magnetic resonance spectroscopy, 11, 12f–13f, 13
McKusick's OnLine Mendelian Inheritance in Man
resource, 178
MDM2 gene
in cell cycle control, 216
in glioblastoma multiforme development, 207f, 208
Melanoma, brain tumors associated with, 172t
Meningiomas, risk of seizure with, 151
Metastases, risk of seizure with, 151
C-L-methylmethionine, in radionuclide imaging, 9
Minigemistocytes, in oligodendrogliomas, 45
Misdifferentiation hypothesis of tumorigenesis, 199, 201,
202f
Mixed gliomas, classification and pathobiology of,
52–53
Mixed neuronal and glial tumors, 57 60
desmoplastic infantile ganglioglioma, 59
dysembryoplastic neuroepithelial tumor, 59 60
ganglioglioma, 57–59
Mixed oligoastrocytomas
imaging studies of, 14–16, 15f–16f
molecular genetics of, 210–211, 211f
Molecular genetics, 193–224. See also Genetics
of apoptosis, 217, 220f–221f
brain development and, 193–198
of cell cycle control, 213–217
of central neurocytomas, 56
of desmoplastic cerebral astrocytoma, 42
of diffuse astrocytomas, 36
of ependymomas, 51
of glioma progression, 204–213
in astrocytomas, 204–209, 205f, 207f, 209f
developmental pathways in, 194f, 204
in ependymomas, 211–213, 212f
in mixed oligoastrocytomas, 210–211, 211f
in oligodendrogliomas, 209–210, 210f
of myxopapillary ependymoma, 51
of oligodendrogliomas, 47–48
of pilocytic astrocytomas, 41
of pleomorphic xanthoastrocytomas, 38
of tuberous sclerosis, 175
of tumorigenesis, 199–202
cell growth regulation and, 201–202, 202f–203f
clonal evolution in, 199, 200f–201f
dedifferentiation hypothesis in, 199, 200f–201f
misdifferentiation hypothesis in, 199, 201, 202f
Motor strip of brain, presurgical localization of, 74–75,
75f
Multipotent cells. See Brain development
Mutism, postoperative, after cerebellar astrocytoma
surgery, 107

Myxopapillary ependymoma, classification and
    pathobiology of, 51

N

Neck pain, in cerebellar astrocytomas, 103
Neurocognitive effects, of radiation therapy, 92 93
Neurocytomas, central. See Central neurocytomas
Neurofibromatosis type 1
    autosomal dominant inheritance in, 175–176
    brain stem gliomas related to, 43
    brain tumors associated with, 172t
    dysembryoplastic neuroepithelial tumors related to,
        113
    optic pathway gliomas related to, 43
Neurofibromatosis type 2
    autosomal dominant inheritance in, 176
    brain tumors associated with, 172t
    ependymomas related to, 51
Neurologic deficits
    after cerebellar astrocytoma surgery, 108
    in cerebellar astrocytomas, 104
    in ganglioglioma, 116
    as outcome predictor, in oligodendrogliomas, 46
Neuronal cell tumors
    central neurocytomas, 55–57
    cerebellar dysplastic gangliocytomas, 54–55
    classification and pathobiology of, 53–57
    gangliocytomas, 53–54
    mixed neuronal and glial tumors, 57 60
Neurotrophin-3 (NT3), in brain development, 195f, 196
NF. See Neurofibromatosis type 1; Neurofibromatosis
        type 2
NF-2 gene, mutation of, 212
Nonmaleficence principal, in genetic counseling, 177
Nowell's theory of clonal evolution, 199, 200f–201f

O

O-2A progenitor cells
    in adult brains, 197, 198
    in fetal brains, 195f, 196
Observation vs. treatment. See Deferred treatment
Occipital lobes
    operability of, 73, 73t
    seizures in, 157–158
Oligoastrocytomas
    mixed
        genetic mutations in progression of, 210–211, 211f
        imaging studies of, 14–16, 15f–16f
    scizures in, case study of, 185–187, 186f
Oligodendrogliomas
    chemoradiation therapy of, 99–100
    classification and pathobiology of, 43–48
    diagnosis of, 45
    gemistocytic astrocytomas vs., 37
    genetic mutations in progression of, 209–210, 210f
    GFAP-positive cells in, 45
    histologic grading of, 46
    imaging studies of, 14–16, 15f–16f
    incidence of, 43
    magnetic resonance spectroscopy of, 12f–13f
    methylmethionine update of, 9
    molecular genetics of, 47–48
    morphologic features of, 44
    neuronal markers in, 45
    O-2A progenitor cell in, 47

prognostic factors in, 46, 136
proliferative activity of, 46–47
radiation therapy of
    postoperative, 84, 85t
    for seizures, 183
seizures in
    case studies of, 181–185, 182f, 184f
    risk of development of, 151, 151t
    spinal, 44
Oligodendromatosis, 44
Oncogenes, activating mutations of, 201–202, 202f–203f
OnLine Mendelian Inheritance in Man (OMIM) resource,
    178
Optic pathway gliomas
    classification and pathobiology of, 43
    MR image of, 7f
Outcome
    measurement of, 234
    of radiation therapy. See Radiation therapy, outcome of
    of surgical treatment, 78 79, 108, 144

P

p16 gene mutations, cell cycle effects of, 214–215
p16-CDK4/cyclinD-Rb1 axis, in cell cycle control,
    214–215
p21 gene
    in cell cycle control, 216
    in gene therapy, 223
p21-p53-MDM2/PAX5 axis, in cell cycle control,
    215–217
p53 gene
    abnormalities of
        in astrocytomas, 215
        in diffuse astrocytomas, 36
        in oligodendrogliomas, 47
        in pilocytic astrocytomas, 41
    in apoptosis induction, 217, 219
        genetic alterations in, 221
    in gene therapy, 223
    lack of abnormalities, in ependymomas, 212
p53 protein
    in cell cycle control, 215
    in p21-p53-MDM2/PAX5 axis, 215–217
Papilledema, in choroid plexus papillomas, 112
Papova virus, ependymoma related to, 51
Parietal lobes
    operability of, 73, 73t
    seizures in, 157, 157f
Pathobiology. See Classification and pathobiology
PAX5 gene
    in cell cycle control, 216–217
    in glioblastoma multiforme development, 207f, 208
PCV (procarbazine, vincristine, and lomustine)
        chemotherapy, 99–100
Penetrance, of disease-causing genotype, 175
Phenotype, 173
Pilocytic astrocytomas
    in adults, 118–120
    chemotherapy of, 120
    classification and pathobiology of, 39–41
    clinical presentation of, 119
    diffuse astrocytomas vs., 42
    histologic findings in, 40
    imaging studies of, 7, 10f–11f
    immunoreactivity of, 40

Pilocytic astrocytomas (*contd.*)
  malignant transformation of, 40, 120
  management of, 119–120
  microscopic features of, 40
  molecular genetics of, 41
  multicentric spread of, 120
  prognosis in, 136
  radiation therapy of, 91, 119–120
  recurrence of, 120
  surgical treatment of, 119, 144
  vascularity of, 39–40
Platelet-derived growth factors (PDGF)
  in brain development, 195f, 196
  in malignant progression
    of astrocytomas, 205
    of ependymomas, 212
Pleomorphic xanthoastrocytomas
  anaplastic progression of, 38
  classification and pathobiology of, 37–38
  imaging studies of, 13–14, 14f, 121
  immunoreactivity of, 38
  incidence and clinical presentation of, 120–121
  malignant transformation of, 121
  management of, 121–122
  microscopic features of, 37–38
  prognosis in, 38, 136
  radiation therapy of, 91, 121
  recurrence of, 121
Positron emission tomography (PET)
  of astrocytomas, 8
  in detection of malignant degeneration of gliomas,
    140–141
  [18]F Fluorodeoxyglucose (FDG) tumor uptake in, 141
Potassium, in glioma-related epilepsy, 150, 150f, 151
Practice parameters (guidelines), for glioma therapy,
    231–233
  biopsy in, 233
  development of, 231–232, 232f
  evidenced-based criteria for, 232–233
  observation vs. treatment in, 233
  radiation therapy in, 233
  surgical resection in, 233
Predisposition testing, in genetic counseling, 177
Prenatal diagnosis, in genetic counseling, 176–177
Procarbazine, vincristine, and lomustine (PCV)
    chemotherapy, 99–100
Progenitor cells. See Brain development
Programmed cell death. See Apoptosis
Proliferation markers, as prognostic indicators, 140
Protoplasmic astrocytomas
  differential diagnosis of, 37
  pathology of, 35, 36–37
PTEN/MMAC-1 gene mutation, in Cowden's disease,
    207

R
Radiation necrosis
  clinical presentation and outcome of, 95, 94f 95f
  incidence of, 93, 95
  tumor recurrence vs., 96
Radiation therapy, 81–96
  of astroblastoma, 111–112
  brachytherapy in, 92, 164
  of central neurocytomas, 92, 118

chemotherapy combined with, for
    oligodendrogliomas, 99–100
  of choroid plexus papilloma, 113
  chromic phosphate (^{32}P) therapy in, 92
  delayed
    after biopsy or cytoreductive surgery, 143–144
    vs. early therapy, natural history and outcome
      with, 81–82, 82t
  of ependymomas, 123–124
  for epilepsy and seizures, 84, 86, 163–164
  for favorable low-grade glioma variants, 91–92
  of ganglioglioma, 91, 117
  of low-grade glioma, 82–83
  neurocognitive effects of, 92 93
  of oligodendroglioma, 84, 85t, 183
  outcome of
    age factors in, 84
    in epilepsy, 84, 86
    in high-dose vs. low-dose therapy, 86, 90, 90f
    malignant degeneration and, 86
    in partial-brain vs. whole-brain radiation, 86, 93
    in supratentorial gliomas, 82, 83t, 84
    in supratentorial oligodendrogliomas, 84, 85t
  of pilocytic astrocytomas, 91, 119–120
  of pleomorphic xanthoastrocytomas, 91, 121
  postoperative, 82 90
  practice parameters for, 233
  radionecrosis due to, 93, 94f 95f, 95
  stereotactic, 92
  of subependymomas, 92, 125
  toxicity of, 92 95, 94f 95f, 142
  treatment planning for (conformal radiation),
    86, 87f 90f
  tumor recurrence after, 95 96
Radiography. See Imaging studies
Radionuclide imaging, of astrocytomas, 8–10
RB1 gene mutations
  cell cycle effects of, 213–214
  in progression of anaplastic astrocytomas, 206
Regional astrocytomas, 42–43
Ringertz classification system, 34
Rosenthal fibers, in cerebellar astrocytomas, 105, 108

S
St. Anne-Mayo Clinic grading system, 34, 137, 140
Seizures. See Epilepsy and seizures
Shunt, ventricular peritoneal, 106, 112
Signet ring cells, in oligodendrogliomas, 45
Simian virus (SV40), in initiation of
    ependymomas, 213
Single photon emission computed
    tomography (SPECT)
  of dysembryoplastic neuroepithelial tumor, 20
  thallium-201 in, 9–10
Somatostatin, in glioma-related epilepsy, 150, 150t
Spectroscopy, magnetic resonance, 11, 12f–13f, 13
Speech centers, presurgical localization of, 74, 75 76
Spinal cord
  astrocytomas of, 42–43
  ependymomas of, 48
  myxopapillary ependymoma of, 51
  oligodendrogliomas of, 44
  subependymomas of, 52
Status epilepticus, 151

Stem cells, multipotent
  in brain development, 193, 194f–195f, 196
  neoplastic transformation of, 201
Stereotactic biopsy
  in classification of neoplasms, 33–34
  correlation with surgical specimens, 33–34
  of low-grade gliomas, 143, 145, 145f
    radiation therapy after, 143
  with MRI and CT, 72
  risks of, 71–72, 143
  technique of, 72
Stereotactic imaging systems
  in cerebellar astrocytoma surgery, 107
  for surgical therapy, 74, 76 77
Stereotactic radiation therapy, 92
Subependymal giant cell astrocytomas
  associated with tuberous sclerosis, 38, 122
  classification and pathobiology of, 38–39
  imaging studies of, 18, 122
  management of, 122
  prognosis in, 39
  radiation therapy of, 92
Subependymomas
  classification and pathobiology of, 51–52
  imaging studies of, 16–18, 17f, 124
  incidence and clinical presentation of, 124
  management of, 124–125
  radiation therapy of, 92, 125
  recurrence of, 125
Suicide genes, 222
Supratentorial astrocytomas
  classification and pathobiology of, 42
  cystic changes in, imaging studies of, 7, 9f
  diagnostic imaging of, 138
Surgical treatment, 71–79
  approach to, 72f
  of astroblastoma, 111–112
  biopsy preceding, 71–72, 143
    proposed classification scheme based on, 73
  brain shifts during, 77
  Broca and Wernicke area location in, 75
  causes of morbidity in, 74
  of central neurocytomas, 118
  of cerebellar astrocytomas, 105–108
    in children, 105–108, 107f
    emergency ventriculostomy in, 105–106
    incisions and dissection in, 106–107, 107f
    outcome of, 108
    patient positioning in, 106
    postoperative ventriculostomy management in, 107–108
    tumor removal in, 107
  of choroid plexus papillomas, 113
  cortical motor mapping in, 76, 117
  for debulking of tumor, 144
  of dysembryoplastic neuroepithelial tumors, 114
  of ependymomas, 123–124
  for epilepsy, 144, 161–163, 158 (see insert)
  of fibrillary astrocytoma, case studies of, 189
  functional MRI in, 76
  of gangliocytomas, 115
  of ganglioglioma, 116–117
  indications for, 73 74, 143, 144
    controversial, 74

of Lhermitte-Duclos disease, 115
motor strip localization in, 74–75, 75f
near eloquent areas, 74–76, 75f
of oligoastrocytoma, case studies of, 187
of oligodendroglioma, case studies of, 183, 185
operable brain regions, 73, 73t
outcome of
  in cerebellar astrocytomas, 108
  in low-grade vs. high-grade tumors, 78 79
  tumor biology as predictor of, 144
of pilocytic astrocytomas, 119, 144
of pleomorphic xanthoastrocytomas, 121
practice parameters for, 233
rationales for, 71
seizures after, 158–159
speech centers localization in, 74, 75 76
of subependymal giant cell astrocytomas, 122
of subependymomas, 124–125
three-dimensional imaging in
  intraoperative MRI in, 77 78
  point-based registration systems in, 76 77
  stereotactic systems in, 74, 76 77
  ultrasound in, 77, 78f
timing of, 142–144
tumors with potential for cure, 72, 73t
SV40 virus, in initiation of ependymomas, 213

T
T1 astrocyte progenitor cells, 195f, 196
Tamoxifen, as antiproliferative agent, 100
Tegretol (carbamazepine), 160
Telomerase expression, in oligodendrogliomas, 47
Temporal lobes
  ganglioglioma in, 116
  operability of, 73, 73t
  seizures in, 155–157, 155f–156f
Thalidomide, as angiogenesis inhibitor, 100
Thallium-201 single-photon-emission computed
    tomography (SPECT), 9–10
Three-dimensional imaging systems, for surgical therapy,
    74, 76 78, 78f
TNF. See Tumor necrosis factor (TNF)
TP53 gene. See p53 gene
Transforming growth factors, in progression of
    ependymomas, 212
Tuberous sclerosis
  autosomal dominant inheritance in, 175
  brain tumors associated with, 172t
  subependymal giant cell astrocytomas related to, 38,
    122
Tumor necrosis factor (TNF)
  in Fas ligand/TNF-induced apoptosis, 217, 220f–221f
    genetic alterations in, 219, 220f–221f, 221
  in gene therapy, 223
Tumor suppressor genes
  inactivating mutations of, 201–202, 202f–203f
  location of
    on chromosome 10, 206–207
    on chromosome 19, 206
  loss of, in ependymomas, 212

U
Ultrasonography, intraoperative, 77, 78f, 107
Urinary incontinence, postictal, 185

V

Vascular malformations, pilocystic
    astrocytomas vs., 39–40
Ventricular peritoneal shunt
    in cerebellar astrocytoma, risk of uncontrolled
        CSF drainage via, 106
    in choroid plexus papilloma surgery, 112
Ventriculostomy, in cerebellar astrocytoma
    emergency placement of, 107–108
    postoperative management of, 107–108
    risk of uncontrolled CSF drainage and, 106
Viruses
    as gene therapy vectors, 222
    papova, ependymoma related to, 51
    SV40, in initiation of ependymomas, 213

Vomiting, in cerebellar astrocytomas, 104
Von Hippel-Lindau syndrome, brain tumors associated
    with, 172t
von Recklinghausen disease. See Neurofibromatosis type 1

W

Wernicke's area, presurgical localization of, 75
World Health Organization classification
    correlation with diagnostic imaging, 5
    correlation with proliferative indices, 137, 140
    of diffuse astrocytomas, 34
    grading system in, 136–137

X

X-linked inheritance, 174f, 176